DANFORTH'S HANDBOOK OF

OBSTETRICS
AND GYNECOLOGY

DANFORTH'S HANDBOOK OF
OBSTETRICS AND GYNECOLOGY

James R. Scott, M.D.
Professor and Chairman
Department of Obstetrics and Gynecology
University of Utah School of Medicine
Salt Lake City, Utah

Philip J. DiSaia, M.D.
The Dorothy Marsh Chair in Reproductive Biology
Professor
Department of Obstetrics and Gynecology
University of California at Irvine, College of Medicine
Orange, California

Charles B. Hammond, M.D.
E. C. Hamblen Professor and Chairman
Department of Obstetrics and Gynecology
Duke University School of Medicine
Durham, North Carolina

William N. Spellacy, M.D.
Professor and Chairman
Department of Obstetrics and Gynecology
University of South Florida College of Medicine
Tampa, Florida

John D. Gordon, M.D.
Clinical Fellow
Reproductive Endocrinology Center
University of California, San Francisco
San Francisco, California

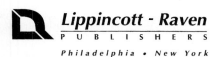

Lippincott - Raven
P U B L I S H E R S
Philadelphia • New York

Acquisitions Editor: Lisa McAllister
Assistant Editor: Emilie Linkins
Production Editor: Sharon McCarthy
Production Manager: Janet Greenwood
Indexer: Page Two Associates, Inc.
Compositor: Page Two Associates, Inc.
Printer/Binder: R.R. Donnelley & Sons

Library of Congress Cataloguing-in-Publications Data

Danforth's handbook of obstetrics and gynecology / [edited by] James R.
Scott ... [et al.]. — 1st ed.
    p.   cm.
    Smaller version of: Danforth's obstetrics and gynecology. 7th ed. c1994.
    ISBN 0-397-51281-3
    1. Gynecology—Handbooks, manuals, etc. 2. Obstetrics—Handbooks,
manuals, etc. I. Danforth, David N., 1912– . II. Scott, James R., 1937– .
III. Danforth's obstetrics and gynecology.
    [DNLM: 1. Genital Diseases, Female—handbooks. 2. Obstetrics—
handbooks.]
RG110.D36 1995
618—dc20
DNLM/DLC
for Library of Congress   95-21882
                                                              CIP

9 8 7 6 5 4 3 2 1

◆ Contributors

Karlis Adamsons, M.D., Ph.D.
San Juan, Puerto Rico

Kevin E. Bachus, M.D.
Durham, North Carolina

Robert W. Bendon, M.D.
Louisville, Kentucky

Alfred E. Bent, M.D.
Baltimore, Maryland

Marc A. Bernhisel, M.D.
Tampa, Florida

D. Ware Branch, M.D.
Salt Lake City, Utah

Beth A. Brindley, M.D.
Detroit, Michigan

Jonn R. Brumsted, M.D.
Burlington, Vermont

Ronald A. Chez, M.D.
Tampa, Florida

Steven L. Clark, M.D.
Salt Lake City, Utah

Grace M. Couchman, M.D.
Durham, North Carolina

William T. Creasman, M.D.
Charleston, South Carolina

Dwight P. Cruikshank, M.D.
Milwaukee, Wisconsin

John O.L. DeLancey, M.D.
Ann Arbor, Michigan

Julian E. DeLia, M.D.
Milwaukee, Wisconsin

Philip J. DiSaia, M.D.
Orange, California

Mitchell P. Dombrowski, M.D.
Detroit, Michigan

Robert D. Eden, M.D.
Palm Springs, California

David A. Eschenbach, M.D.
Seattle, Washington

John I. Fishburne Jr., M.D.
Oklahoma City, Oklahoma

Thomas J. Garite, M.D.
Orange, California

Paul R. Gindoff, M.D.
Washington, District of Columbia

Laura T. Goldsmith, Ph.D.
Newark, New Jersey

Ralph B.L. Gwatkin, Ph.D.
Cleveland, Ohio

Charles B. Hammond, M.D.
Durham, North Carolina

William R. Keye, Jr., M.D.
Royal Oak, Michigan

Neil K. Kochenour, M.D.
Salt Lake City, Utah

L. Stanley James, M.D.
New York, New York

Douglas J. Marchant, M.D.
Providence, Rhode Island

Daniel R. Mishell, Jr., M.D.
Los Angeles, California

Margaret J. Nachtigall, M.D.
New Haven, Connecticut

Jennifer E. Niebyl, M.D.
Iowa City, Iowa

David L. Olive, M.D.
New Haven, Connecticut

Donald R. Ostergard, M.D.
Long Beach, California

Michael T. Parsons, M.D.
Tampa, Florida

Martin M. Quigley, M.D.
Gulf Breeze, Florida

Elvoy Raines, M.D., M.P.H.
Washington, District of Columbia

Kathryn L. Reed, M.D.
Tucson, Arizona

Daniel H. Riddick, M.D., Ph.D.
Burlington, Vermont

Daniel K. Roberts, M.D., Ph.D.
Wichita, Kansas

Kenneth J. Ryan, M.D.
Boston, Massachusetts

Lisa Barrie Schwartz, M.D.
New Haven, Connecticut

James R. Scott, M.D.
Salt Lake City, Utah

Alejandro R. Soffici, M.D.
Santa Barbara, California

Robert J. Sokol, M.D.
Detroit, Michigan

William N. Spellacy, M.D.
Tampa, Florida

Robert J. Stillman, M.D.
Washington, District of Columbia

Richard L. Sweet, M.D.
Pittsburgh, Pennsylvania

Michael W. Varner, M.D.
Salt Lake City, Utah

Joan L. Walker, M.D.
Oklahoma City, Oklahoma

Kenneth Ward, M.D.
Salt Lake City, Utah

Gerson Weiss, M.D.
Newark, New Jersey

Harold C. Wiesenfeld, M.D.
Pittsburgh, Pennsylvania

Frank J. Zlatnik, M.D.
Iowa City, Iowa

◆ Preface

The changes in health care and emphasis on protocols, cost effectiveness, and evidence-based medicine call for new and innovative approaches to learning. This may be one reason *Danforth's Obstetrics and Gynecology* is used by practicing physicians worldwide as an important reference book. However, we wanted to produce a smaller version that would allow rapid access to the entire specialty and which could be easily carried by medical students, housestaff, and other physicians directly involved in patient care. To do this, I enlisted the aid of John Gordon, M.D. who had organized a housestaff manual while a resident in obstetrics and gynecology. Since John is not far removed from that experience, he had the right perspective and was able to capture the essence of what is important "in the trenches." The co-editors and I have reviewed the completed outlines for each chapter. John put a tremendous amount of time and effort into this project, and we are indebted to him for the final product. We are pleased with the result and hope that you find the Handbook useful. We hope this will become a permanent fixture that will be revised each time the textbook is updated. Finally, we also appreciate the valuable assistance of Emilie Linkins and Lisa McAllister at Lippincott-Raven Pubishers in completing this handbook.

James R. Scott

◆ Contents

1

◆ Clinical Anatomy of the Female Genital Tract

BONY PELVIS

Individual components (Fig. 1-1)
- innominate bones
  - fused ischium, ilium, and pubis
  - form anterior/lateral aspect
- sacrum, coccyx
  - form posterior aspect

Plane of inlet rests at 60 degrees with horizontal (Fig. 1-2)
- axis of sacrum about 110 degrees with lumbar spine

Median and lateral notches
- median subpubic notch
  - formed by union of pubic rami at symphysis
  - traversed by urogenital apparatus
- lateral sciatic notch
  - lateral margin of sacrum and coccyx and ischial tuberosity
  - greater and lesser foramen defined by sacrospinous, sacro-tuberous ligaments

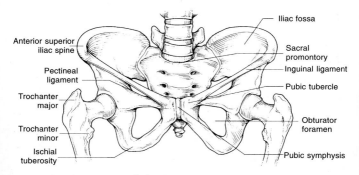

Figure 1-1. Anterior view of the pelvic bones.

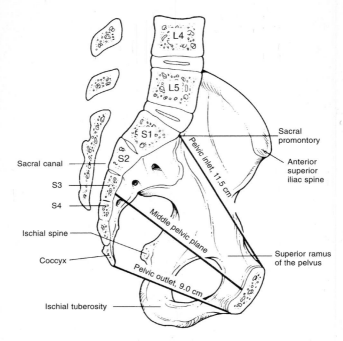

Figure 1-2. Lateral view of the pelvic bones.

Function of bony pelvis
- protect pelvic viscera
- support vertebral column
- facilitate locomotion

Gender-specific female pelvic characteristics
- inlet oval
- regular outline
- sacral promontory less prominent
- sacrum shorter, less curved
- ilial flares flatter
- pelvic cavity broader, shallower
- acetabular and ischial tuberosities set further apart
- bony walls become more vertical
- subpubic angle broader

Pelvic diameters are of practical importance (see Chapter 6)
- transverse diameter
  - inlet 13 to 14 cm
  - outlet 10 to 12 cm
- anteroposterior diameter

- pelvic inlet 11.5 cm
- middle pelvic plane 12 cm
- outlet 9 cm
- oblique diameter 12.5 cm

PELVIC VISCERA

◆ Broad Ligament

Tent-like reflection of peritoneum (Fig. 1-3)
Irregular quadrilateral outline
Contents
- fallopian tube
- ovary
- round ligament
- uterine and ovarian vessels
- nerves, lymphatics, and fatty tissue
- ureter

◆ Ureter

Emerges from behind ovary and under its vessels
Passes behind uterine and superior and middle vesicle arteries
Courses near lateral fornix of vagina
- passes 8 to 12 mm from cervix
Enters bladder
- ureters 5 cm apart
- oblique direction through muscularis
  - constitutes a valvular arrangement; no true valve is present
- ureteral orifices 2.5 cm apart
Histologic appearance
- 3-mm thick wall with three layers

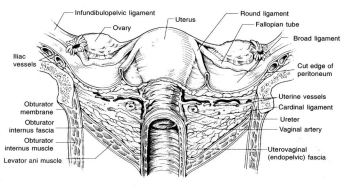

Figure 1-3. Ligamentous, fascial, and muscular support of the pelvic viscera.

- connective tissue
- muscle (external circular and internal longitudinal)
- mucous membrane

Blood supply
- direct branch hypogastric in pelvic portion
  - anastomosis with iliolumbar superiorly
  - vesicle and middle hemorrhoidal inferiorly

◆ Bladder

Located anteriorly in pelvis
Peritoneum passes over the uterus posteriorly
Normal uterus rests on superior surface of the empty bladder
Mucous membrane
- rose-colored transitional epithelium
- irregular folds (rugae)
- trigone
  - internal urethral orifice
  - two ureteral orifices

Blood supply
- branches of hypogastric artery
  - superior vesicle from terminal branch hypogastric (umbilical)
  - middle vesicle from superior vesical or umbilical
  - inferior vesical directly from hypogastric

◆ Urethra

Small tube 2.5 to 5 cm long
Average caliber 2 to 8 mm
Skene glands open close to posterior margin of orifice
Pelvic portion
- 2 to 3 cm long
- begins at vesicle orifices 2 to 3 cm behind symphysis
- terminates at point of penetration of urogenital diaphragm
- internal sphincter surrounds urethra at vesicle neck
Perineal portion
- 1 cm long
- urogenital diaphragm to below subpubic angle
- opens into vestibule

◆ Vagina

Tubular structure extends from introitus to cervix
Traverses urogenital diaphragm
Extends through genital hiatus of levator ani
Lies in horizontal plane
- anterior wall (9 cm) shorter than posterior wall (10 cm)
Blood supply
- hypogastric artery
- uterine arteries

- middle rectal artery
- inferior vaginal branch of internal pudendal

Ligamentous attachments
- lower third
  - pelvic diaphragm
  - urogenital diaphragm
  - perineal body
- middle third
  - pelvic diaphragm
  - cardinal ligaments
- upper third
  - levator plate
  - cardinal ligaments
  - uterosacral ligaments

◆ Perineum

Divided into urogenital triangle and anal triangle (Fig. 1-4)
Vestibule
- opening through which urethra and vaginal introitus pass externally

Clitoris
- part of perineum and vestibule

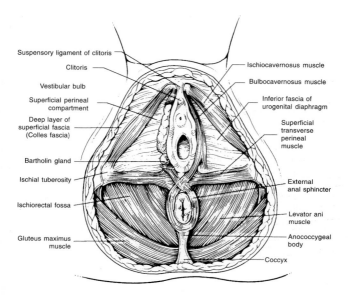

Figure 1-4. Anatomy of the perineum beneath the skin.

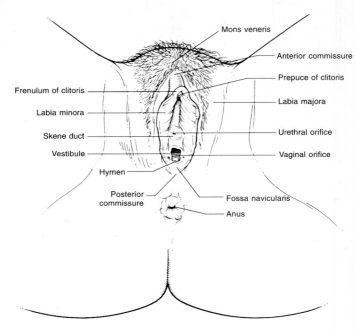

Figure 1-5. Anatomy of the external genitalia.

Blood supply
- internal pudendal artery
- branch of hypogastric (internal iliac)

Innervation
- perineal branch of pudendal
- perineal branch of posterior femoral cutaneous nerve (S2 to S3)
- ilioinguinal, genitofemoral nerves

Fascial layers
- deep layers cover muscles (Colles)
- superficial layers contiguous with Scarpa and Camper loose connective tissue planes
  - infection can spread as cellulitis or necrotizing fascitis

◆ Vulva (Fig. 1-5)

Mons pubis

Labia majora
- extend from mons to posterior fourchette
- homologous to scrotum

Labia minora
- between vaginal opening and labia majora
- form the prepuce and frenulum of clitoris
- homologous to penile urethra and skin of penis

Clitoris
- erectile organ 2 cm long
- attached periosteum by two crura
- covered by prepuce
- exposed portion is the glans
- homologous to glans penis

Urethra
- distal one third stratified squamous epithelium

Skene (paraurethral) glands
- secrete mucus
- homologous to prostate

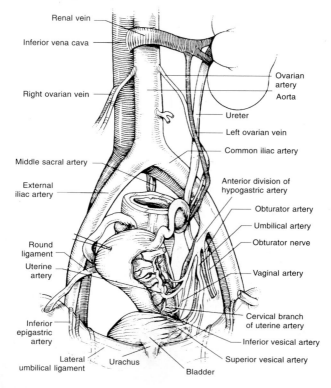

Figure 1-6. Blood supply of the pelvis.

Bartholin (greater vestibular) glands
- lie on posterolateral surface
- covered with cuboidal epithelium
- duct covered with transitional epithelium
- produce mucoid secretion
- homologous to bulbourethral (Cowper) glands in men

◆ Vasculature

Derived from common or internal iliac artery (Fig. 1-6)
Two divisions of internal iliac (hypogastric artery)
1. anterior (seven branches)
   - umbilical and superior vesical
   - uterine
   - vaginal
   - middle rectal
   - obturator (arises from inferior epigastric 40% of time)
   - internal pudendal
   - inferior gluteal
2. posterior (three branches)
   - iliolumbar
   - lateral sacral
   - superior gluteal
Ovarian arteries
- direct branch of aorta
- can by ligated along with hypogastric artery in cases of life-threatening hemorrhage

◆ Lymphatic System

Follows arterial system but does not always drain in the same pattern (Fig. 1-7)
External genitalia, anus, and anal canal
- drain into superficial inguinal nodes
Lower one third of vagina
- drains into sacral nodes and internal common iliac nodes
Cervix
- drains into external or internal iliac and sacral nodes
Lower uterine segment
- drains into external iliac, obturator, and paraaortic nodes
- 10% involvement in stage I endometrial carcinoma
Upper uterus drains into ovarian lymphatics to lumbar nodes
Ovaries drain out of pelvis to lumbar nodes

◆ Nerve Supply

Striated muscle of the vaginal outlet and skin of perineum
- receive somatic motor and sensory fibers via lumbosacral plexus
Pelvic viscera
- autonomic plexuses

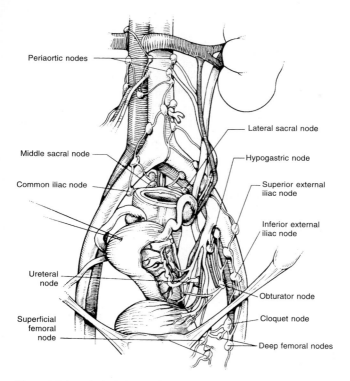

Figure 1-7. Lymphatic drainage of the pelvis.

- symphathetic
  - muscle contraction, vessel constriction
- parasympathetic
  - muscle relaxation, vessel dilation

◇ *Superior hypogastric plexus*
Runs from fourth lumbar vertebra to hollow of sacrum
Descends into base of broad ligament
Joins pelvic plexuses
- motor and sensory nerves from S2 to S4 travel by way of pelvic nerves (nervi erigentes)

◇ *Uterine sensory nerves*
Accompany sympathetic nerves
Enter cord at T11 to T12
- result in referral of pain to abdomen

- cervical afferents referred to lower back and lumbar sacrum region

✧ *Sciatic nerve*
From L5, S2, S3
Exits between ischial spine and inferior border of piriformis muscle
Gives off internal pudendal nerve as it leaves the pelvis (Fig. 1-8)

✧ *Sacral plexus*
Includes lumbosacral trunk and first, second, and third sacral nerves
S3 and S4 supplies levator ani and coccygeus muscle
S4 supplies perineum

✧ *Inferior hypogastric plexus*
Supplies rectum, uterus, vagina, bladder, ureter
Visceral afferent pain pathways connect with cord at T11 to T12 referred pain to dermatomal pattern

✧ *Genitofemoral nerve*
L1 to L2 origin
Courses on belly of psoas muscle

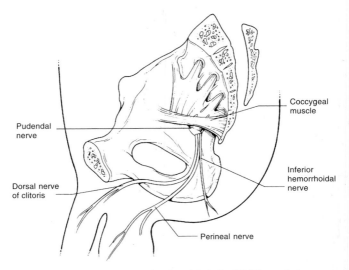

Figure 1-8. The pudendal nerve has its origin in the S2-S4 sacral plexus. As it enters the pudendal canal, it gives off the inferior rectal nerve and then divides into the perineal nerve and the dorsal nerve of the clitoris. The pudendal nerve and its branches innervate the muscles, skin, and erectile tissue of the perineum.

Supplies labia majora
Injury results in sensory changes

✧ *Obturator nerve*
L2 to L4 origin
Passes posterior to iliac vessels
- lateral to hypogastric vessels
Motor branches
- adductor of leg, hip, knee, medial thigh
  - injury results in loss of thigh adduction
    - loss of power in internal and external rotation
    - sensory losses

2

◆ Embryology and Developmental Defects of the Female Reproductive System

ORIGIN AND MIGRATION OF GERM CELLS

Germ cells migrate into genital ridge from yolk sac endoderm (Fig. 2-1)
- genital ridges appear in 31- to 35-day-old embryos
- germ cells recognizable by specific characteristics
  - relatively large (12 μm diameter) with clear cytoplasm
  - spheroid nucleus
  - high affinity for toluidine blue dye
  - high level of alkaline phosphatase activity

Move by ameboid motion
- probably follow chemotactic signal

GENETIC DETERMINATION OF GONADAL SEX

◆ Testis-Determining Factor (TDF)

Sex determined by presence or absence of Y chromosome
TDF produced by region near top of short arm of Y chromosome
Explains the presence in nature of XX males and XY females
Exact mechanism of action unknown
Appears to require cooperation of one or more autosomal genes

◆ Ovarian-Determining Gene

Assumption that ovarian development occurs by default is an oversimplification
Female development requires proliferation of secondary (cortical) sex cords (Fig. 2-2)

OOGENESIS

◆ Oogenesis and Atresia

At 3 weeks of development, a few hundred germ cells exist (oogonia)
By 20 weeks gestation, seven million germ cells (Fig. 2-3)

Most become atretic

Some begin meiosis (oocytes)
- remain arrested at prophase within primordial follicles (Fig. 2-4)
- much longer prophase arrest (50 years) than any other cell in the body

◆ Oocyte and Follicular Maturation

Groups of oocytes resume meiosis periodically
- germinal vesicle forms
- primary oocyte increases in diameter
- cortical granules produced
- granulosa cells multiply

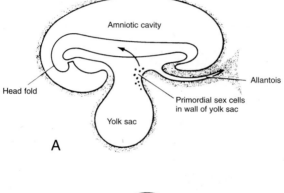

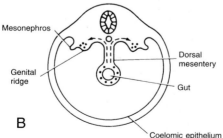

Figure 2-1. Migration of the primordial germ cells. (**A**) Sagittal section shows the origin of the germ cells in the yolk sac endoderm. (**B**) Transverse section shows the path of germ cell migration through the mesentery of the hindgut to the genital ridges. (Snell RS. The genital system. In: Clinical embryology for medical students. 2nd ed. Boston: Little, Brown & Co., 1975.)

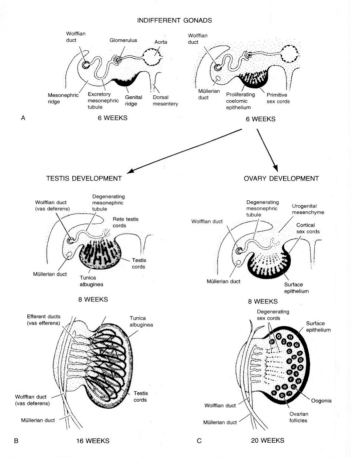

Figure 2-2. Differentiation of human gonads shown in transverse sections. (**A**) Indifferent stages, showing proliferation of the primitive sex cords. (**B**) Male development, showing persistence of the primitive sex cords that develop into the testicular ducts. (**C**) Female development, showing degeneration of the primitive sex cords, which are replaced by secondary (cortical) sex cords that proliferate from the surface epithelium. (Gilbert SF. Developmental biology. 3rd ed. Sunderland, MA: Sinauer, 1991:762.)

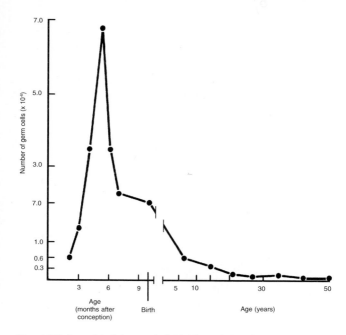

Figure 2-3. Age-related changes in the total population of germ cells in the human ovaries. The increase during the first half of pregnancy is rapid, followed by an equally rapid atresia of most of the germ cells. (Baker TG. Radiosensitivity of mammalian oocytes with particular reference to the human female. Am J Obstet Gynecol 1971;110:746.)

Transfer of cAMP is thought to keep oocyte in germinal vesicle stage
Germinal vesicle breakdown occurs just before ovulation
First polar bodies/secondary oocyte (Fig. 2-5)
Fewer than 0.1% of oocytes complete full maturation process

◆ Gene Expression During Oogenesis

RNA synthesis occurs in oogonia and oocytes at various stages of meiotic prophase
- some gene products support oocyte maturation
- other gene products remain dormant

Embryonic transcription is required in humans after a few divisions
Specific genes studied
- c-mos protooncogene

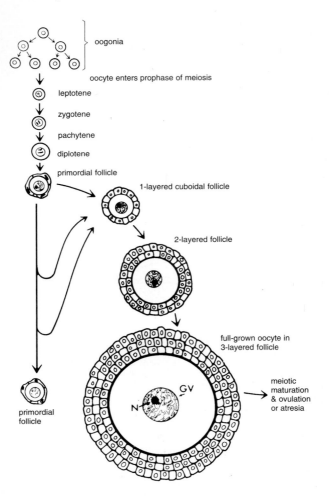

oogonia

oocyte enters prophase of meiosis

leptotene

zygotene

pachytene

diplotene

primordial follicle

1-layered cuboidal follicle

2-layered follicle

full-grown oocyte in
3-layered follicle

N — GV

meiotic
maturation
& ovulation
or atresia

primordial
follicle

Figure 2-4. Development of the female germ cells from oogonia to secondary oocytes and the concomitant stages of follicular development. Primary oocytes can remain for years in primordial follicles before beginning oocyte and follicular development. (Bachvarova R. Gene expression during oogenesis and oocyte development in mammals. In: Browder LW, ed. Developmental biology, a comprehensive synthesis. New York: Plenum Press, 1985.)

- octamer-binding gene (oct-3)
- c-kit protooncogene
- tissue plasminogen activator (tPA) gene
- sperm receptor (ZP3) gene
  - exclusively in oocytes
  - located on chromosome 5
  - regulated by cis-acting sequence in 5'-flanking region

PHENOTYPIC SEXUAL DIFFERENTIATION

Human sexual differentiation and development are simple and logical

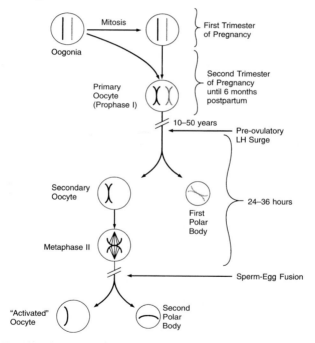

Figure 2-5. Meiosis. For simplicity, only a single pair of chromosomes is shown. During the first half of pregnancy, germ cells replicate by mitosis. Meiosis begins when the chromosomes are duplicated without cytoplasmic division occurring. The primary oocyte becomes arrested at this stage (i.e., prophase of meiosis I) until follicular development begins, usually years later. In response to the preovulatory release of luteinizing hormone, the duplicated pairs of chromosomes are separated into the secondary oocyte or the first polar body. After fertilization, meiosis is completed with division of the duplicated chromosomes into the oocyte or the second polar body.

Early embryo is bipotential
Without biochemical intervention, female phenotype develops
Male development requires two factors
1. active secretion of testicular androgens
2. nonsteroidal müllerian inhibitor factor (MIF)
   • results in regression of female internal ductal system

◆ Development of the Internal Genitalia

Close relationship between genital and urinary systems (Fig. 2-6)
Humans develop three urinary systems in succession
1. pronephros (third to fourth weeks)
2. mesonephros (fourth week)
3. metanephros (sixth week)
Male system expropriates the mesonephric (wolffian) duct
Female embryo develops paramesonephric (müllerian) duct (Fig. 2-7)
   • distinct and separate from primitive urinary tract
   • degenerates in male embryo under the influence of MIF

AGE	GLANDS	URINARY TRACT	♂ DUCTS ♀		EXTERNAL GENITALIA
3-4 weeks	PRIMORDIAL GERM CELLS	PRONEPHROS (nonfunctional) Tubules and Ducts	PRONEPHRIC		
4-9 weeks		MESONEPHROS or WOLFFIAN BODY (temporary function) Tubules and Ducts	MESONEPHROS or WOLFFIAN		CLOACA
5th week	UROGENITAL RIDGE				
6th week	INDIFFERENT GONAD: GERMINAL AND CORE EPITHELIUM	METANEPHROS or KIDNEY (permanent) Tubules and Ducts	PARAMESONEPHRIC or MÜLLERIAN		CLOACA SUBDIVIDES — — — — — GENITAL TUBERCLE
7th week	MALE TYPE CORDS				ANAL AND URETHRAL MEMBRANES RUPTURE
8th week	TESTIS AND OVARY				
9th week			MÜLLERIAN DUCTS FUSE AT TUBERCLE		URETHRAL AND LABIOSCROTAL FOLDS,
10th week			MÜLLERIAN DUCTS DEGENERATE	WOLFFIAN DUCTS DEGENERATE	PHALLUS AND GLANS
11th week			SEMINAL VESICLES, EPIDIDYMIS, VAS DEFERENS		
12th week	OVARY DESCENT COMPLETE			WALLS FORM	SEX DISTINGUISHABLE
5 months	TESTIS AT INGUINAL RING			SINUS EPITHELIUM GROWS IN VAGINAL CLEFT	
8 months	TESTIS DESCENT			RAPID UTERINE GROWTH	
TERM	COMPLETE				

Figure 2-6. Interrelations and time sequence of events in the development of the male and female genitourinary systems.

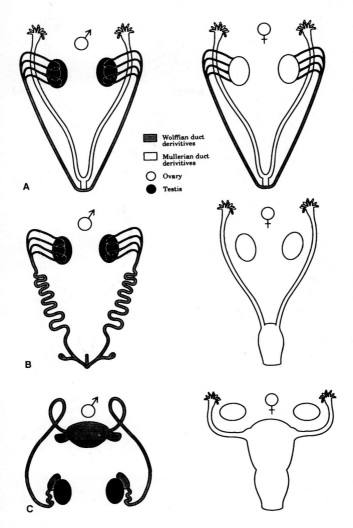

Figure 2-7. Development of the internal genital ducts. (**A**) Indifferent stage. (**B**) Intermediate stage. (**C**) Definitive female and male.

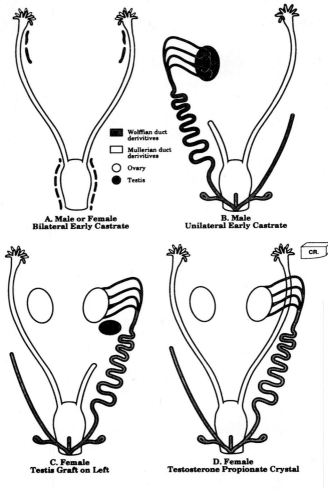

Figure 2-8. Classic rabbit experiments performed by Alfred Jost. (**A**) Female sexual development in the absence of a functional gonad. (**B**) Normal male sexual differentiation ipsilateral to the testis and female sexual development contralateral to the testis in a male fetus castrated on one side. (**C**) Male differentiation (including müllerian regression) ipsilateral to a testis graft in a female fetus with normal female development contralateral to the graft. (**D**) Male ductal differentiation without müllerian regression ipsilateral to a testosterone proprionate implant (CR) in a normal female fetus.

◆ Development of the External Genitalia

Cloaca initially serves as terminus for intestinal, urinary, and reproductive tracts
- during the sixth week, urorectal septum divides cloaca
  - anterior urogenital sinus
  - posterior rectum
- urogenital sinus develops further
  - urinary system (urethra, bladder)
  - genital system (vagina)
- before 12 weeks, sex is determined only by histologic examination of gonads

ANOMALIES OF INTERNAL SEXUAL DEVELOPMENT

Classic rabbit experiments of Alfred Jost demonstrated the process of development (Fig. 2-8)

Anomalous female internal genitalia subdivided into four areas (with examples noted)
1. failure of formation of the primordial ducts
   - müllerian agenesis
2. failure of fusion of the primordial ducts
   - uterus didelphys
3. failure of dissolution of the septum between the fused ducts
   - medium septum

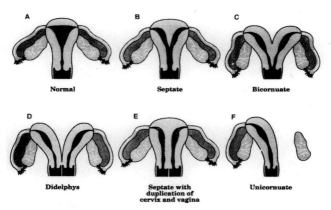

Figure 2-9. Common clinical manifestations of abnormalities of müllerian duct development. (**A**) Normal female. (**B**) Septate uterus (i.e., failure of dissolution of septum). (**C**) Bicornuate uterus (i.e., failure of fusion of mid-müllerian ducts). (**D**) Didelphys anomaly (ie., complete failure of fusion). (**E**) Septate uterus with duplication of cervix and vagina (i.e., combined failure of fusion and dissolution of septum). (**F**) Unicornuate uterus (i.e., failure of formation of one müllerian duct.)

4. failure of structures to disappear
- Gartner duct cyst

Common developmental abnormalities of the first three types are seen in Figure 2-9

MANAGEMENT OF INTERNAL SEXUAL ABNORMALITIES

◆ Müllerian Agenesis or Dysgenesis

Complete agenesis is relatively common
Vaginal agenesis often is not diagnosed until puberty
- must determine presence or absence of uterus
- progressive dilation often very successful in forming neo-vagina

High incidence of associated urinary tract anomalies
Absence of outflow tract is difficult to manage
- may require multiple surgical procedures
- hysterectomy with ovarian conservation may be considered

Failure of one duct to develop results in hemiuterus
- no correction required
- may predispose to preterm delivery

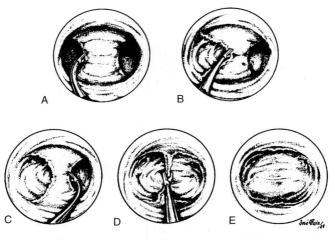

Figure 2-10. Hysteroscopic technique for septal incision. (**A**) If the septum is broad, one blade of the scissors cuts into the substance of the septum, and the other blade remains free in the cavity. (**B**) If the fundus is reached on one side, the other side is transected in a similar manner. (**C**) The center, now thinned, of the septum is transected. (**D**) The upper portion septum is cut. (**E**) The operation is finished. (Baggish MS, Barbot J, Valle RF. Diagnostic and operative hysteroscopy: a text and atlas. Chicago: Year Book, 1989:171.)

◆ Uterine Cavity Duplication

Bicornuate uterus less common
* not usually associated with infertility or pregnancy loss

Septate uterus frequently associated with repetitive pregnancy losses
* easily treated by hysteroscopic resection (Fig. 2-10)
* simultaneous laparoscopy should be performed
* only indication for septum removal is recurrent pregnancy loss or primary infertility with all other factors excluded

ANOMALIES OF EXTERNAL SEXUAL DIFFERENTIATION

◆ Hormonal Causes

Female external development occurs in absence of androgens
Male sexual development requires androgens
* testosterone must be converted to DHT by 5 α-reductase

Female abnormalities from androgen exposure
* congenital adrenal hyperplasia
* androgen-producing adrenal or ovarian tumors

Male abnormalities are more common
* interference with androgen production
* deficit in 5 α-reductase production
* failure in androgen action
  * androgen insensitivity syndrome (complete testicular feminization)

◆ Evaluation of the Infant With Ambiguous Genitalia

Difficult and potentially psychologically devastating event
Three questions must be considered
1. Is there a life-threatening condition that has resulted in the abnormal differentiation?
2. What is the potential for fertility?
3. What is the potential for normal sexual functioning?

Need to immediately rule out salt-losing form of CAH
* check serum 17-OH progesterone
  * level greater than 1000 ng/dL virtually diagnostic

Normal future fertility consistently present only in CAH
5 α-reductase deficiency may present with incomplete masculinization
Size of a phallus may be determining factor in assigning sex
* less than 2.5 cm long, trial of three months of testosterone
  * failure of penis to lengthen should give consideration to sex reversal surgery

3

◆ Physiology of Reproduction

INTRODUCTION

Successful reproduction relies on complex system of communication between hypothalamus, pituitary, ovary, and endometrium

Sexual maturity, ovarian follicular development, and ovulation are dependent on this interplay

Monthly cycle of oogenesis, conception or menstruation depends on pulsatile GnRH release from hypothalamus and episodic pituitary gonadotropin secretion (Fig. 3-1)

HYPOTHALAMUS

Forms lateral walls of the ventral aspect of the third ventricle
* junction between the diencephalon and the telencephalon

Comprised of two types of nerve fibers
1. unmyelinated fibers connecting within hypothalamus involved in peptide synthesis and release
2. ascending myelinated neurons that secrete norepinephrine and serotonin
   * directly regulate GnRH secretion

Parvicellular neurosecretory system within medial hypothalamus closely linked to reproductive function
* two important neural bundles: GnRH and Dopamine

GnRH secretion modified by ascending input into hypothalamus

◆ Hypothalamic Hormones

Pituitary hormone synthesis and secretion directed by five hypothalamic peptides
* GnRH (gonadotropin-releasing hormone)
* CRF (corticotropin-releasing factor)
* GHRF (growth hormone-releasing factor)
* somatostatin
* TRH (thyrotropin releasing hormone)

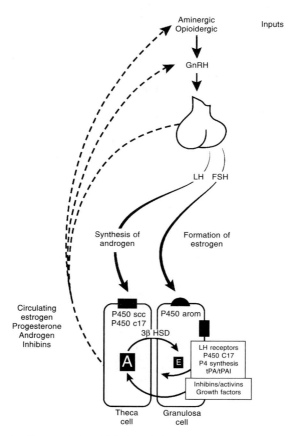

Figure 3-1. Representations of the hypothalamic-pituitary-ovarian interaction in the control of the human menstrual cycle. The pulsatile release of luteinizing hormone (LH) and follicle-stimulating hormone (FSH), mediated by the hypothalmic gonadotropin-releasing hormone (GnRH), induces ovarian theca and granulosa cell steroidogenesis and follicular maturation. The theca cell is endowed with LH receptors, which mediate LH-induced P-450 steroidogenic enzymes and the synthesis of androgens and function as targets of modulators from the paracrine granulosa cells. The multifunctional granulosa cell has the capacity to generate FSH-mediated LH receptors, P-450 C17 enzyme, and progesterone synthesis (P_4). It has the ability to produce locally a variety of autocrine paracrine regulators, such as growth factors and tissue plasminogen activator and inhibitors (tPA and tPAI). (Yen SSC, Jaffe RB: Reproductive endocrinology. 3rd ed. Philadelphia: WB Saunders, 1991:291.)

GnRH
- decapeptide
- pulsatile release 60 to 90 minute cycle
  - stimulates pulsatile release of FSH and LH
- circulatory half life = 2 to 4 minutes
- pulse amplitude and frequency important
- agonists downregulate the axis (mimic menopausal condition at ovary)

CRF
- controls pituitary secretion of ACTH
- major role is mediating response to stress/hypoglycemia
- release inhibited by circulating cortisol

GHRF
- triggers episodic GH secretion and release from anterior pituitary
- GH regulates many growth functions
  - stimulated by GHRF
  - tonic inhibition from somatostatin
- GHRF inhibited by IGF-1 and IGF-2 action

Somatostatin
- inhibits release of GH, TSH, GI hormones
- reduces intestinal blood flow, may suppress immune function

TRH
- stimulates TSH release
- critical for thyroid regulation
- inhibited by negative feedback from thyroid hormones

◆ **Regulation of Hypothalamic Function**

GnRH secretion regulated by central and peripheral feedback
- central action of neurotransmitters

GnRH can upregulate the concentration of its own receptors
- high pulse frequency or tonic exposure decreases receptor number

PITUITARY

◆ **Regulation of Pituitary Function**

Largely under hypothalamic control, modified by ovarian steroid feedback

Hypothalamic factors travel through the hypophyseal portal system

Pituitary is major site of steroid feedback action
- biphasic feedback results in preovulatory gonadotropin surge

Ovarian factors
- inhibin
  - α and β subunit protein produced by granulosa cells
  - potent inhibitor of FSH release
- activin

- BB homodimer
- stimulates FSH release

Control of prolactin synthesis and secretion is different
- mediated by dopamine
- tonic inhibitory control

◆ Anterior Pituitary Function (LH, FSH, Prolactin)

◇ *LH and FSH*

Glycoprotein dimers secreted by gonadotrophs

β subunits are distinctive

Menopausal levels chronically elevated
- extraction from urine useful in fertility treatments

◇ *FSH*

Stimulates follicular maturation

Stimulates granulosa cells to aromatize androgens to estradiol

Peak secretion with midcycle LH surge

Critical sequence for follicular and granulosa cell stimulation

FSH → FSH and estradiol → FSH, LH, and estradiol

◇ *LH*

Stimulates theca cell androgen production

Stimulates ovum maturation (meiosis)

Ovulation

Luteinization of granulosa cells

Progesterone production

Corpus luteum formation

◇ *Prolactin*

Single polypeptide secreted by lactotrophs
- homology with GH, hPL (human placental lactogen)

Affects numerous metabolic processes
- mammary gland development
- stimulation of milk secretion
- maintenance of newly formed LH receptor sites in folliculo-
genesis

◆ Posterior Pituitary Hormones

◇ *Vasopressin (ADH)*

Synthesized as prohormone

Bound to neurophysin (large transport peptide)

Responsible for volume regulation and osmolarity

Probably regulated by anterior hypothalamic osmoreceptor

◇ *Oxytocin*

Also synthesized as prohormone and bound to neurophysin

Primarily involved in labor and lactation
- uterine action
- mammary myoepithelial action

Control of secretion

Primarily regulated by cholinergic and noradrenergic neurotransmitters and opiod peptides

Also influenced by estrogen, TRH, and angiotensin II

OVARY

Primordial germ cells originate from yolk sac endoderm

Migrate to genital ridge by 5 weeks gestation

Maximum number of germ cells 6 to 7 million at 20 weeks
gestation

- follicular atresia reduces this to 1 to 2 million at birth
- 300,000 at time of puberty

◆ Ovarian Hormones

Three lipid-related-steroids: estrogens (C18), androgens (C19),
progestins (C21)

- all share perhydrocyclopentanophenanthrene ring
- synthesized from cholesterol (Fig. 3-2)

◆ Regulation of Ovarian Function

✧ *Follicular phase*

10 to 14 day complex, orderly cascade resulting in rich estradiol
microenvironment

Primordial follicle

- oocyte surrounded by granulosa cell precursors

Primary follicle

- oocyte surrounded by single layer of cuboidal granulosa cells
- zona pellucida formed from mucopolysaccharide secretions
  of granulosa cells

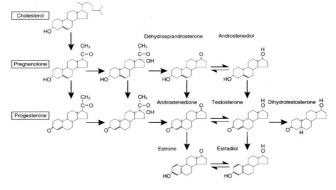

Figure 3-2. General scheme for the synthesis of estrogens and androgens.
(Yen SSC, Jaffe RB. Reproductive endocrinology. 3rd ed. Philadelphia: WB
Saunders, 1991:159.)

Secondary follicle
- primary oocyte arrested in first prophase of first meiotic division
- several layers of granulosa cells

Tertiary follicle
- formation of antrum (steroid-rich follicular fluid)
- two to three layers of granulosa cells
- formation of cumulus oophorus
- large preovulatory follicle = graafian follicle

Follicular development dependent on gonadotropins
FSH induces receptor upregulation on granulosa cells
- aromatase converts androgens to estrogens
  - estrogens further stimulate granulosa cells

LH stimulates theca cells production of androstenedione

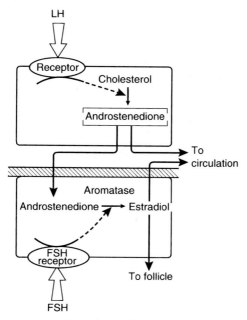

Figure 3-3. Coupling of granulosa and theca cells in the two-cell, two-gonadotropin theory of follicular estrogen production. (FSH, follicle-stimulating hormone; LH, luteinizing hormone; Ryan KJ, Berkowitz R, Barbieri R, eds. Kistner's gynecology, principles and practice. 5th ed. Chicago: Year Book, 1990.)

- two-cell, two-gonadotropin theory
- delicate balance
  - low levels of androstenedione promote aromatase
  - high levels promote follicular atresia (Fig. 3-3)

Preovulatory events
- dominant follicle has increased estradiol production
  - associated with falling FSH
- peak estradiol 24 to 36 hours prior to ovulation
- progesterone production also shows increase 12 to 24 hours prior to ovulation

✧ *Ovulation*

Preovulatory LH and FSH surge
- precedes ovulation by as much as 36 hours

Mechanism of ovulation is complex
- not simply a pressure phenomenon

✧ *Luteal phase*

Granulosa cells reorganize to form corpus luteum

Increased progesterone synthesis

Rapid vascularization

Negative feedback on gonadotropin pulse generator

Corpus luteum dependent on tonic LH support

Luteolysis occurs in 14 ± 2 days if no pregnancy occurs
- hCG maintains luteal function by binding to LH receptor
- luteoplacental shift occurs by 8 weeks gestation
- if no pregnancy then progesterone and estradiol levels drop allowing for new follicular growth

PUBERTY

Developmental period during which sexual maturity is attained

Under strict neuroendocrine control
- relies on increase in pulse amplitude of GnRH

◆ Neuroendocrine Development

GnRH pulsatile secretion
- detectable after 20 weeks gestation
- gradually decreases in first year of life
- nadir at 6 to 8 years
- initiation of puberty driven by increase in pulse amplitude
  - no change in pulse frequency

Prolactin detected as early as 12 weeks gestation
- during puberty levels rise to adult levels in girls

Growth hormone
- increase in episodic release and in volume
- necessary for skeletal, muscle growth

Adrenal androgen
- increase in adrenal steroids (adrenarche) occurs as early as 7 to 8 years

Stage 1. Infantile or preadolescent stage that persists from infancy; areola not pigmented, only papilla are elevated.

Stage 2. Breast bud stage that is the first indication of pubertal changes. The areola diameter enlarges; breast and papilla are elevated in a small mound.

Stage 3. Breast and areola enlarge further, with a continuous round contour.

Stage 4. Areola and papilla enlarge and project to form a secondary mound above the remaining breast.

Stage 5. Mature adult breast develops, with resolution of the secondary mound to achieve a smooth, rounded contour with projection of the papilla only.

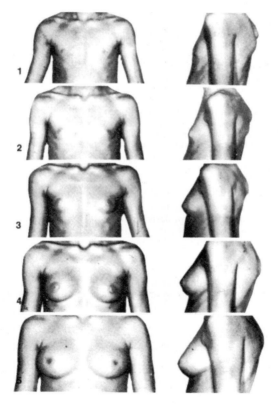

Figure 3-4. Tanner stages of breast development. (Tanner J.M. Growth at adolescence. 2nd ed. Oxford: Blackwell Scientific, 1962)

- precocious puberty does not result from premature acceleration of adrenal axis
- adrenarche and gonadarche are independent events

◆ Sexual Maturation and Growth During Puberty

Mean age of onset of puberty 11 years
- precocious <7.5 years
- delayed >14 years

Breast development typically the first physical manifestation of puberty

Orderly progression through Tanner stages (Fig. 3-4)
- breast development varies greatly—based on nutrition and genetics
- progression from stage 2 to 5 takes 4 years on average
  - some women never reach Stage 5 until 1st pregnancy or later
- hormonal stimulation required for endocrine function of the breast
  - estrogen for ductal growth
  - progesterone and prolactin for lobuloalveolar development

◆ Pubic Hair Development (Fig. 3-5)

Influenced by pubertal increase in adrenal androgens
Breast development and pubic hair development do not necessarily begin at same time
Pubic hair may appear first but usually follows thelarche

◆ Acceleration of Linear Growth

Usually precedes menarche
Associated with early puberty in girls
- boys' peak height velocity occurs 2 years later

Governed by GH and gonadal sex steroids

◆ Bone Development

Useful index of development
Correlates more closely with menarche than chronologic age

◆ Body Composition

Women acquire two times as much body fat
Men have 1.5 times increase in lean body mass, muscle mass, skeletal mass

MENSTRUAL CYCLE

◆ Characteristics

Mean age of menarche 12.3 to 12.8 years
Menstrual cycle standard length 28 days (range 26 to 30 days)

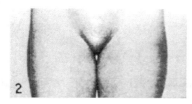

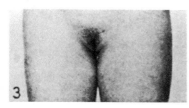

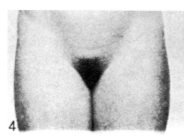

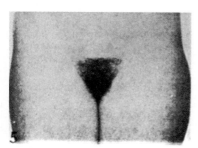

Stage 1.
Infantile or preadolescent with no pubic hair.

Stage 2.
Sparse or growth of long, slightly pigmented, downy hair, primarily on labia majora.

Stage 3.
Amount of hair increases, with some spread to mons pubis, and becomes coarser, darker, more curly.

Stage 4.
Adult-type hair covering a smaller area than in most adults, with no spread to medial thigh.

Stage 5.
Adult distribution of coarse hair with some spread to medial surface of the thighs, characteristic of normal female escutcheon.

Figure 3-5. Standards for evaluating pubic hair development. (Tanner J.M. Growth at adolescence. 2nd ed. Oxford: Blackwell Scientific, 1962)

First day of bleeding = Day 1 of cycle
Menstrual flow usually 4 to 6 days, 25 to 60 mL total blood loss

◆ Histologic Phases

◇ *Early proliferative*
Endometrium <2 mm thick, low columnar
Glands tubular, straight, narrow

◇ *Late proliferative*
Glands hypertrophy
Increase in stromal ground substance

◇ *Secretory (Fig. 3-6)*
Stromal edema
Epithelium with glycogen-rich basal vacuoles

◇ *Mid-late secretory*
Tortuous glands
Secretory debris

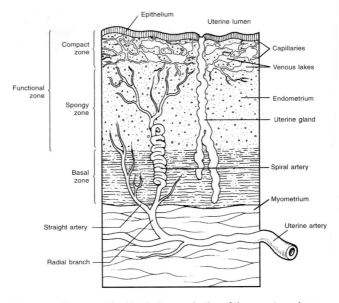

Figure 3-6. Diagram of the histologic organization of the secretory-phase human endometrium. (Blandau RJ. Weiss-Greep histology. 4th ed. New York: McGraw-Hill, 1977:911.)

✧ *Premenstrual*
Stromal infiltration by polymorphonuclear and mononuclear leukocytes

◆ Mechanism of Menstruation

Prostaglandins accumulate
Inadequate perfusion for upper one half to one third of endometrium
Disruption of lysosomes contribute to cellular destruction, tissue necrosis, and endometrial sloughing
- phospholipases liberate arachidonic acid
- increased prostaglandin concentration leading to uterine contractions

MENOPAUSE

Ovary gradually loses responsiveness to FSH/LH
Early follicular phase FSH levels increase
LH levels unaffected
Rise in FSH possibly related to decreased inhibin production
Cessation of ovarian follicular maturation defines menopause
Postmenopausal ovary has minimal estrogen production but significant testosterone and androstenedione

4

◆ Normal and Abnormal Placental Development

INTRODUCTION

Placental examination indicated after every delivery
- systematic examination required
- only 5% to 15% of placentas require full pathologic analysis

Correlation of clinical outcome with placental pathology still evolving

PLACENTAL ANATOMY AND PHYSIOLOGY

◆ Gross Placental Development

Entire surface of chorion covered with villi in early pregnancy
Differential growth evident by third month
- chorion laeve (abembryonic side)
- chorion frondosum (future formal placenta)

Term placenta
- round or oval
- 15 to 20 cm diameter
- 2 to 3 cm thick
- weight 450 to 550 g
- maternal surface 12 to 20 subdivisions (cotyledons)

◆ Normal Placental Histology

Primary villi replaced by tertiary villi (contain blood vessels)
Covered by double layer of epithelium
- inner cytotrophoblast (Langerhans layer)
- outer syncytiotrophoblast

Two functional layers develop in decidua (Fig. 4-1)
1. inner layer (Rohr layer)
2. outer layer (Nitabuch layer)
   - may have immunoprotective function

Three types of villi
1. stem villi
2. intermediate villi
3. terminal villi
   - site of maternofetal exchange

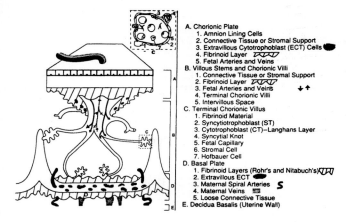

A. Chorionic Plate
  1. Amnion Lining Cells
  2. Connective Tissue or Stromal Support
  3. Extravillous Cytotrophoblast (ECT) Cells
  4. Fibrinoid Layer
  5. Fetal Arteries and Veins
B. Villous Stems and Chorionic Villi
  1. Connective Tissue or Stromal Support
  2. Fibrinoid Layer
  3. Fetal Arteries and Veins
  4. Terminal Chorionic Villi
  5. Intervillous Space
C. Terminal Chorionic Villus
  1. Fibrinoid Material
  2. Syncytiotrophoblast (ST)
  3. Cytotrophoblast (CT)–Langhans Layer
  4. Syncytial Knot
  5. Fetal Capillary
  6. Stromal Cell
  7. Hofbauer Cell
D. Basal Plate
  1. Fibrinoid Layers (Rohr's and Nitabuch's)
  2. Extravillous ECT
  3. Maternal Spiral Arteries
  4. Maternal Veins
  5. Loose Connective Tissue
E. Decidua Basalis (Uterine Wall)

Figure 4-1. Schematic view of a placental unit and the components of identified segments. (Novak RF. A brief review of the anatomy, histology, and ultrastructure of the full-term placenta. Arch Pathol Lab Med 1991; 115:654.)

◆ Fetal and Maternal Placental Circulation

Vascular system appears by the middle of the third week in embryo
- by 5 to 6 weeks yolk-sac-derived erythroblasts arrive in villous vessels

Umbilical ring constricts
- only umbilical vessels remain by the end of the third month

Umbilical cord
- 30 to 100 cm long
- 2 cm diameter
- three vessels
  - single vein
    - carries oxygenated blood to fetus
  - paired arteries
    - branches of hypogastric artery
- umbilical blood flow
  - 500 mL/min at term
- uteroplacental blood flow
  - 600 mL/min at term
  - total intervillous space
    - 150 mL at term
    - replenished 3 to 4 time per minute
  - no vascular control mechanism
    - control proximal to uteroplacental arteries

◆ Fetal Membranes

Chorion and amnion have different anatomic origins
Growth continues until 28 weeks
- enlargement by stretching after 28 weeks

Strength
- amnion is one third as thick as chorion, but tensile strength is greater than chorion

Twins (Fig. 4-2)
- membranes have profound clinical importance

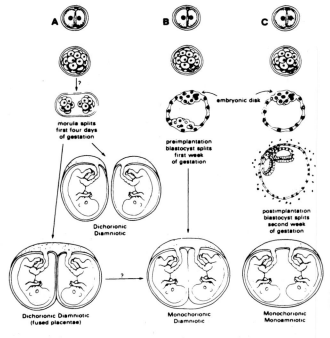

Figure 4-2. The evolution of placentation in monozygotic twins. (**A**) Splitting of the developing embryo before 4 days results in separate amnions and chorions. These may implant in the endometrium at a distance or close together, where the placentas may fuse. The dividing septum in the latter case consists of four layers. (**B**) The preimplantation blastocyst splits before amnion development, during the late first week or early second week. The chorion envelops both fetuses, but they have separate amnions. The septum contains two layers. (**C**) Splitting after implantation and amnion differentiation results in no septum. Later splits result in conjoined twins. (Hafez ESE, Evans TN. Human reproduction conception and contraception. Hagerstown: Harper & Row, 1973.)

◆ Postpartum Placental Examination

All placentas should be examined grossly
Pathologic examination indicated in certain cases (Table 4-1)
Umbilical cord
- length, insertion site, vessels, knot

Fetal surface
- course of vessels

Membranes
- color, opacity, insertion site, chorionic plate
- meconium, infarction, amnion nodosum

Maternal surface
- missing cotyledons
- old clot/infarction

GROSS ABNORMALITIES OF THE PLACENTA

◆ Placentomegaly

>600 g unfixed
Many etiologic factors
- diabetes
- anemia
- chronic infection

**TABLE 4-1. Indications for Placental Processing and
Examination by a Pathologist**

Maternal Indications
Diabetes mellitus
Chronic hypertension
Pregnancy-induced hypertension
Preterm delivery (<35 wk)
Postterm delivery (>42 wk)
Unexplained fever
Previous poor obstetric history
No or minimal prenatal care
Substance abuse
Unexplained elevation of α-fetoprotein

Fetal Indications
Stillborn
Neonatal death
Multiple gestation
Intrauterine growth retardation
Congenital anomalies
Hydrops fetalis
Admission to neonatal intensive care
Low 5-minute apgar (<6) or umbilical artery pH (<7.20)
Meconium-stained fluid
Polyhydramnios or oligohydramnios

- blood group incompatibility
- twin-twin transfusion syndrome
- congenital neoplasm

◆ Multiple Placental Discs

Accessory lobes
- succenturiate placenta
  - completely separate from main lobe
- bipartite placenta
- duplex placenta
  - no main lobe identified

◆ Placenta Membranacea

Attaches to entire surface of uterus
- may result from too-shallow implantation
Increased risk for bleeding, prematurity

◆ Extrachorial Placentas

Membranous chorion does not insert at periphery of villous chorion
Circumarginate
- membranes arise without bulky folding

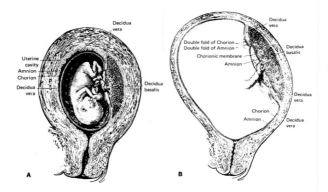

Figure 4-3. Placenta circumvallata. (**A**) At 12 weeks of gestation, the maternal surface of the placenta is in contact with the decidua basalis. The fetal surface is composed of a central chorionic membrane and, at the periphery, an extrachorionic zone covered by decidua. Fetal membranes are reflected at the margin of the central portion, producing a circumvallate ring.(**B**) In late pregnancy, a well-developed annulus can be seen. Notice the relations between the chorionic membrane and extrachorionic decidua and the duplication of membranes. (Williams JW. Placenta circumvallata. Am J Obstet Gynecol 1927;13:1.)

Circumvallate (Fig. 4-3)
• arise from an elevated cup-like fold

◆ Amnion Nodosum

Fetal surface covered by elevated nodules <5 mm diameter
Pathognomonic for oligohydramnios

◆ Amniotic Bands

Two pathologic categories (Fig. 4-4)
Can result in severe fetal deformation (Table 4-2)

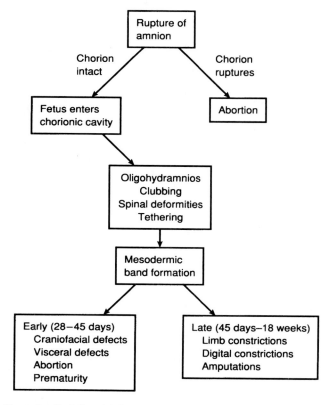

Figure 4-4. Evolution of defects from amnion disruption. Early rupture typically produces deformities and malformed structures with later ruptures. (Seeds JW, Cefalo RC, Herbert WN. Amniotic band syndrome. Am J Obstet Gynecol 1982; 144:24.)

TABLE 4-2. Abnormalities Associated With Amnion Disruption

Multiple and Asymmetric Limb Defects
Constriction rings of limbs or digits
Amputation of limbs or digits
Pseudosyndactyly
Abnormal dermal ridge patterns
Simian creases
Clubbed feet

Craniofacial Defects
Multiple and asymmetric encephalocele
Anencephaly
Facial clefting (e.g., lip, palate)
  Embryologically appropriate
  Embryologically inappropriate
Severe nasal deformity
Asymmetric microphthalmia
Incomplete or absent cranial calcification

Visceral Defects
Gastroschisis
Omphalocele

◆ Infarcts and Placental Ischemia

Single spiral artery is end artery for a portion of placenta
- infarcts typically pyramidal in shape
  - more significant if central area is >3 cm
  - fetus can tolerate as much as 30% infarction if placental flow is otherwise normal
    - 5% to 10% infarction may cause poor perinatal outcome in presence of uteroplacental insufficiency
  - commonly occurs with PIH or underlying vasculopathy (SLE, diabetes)

Maternal floor infarct
- pathogenesis unknown
- 3- to 6-mL band of fibrinoid exudate covers maternal surface
- massive intervillous fibrin deposition
- 50% of women have had previous spontaneous abortion or stillbirth
  - high recurrence rate

UMBILICAL CORD ABNORMALITIES

◆ Variations in Length

Function determining cord length is not well understood
- short cords could be result of impaired fetal movement
  - can result in labor complications

- Long cords are associated with fetal heart rate abnormalities
  - nuchal cord (one fifth of all deliveries)
    - fetal injury in extreme cases

◆ True Knots

Found in 1% of pregnancies
Most are loose
Tight knots could result in adverse outcomes

◆ Abnormal Cord Insertion

Usually central or paracentral insertion
- high rate of eccentric insertions in twins
Velamentous insertion
- fetal vessels can be torn in labor
Insertia funiculi furcata
- rare anomaly with lack of Wharton jelly in portion of cord proximal to insertion of placenta

◆ Single Umbilical Artery

Incidence 0.25% to 1.0%
- increased in infants of diabetic mothers, twins
- acardiac monster
- sirenomelia (embryopathy from vascular shunting)
Always check mid-point of cord to eliminate false impression of single artery from fusion of two arteries
Perinatal outcome worse
- 1/4 have associated anomalies
  - renal
  - tracheoesophageal fistula
  - CNS abnormalities

◆ Twinning and Multiple Gestation

Increasing rate of multiple births
Natural reduction does occur
Determines zygosity by examination of placenta
- monozygosity incurs certain risks
  - vascular connections resulting in twin-twin transfusion syndrome
  - in utero death of one twin
    - stuctural lesions can occur in survivor (Table 4-3)

◆ Miscellaneous Lesions

Cysts of all sizes can be found
- occasionally 1 cm, rarely 5 cm
- lined by X cells
  - extravillous trophoblastic cells
- clear fluid

Hemangiomas, chorioangiomas occur in 1/5000 deliveries
- can be associated with fetal complications (acute polyhydramnios)

Malignant neoplasms
- rare but have been reported

MICROSCOPIC ABNORMALITIES OF THE PLACENTA

◆ Inflammation

Chorioamnionitis occurs in more than 20%
- usually ascending infection often with prolonged ruptured membranes but can occur in intact membranes
- can occur in patients without clinical signs or symptoms (pathologic diagnosis only)
  - consider a serious maternal infection if no clinical basis for chorioamnionitis exists
    - syphilis
    - listeriosis
    - malaria
    - Chagas disease
    - tuberculosis
- inflammatory cells enter from maternal side

Funisitis (umbilical cord inflammation) indicates prolonged and severe infection

Intervillositis suggests listeriosis

TABLE 4-3. Abnormalities in Children Whose Monozygotic Co-twin Died in Utero

---

Central nervous system defects
  Cerebellar necrosis
  Hydranencephaly
  Porencephaly
  Multicystic encephalomalacia
  Hydrocephalus
  Microcephaly
  Spinal cord transection
Gastrointestinal defects
  Small bowel atresia
  Colonic atresia
  Appendiceal atresia
Renal defects
  Congenital renal cortical necrosis
  Horseshoe kidney
Hemifacial microsomia
Aplasia cutis congenita
Terminal limb defects

Hoyne HE, Higginbottom MC, Jones KL. Vascular etiology of disruptive structural defects in monozygotic twins. Pediatrics 1981;67:81.

Villitis associated with poor fetal outcome
* CMV
* parvovirus
* toxoplasmosis
* syphilis
* unknown 7% to 14%
    * associated with a risk of recurrence

◆ Disorders of Villous Maturation

Naturally accelerated in conditions associated with maternal uteroplacental vascular insufficiency

Maturity delayed in diabetes, nonimmune hydrops, severe anemia, syphilis

Dysmature development in karyotypically abnormal fetuses

◆ Fetal Nucleated Erythrocytes

Do not occur in normal pregnancies beyond the second trimester
* their release indicates an abnormal condition
    * blood group incompatibility
    * chronic intrauterine infection
    * chronic fetomaternal transfusion
    * fetal hypoxia

◆ Meconium Staining

Meconium exacerbates preexisting chorioamnionitis
* necrosis of amniotic epithelium

Can probably affect umbilical vessel vascular tone

Timing of passage of meconium
* acute staining characterized by green discoloration
* subacute staining brown-green discoloration
* muddy brown staining indicates meconium expressed for at least 3 hours

5

◆ Normal Pregnancy and Prenatal Care

OBJECTIVES OF PRENATAL CARE FOR THE PATIENT

To increase patient well-being before, during, and after pregnancy
To improve self-image and capability for self-care
To reduce maternal morbidity/mortality
To decrease fetal loss and unnecessary pregnancy interventions
To reduce risk to health before subsequent pregnancies and beyond childbearing years
To promote development of parenting skills

OBJECTIVES FOR PRENATAL CARE AND CARE OF THE INFANT

To increase the child's well-being
To reduce preterm birth, intrauterine growth retardation, congenital anomalies, and failure to thrive
To promote healthy growth and development, immunization, and health supervision
To reduce neurologic, developmental, and other morbidities
To reduce child abuse, neglect, injuries, preventable acute and chronic illnesses

OBJECTIVES OF PRENATAL CARE FOR THE FAMILY DURING PREGNANCY AND FIRST YEAR OF LIFE

To promote family development and positive parent-infant interaction
To reduce unintended pregnancies
To identify behavior disorders leading to child neglect and family violence

PRINCIPLES AND DEFINITIONS OF VITAL STATISTICS

Live Birth   Expulsion or extraction of a product of human conception from the mother regardless of gestational age which shows evidence of life (sustained heart beat, respiration)

Fetal Death or Stillbirth   Death before complete expulsion or extraction of a product of human conception from the mother excluding pregnancy termination

Early Neonatal Death   Death of a live born infant during 7 days of life

Late Neonatal Death   Death of infant after 7 days but before 29 days of life

Perinatal Death   Combination of fetal deaths and neonatal deaths

Maternal Mortality   Death of a woman from any cause related to or aggravated by pregnancy or its management up to 40 days after the termination of pregnancy

Direct Obstetric Death   Result of obstetric complication of pregnancy, labor, or puerperium

Indirect Obstetric Death   Result from a preexisting disease or a disease that developed during pregnancy, labor, or the perperium where physiologic effects of pregnancy were partially responsible

Fetal Death Rate (Stillborn Rate)   Number of stillborn infants/1000 infants born

Neonatal Mortality Rate   Number of fetal deaths plus neonatal deaths/1000 total births

PRECONCEPTIONAL COUNSELING

◆ Maternal Disease That Adversely Affect Pregnancy

✧ *Diabetes*
Major malformations significantly more common
- metabolic control of paramount importance

✧ *Phenylketonuria (PKU)*
Elevated maternal levels of phenylalanine result in fetal defects
- microcephaly
- IUGR
- congenital heart disease
- subsequent mental retardation

Preconceptual lowering of phenylalanine levels is important in preventing this syndrome

◆ Maternal Disease Adversely Affected by Pregnancy

Cardiac diseases
Thromboembolic diseases
Marfan syndrome

◆ History of Poor Pregnancy Outcome

Preconceptional evaluation and therapy
- antiphospholipid antibodies
- lupus anticoagulant
- heparin, steroid, or low-dose aspirin treatment may be indicated

◆ Maternal Medications That Adversely Affect Pregnancy

See Chapter 13

◆ Immunizations

Congenital rubella infection has devastating sequelae
Preconceptional assessment of immunity with vaccination may be helpful

◆ Social Habits That Adversely Affect Pregnancy

See Chapter 13

◆ Genetic Risks

See Chapter 12

◆ Nutritional Counseling

Early treatment of eating disorders is appropriate before conception
Folate may decrease risk of neural tube defects

DIAGNOSIS OF PREGNANCY

◆ Positive Evidence of Pregnancy

◇ *Fetal heart rate*

Can be detected by transvaginal ultrasound 4 weeks after conception
• 6 weeks after conception by transabdominal ultrasound
Auscultation
• Doppler 10 to 12 weeks
• fetoscope 17 to 19 weeks

◇ *Fetal movement*

After 19 weeks, intermittent movements are perceived by the mother

◇ *Visualization of the fetus*

Gestational sac visualized by 5 to 6 weeks after LMP by transvaginal ultrasound
After 16 weeks, fetus can be seen on pelvic x-rays

◆ Probable Evidence of Pregnancy

◇ *Enlargement of the abdomen*

Pelvic organ before 12 weeks
Palpable abdominal organ after 12 weeks

◇ *Uterine changes*

Hegar sign

Palpable softening of the lower part of the corpus
Appears at the sixth week of gestation

✧ *McDonald sign*
Uterine body and cervix can be flexed against each other
Depends on localized softening

✧ *Cervical changes*
Goodell sign
Softening of the cervix

✧ *Chadwick sign*
Blue violet hue to the cervix

✧ *Endocrine tests*
Determination of human chorionic gonadotropin (hCG)
Levels
• 100 mIU/mL by first day of missed LMP
• increases exponentially
• peaks at 70 days
• falls until 120 days then remains at 5 to 20 mIU/mL
Pregnancy tests
• enzyme-linked immunoassays (ELISA)
• sensitive down to 25 mIU/mL

◆ **Presumptive Evidence of Pregnancy**

✧ *Cessation of menses*
Reliable in reproductive-aged women with previously regular
    menses

✧ *Breast changes*
Shortly after missed period several symptoms appear
• heavy sensation
• tingling and soreness

✧ *Vaginal mucosa and skin changes*
Mucosa becomes congested, blue-violet hue
Increased pigmentation, abdominal striae common

✧ *Nausea*
One half of pregnant women experience nausea in early preg-
    nancy
Usually appears between 2 and 12 weeks
• subsides in most cases 6 to 8 weeks later
Commonly more severe in the morning

✧ *Bladder irritability*
Common early in pregnancy
Usually resolves by second trimester

✧ *Fatigue*
Can be a severe symptom of early pregnancy

Etiology unclear
Usually resolves by 20th week

✧ *Perception of fetal movement*
Peculiar sensation described as "fluttering"
16 to 18 weeks in a multiparous patient; several weeks later in a
primiparous patient

◆ **Diagnosis of Fetal Death**

Failure of uterine growth
Regression of signs of pregnancy
Positive endocrine tests do not necessarily mean a continuing
viable pregnancy
Real-time ultrasound is primary method of establishing diagno-
sis of fetal death
Two independent observers should document lack of cardiac
activity
Radiologic signs of fetal death
Spalding sign: overlapping of fetal cranium with exaggerated
curvature of spine
Robert sign: presence of gas in fetal abdomen

ESTIMATION OF DURATION OF PREGNANCY

◆ **Naegle Rule**

Convenient method of determining estimated date of confinement (EDC)
Add 7 days to LMP, subtract 3 months and add 1 year

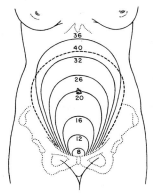

Figure 5-1. The height of the fundus at comparable gestational dates
varies greatly among patients. Those shown are the most common. A
convenient rule of thumb is that, at 20 weeks of gestation, the fundus is
usually at or slightly above the umbilucus.

◆ Timing From Quickening

Maternal perception of fetal movement occurs usually between 16 and 18 weeks

◆ Height of the Fundus

Can be used to evaluate gestational age (Fig. 5-1)
- 12 weeks: uterus felt above the pubic symphysis
- 16 weeks: uterus rises to half the abdomen
- 20 weeks: uterus present at the level of umbilicus
- 36 weeks: uterus just below the ensiform cartilage

Deviations from expected rate of growth can alert the physician to abnormalities

PRENATAL CARE DURING THE FIRST VISIT

◆ Initial History and Physical Examination

Should follow a standardized routine
Typical timetable for low-risk pregnancy

◇ *12 Weeks*
Check fetal heart tones with Doppler

◇ *14 to 16 Weeks*
Assess growth
Order genetic tests as indicated
- amniocentesis
- maternal serum α-fetoprotein (MSAFP)

Review prenatal labs

◇ *20 Weeks*
Auscultate with fetoscope
Reassess gestational age if clinical dates not established
Consider ultrasound

◇ *24 Weeks*
Begin maternal education

◇ *28 Weeks*
Administer Rh immune globulin as indicated
Perform gestational diabetes screen
Risk assessment as indicated

◇ *30 to 40 Weeks*
Observe for complications
Repeat hemoglobin
Initiate fetal surveillance as indicated

◇ *41 Weeks*
Plan for postdate pregnancy

◆ Initial Laboratory Studies

CBC
Blood group with Rh type
Serologic test for syphilis
Rubella
Test for hepatitis B
Urine for glucose, protein, ketones, and culture

◆ Patient Education

Patients should be aware of danger signs
- vaginal bleeding
- persistent vomiting
- chills or fever
- dysuria
- abdominal pain or uterine cramping
- swelling of the face or fingers
- CNS or visual disturbances
- oliguria
- leakage of fluid
- decrease in fetal movements
- signs of preterm labor

PRENATAL CARE DURING SUBSEQUENT VISITS

Weight
Blood pressure
Urinalysis
Examination of the abdomen
Other tests

◇ *Maternal serum α-fetoprotein (MSAFP)*

Screening test for neural tube defects at 15 to 19 weeks
Levels peak at 15 weeks

◇ *Elevated maternal serum α-fetoprotein*

Neural tube defect (NTD)
Abdominal wall defects (gastroschisis, omphalocele)
Fetal death
Multiple gestation
Incorrect dates

◇ *Low MSAFP*

Associated with Down syndrome
Combining with urinary estriol and hCG may be better (triple
marker)

◇ *Glucose tolerance testing*

Clinical history inadequate to select for screening
Screening should be done at 28 weeks
- nonfasting

- perform 3 hour GTT if 1 hour is >130 mg/dL (whole blood) or >150 mg/dL (serum)

✧ Hepatitis B screening
Transmission to fetus is higher in patients with HBeAg
- HBIG and HBV should be administered at delivery
  - 85% to 98% effective at preventing neonatal infection

✧ HIV Testing
Best estimate of risk of congenital transmission is 25% to 35%
Can be transmitted via breast milk

✧ Chlamydia Trachomatis
Detected in the cervix in 2% to 13% of pregnant women
Most are not symptomatic
60% to 70% neonatal transmission rate
- conjunctivitis
- pneumonia
Screening of high-risk group for all patients is based on physician discretion
Erythromycin is drug of choice
- partner should be treated as well

✧ Antepartum Rh immune globulin
See Chapter 24

◆ Principles and Definitions
Requirement: minimal amount of specific nutrient necessary to prevent a deficiency state
Allowance: proportionally increased amount to account for individualized variation in need, absorption, metabolism
National Research Counsel recommended dietary allowances (RDA) (see Table 5-1)

◆ Energy and Weight Gain

✧ Energy requirements
Basal energy needs increase approximately 20%
- 300 kcal/day increase
- total pregnancy: 80,000 kcal
Minimal expenditure in early pregnancy
- increases sharply at end of first trimester

✧ Weight gain
Pregnancy weight gain and prepregnancy weight correlate with birth weight
Weight gain of 24 to 28 lb (11 to 13 kg) commonly recommended
Desirable gain related to prepregnancy weight
    Underweight (BMI <19.9) → 30 lb (13.6 kg)
    Normally proportioned (BMI 19.9-26) → 20 lb (9 kg)
    Overweight (BMI >26 to 29) → 16 lb (7 kg)

TABLE 5-1. Recommended Dietary Allowances for Women of Reproductive Age and for Pregnant and Lactating Women

Nutrient	Nonpregnant Women	Pregnant Women	Increase (%)	Lactating Women	Sources
Energy	2200 kcal	2500 kcal	+14	640 kcal	Protein, fat, carbohydrate
Protein	50 mg	60 mg	+20	65 g	Meats, fish, poultry, dairy
Fat-Soluble Vitamins					
Vitamin A	800 μg	800 μg No change		1300 μg	Dark green, yellow, or orange fruits, vegetables, liver
Vitamin D	5 μg	10 μg	+100	10 μg	Fortified dairy products
Vitamin E	8 μg	10 μg	+25	12 μg	Vegetable oils, nuts, leafy vegetables
Vitamin K		65 μg		65 μg	Green vegetables, dairy products
Water-Soluble Vitamins					
Vitamin C	60 mg	70 mg	+17	95 mg	Citrus fruits, tomatoes
Thiamine	1.1 mg	1.5 mg	+36	1.6 mg	Enriched grains, pork
Riboflavin	1.3 mg	1.6 mg	+23	1.8 mg	Meats, liver, grains
Niacin	15 mg	17 mg	+13	20 mg	Meats, nuts, legumes
Vitamin B$_6$	1.6 mg	2.2 mg	+37	2.1 mg	Poultry, fish, liver, eggs
Folate	180 μg	400 μg	+120	280 μg	Leafy vegetables, liver
Vitamin B$_{12}$	2 μg	2 μg	+10	2.6 μg	Animal proteins
Minerals					
Calcium	800 mg	1200 mg	+50	1200 mg	Dairy products
Phorphorus	800 mg	1200 mg	+50	1200 mg	Meats
Magnesium	280 mg	320 mg	+14	355 mg	Seafood, legumes, grains
Iron	15 mg	30 mg	+100	15 mg	Meats, eggs, grains
Zinc	12 mg	15 mg	+25	19 mg	Meats, seafood, eggs
Iodine	105 μg	175 μg	+17	200 μg	Iodized salt, seafood
Selenium	55 μg	65 μg	+18	75 μg	Seafood, liver, meats

◇ *Protein requirements*
- Estimate requirements by different methods
- RDA provides for an additional 30 g/day
  Mature women: 1.3 g/kg/day
  Adolescents 15- to 18-years-old: 1.5 g/kg/day
  Adolescents <15 years old: 1.7 g/kg/day

◇ *Dietary fasting and food restriction*
Optimal fetal growth dependent on maternal accumulation of certain amount of excess body stores
Fetus cannot protect itself by parasitizing the mother
Pregnant patients with eating disorders are at risk for poor pregnancy outcome

◇ *Iron and folate*
Requirements
- total amount during pregnancy is 1000 mg of iron
- folate requirements are also increased
  - RDA is 800 mg (double that of nonpregnant women)

Effects of Deficiency
- if iron stores are insufficient, hemoglobin and hematocrit will decline
- anemia seen in one third of pregnant women
  - usually iron deficiency
  - rarely folate deficiency
    - adequate folate important in prevention of neural tube defects

Calcium and Vitamin D
- 30 g of calcium accumulated during pregnancy
  - most in fetal skeleton
  - RDA is 1200 mg (one quart of milk)
- vitamin D important in many functions
  - RDA is increased by 5 ng (200 IU)
- osteomalacia can result in cases with short intervals between pregnancies and inadequate calcium and vitamin D intake
- certain drugs can interfere with calcium metabolism
  - heparin
  - phenytoin

REDUCING PSYCHOSOCIAL AND ENVIRONMENTAL RISKS

◆ Smoking
21% to 30% of pregnant women smoke
Associated with IUGR and prematurity

◆ Alcohol Use
Associated with increased rates of
- spontaneous abortion

- perinatal mortality
- IUGR
- low birth weight
- congenital abnormalities (fetal alcohol syndrome)

No known level of alcohol consumption is safe in pregnancy

◆ Drug Abuse

Increasingly a problem especially in inner cities
Complex social problem
Drug treatment programs are recommended

◆ Employment

United States legislation to protect working women has been slow
Little convincing evidence linking work in general to low birth-weight or prematurity.
Conditions should be altered for patients with a history of adverse pregnancy outcome or problem in the index pregnancy

◆ Maternal Stress or Anxiety

Effects of stress are unknown
Improved social support may influence outcome

◆ Family Violence

Pregnancy consistently associated with more frequent violent attacks on women
Reported in all social, economic and education levels
Prenatal risk assessment is appropriate

COMMON COMPLAINTS AND QUESTIONS

◆ Exercise

Uterine oxygen consumption remains constant
- fetal changes are small

Activities should be restricted in those with high-risk conditions
Women should be discouraged from vigorous cardio-vascular conditioning exercises in the third trimester of pregnancy

◆ Immunizations

See Chapter 26

◆ Travel

Avoid sitting for long periods of time without stretching
Plane travel presents no additional risk

◆ Nausea and Vomiting

Common in early pregnancy
Etiology unclear
Hospitalization may be necessary to correct fluid and electrolyte imbalance

◆ Heartburn

Usually from increased gastric acid reflux
Relief provided by antacids
Elevation of the head in bed may be useful

◆ Varicosities

Full length support hose are helpful
Vulvar varicosities may be helped by the use of several perineal pads

◆ Sexual Relations

It is generally accepted that there is no adverse effect
May have adverse effects on high-risk pregnancy
Previous history of preterm labor, premature rupture of membranes increases risk of adverse effect

◆ Vaginal Hygiene

Douching rarely indicated
• never use a bulb syringe
• never place douche bag higher than 2 feet above level of the hip
Tub baths are safe throughout pregnancy

◆ Bowel Habits

Constipation is a common complaint
Liberalized water, vegetable, and fruit intake
Mild laxatives are safe for occasional use
Strong cathartics or enemas should be avoided

◆ Caffeine

CNS stimulant
Generally regarded as safe
No proven deleterious effects when ingested in customary amounts

6

◆ Normal Labor and Delivery

HUMAN GESTATION

Average 266 days from conception or 280 days (40 weeks) from beginning of last menstrual period

Only 5% of pregnancies that continue beyond the second trimester end on the estimated date of confinement (EDC)
- most women deliver within seven days of due date (Table 6-1)

Delayed ovulation/implantation results in overestimation of pregnancies continuing beyond 42 weeks
- in carefully dated pregnancies only 5% remain undelivered 42 weeks from corrected last menstrual period

LABOR

◆ Onset of Labor

Carefully studied in many animal models
- fall in progesterone
- increased estrogen

TABLE 6-1. Term of Pregnancies Delivered at Various Weeks of Gestation

Weeks	Australia* (%, n = 2555)	Iowa† (%, n = 10,244)
37	5.7	5.0
38	11.8	11.7
39	23.2	19.8
40	12.8	35.6
41	18.5	17.5
42	12.9	10.4
Total	99.9	100.0

*Data from Beischer NA, Evans JH, Townsend L, et al. Studies in prolonged pregnancy: the incidence of prolonged pregnancy. Am J Obstet Gynecol 1969;103:476.
†Data from University of Iowa Hospitals, 1982-86.

- fetal cortisol production (sheep)

Human studies are limited
- no decline present in progesterone
- no prelabor surge in fetal cortisol levels

◆ Length of Labor

Three stages of labor
- first stage
  - onset of contractions to full dilation (10 cm)
- second stage
  - complete dilation to delivery of baby
- third stage
  - delivery of baby to delivery of placenta

Parity very important
- nulliparae 8% of labors greater than 24 hours
- multiparae 2% have labors greater than 24 hours

Friedman curve
- based on studies in laboring patients (Table 6-2)
- charts dilatation vs. time in labor

Latent phase
- may last for several hours
  - onset of labor often difficult to assess

Abnormal labors may require physician intervention

COMPONENTS OF LABOR AND DELIVERY

◆ Powers

Relationship between prelabor uterine activity and early labor not fully characterized

TABLE 6-2. Length of Labor

Stage of Labor	Mean	Median	Mode	Limit
Nulliparous				
First stage (h)	14.4	12.3	9.5	
Latent phase (h)	8.6	7.5	6.0	20
Active phase (h)	4.9	4.0	3.0	12
Maximum slope (cm/h)	3.0	2.7	1.5	1.2
Second stage (h)	1.0	0.8	0.6	2.5
Parous				
First stage (h)	7.7	6.5	5.1	
Latent phase (h)	5.3	4.5	3.5	14
Active phase (h)	2.2	1.8	1.5	5.2
Maximum slope (cm/h)	5.7	5.2	4.5	1.5
Second stage (h)	0.2	0.2	0.1	0.8

Early labor
- contractions usually every 5 to 10 minutes, lasting 30 to 45 seconds and 20 to 30 mm Hg of intensity

Advancing labor
- contractions 2 to 3 minutes apart, 50 to 70 seconds in length, and 40 to 60 mm Hg
- traction placed on cervix as upper myometrial fibers shortened
  - cervix "taken up"

In normal labor, fetus descends and patient perceives urge to defecate
- Valsalva and uterine contractions increase descent of fetus and lead to delivery

◆ Passageway

✧ *Bony pelvis*
Predictable sequence of fetal events results in passage through bony pelvis

Anatomy
- four bones
  - sacrum, coccyx, two innominates (each made up of pubis, ischium, and ilium)

Descent is not direct superoinferior journey (Fig. 6-1)

Pelvic Plane

Inlet (top line noted above)
- widest diameter is obstetric conjugate

Mid-pelvis
- narrowest AP diameter important
- transverse diameter (interspinous distance) also crucial to pelvimetry

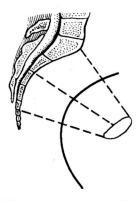

Figure 6-1. The solid line indicates the curve of Carus or axis of the pelvis. Notice that its direction is not superoinferior, but first inferoposterior and finally inferoanterior.

Outlet
- two triangles
  - borders are the inferior pubic symphysis and the sacro-coccygeal junction

✧ *Pelvic types*

Four classic types are recognized
1. gynecoid (Fig. 6-2)
   - best suited for child bearing
   - most common type
2. android (Fig. 6-3)
   - not favorable for delivery
3. anthropoid (Fig. 6-4)
   - AP diameter of inlet greater than transverse diameter
4. platypelloid (Fig. 6-5)
   - least common type (flat)

✧ *Clinical pelvimetry (Table 6-3)*

Not always easy

Three critical pelvic diameters (only one measured directly)
- obstetric conjugate
  - measure diagonal conjugate (Fig. 6-6)
    - exceeds obstetric conjugate by 1.5 to 2 cm
- diameter of mid-pelvis
  - assess prominence of ischial spine
    - prominent spines suggest narrow mid-pelvis
- transverse diameter of outlet
  - assess directly

Other factors
- hollowness of sacrum
- width of sacrosciatic notch
- subpubic angle

TABLE 6-3. Features Determined by Clinical Pelvimetry Related to Pelvic Type

Features	Gynecoid	Android	Anthropoid	Platypelloid
Promontory reached (diagonal conjugate ≤12 cm)	−	±	−	+
Sacrum flat/forward versus curved	−	+	−	+
Spines prominent	−	+	+	−
Sacrosciatic notch narrow (≤2 fingerbreadths)	−	+	−	−
Subpubic arch narrow (acute angle)	−	+	+	−

+, present: −, absent: ±, variable.

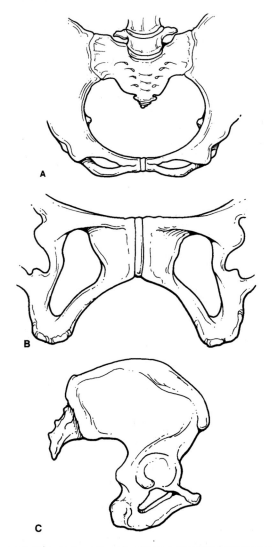

Figure 6-2. Typical gynecoid pelvis. (**A**) Inlet view. The pelvis is almost round. (**B**) Lateral view. (**C**) Subpubic arch view. The sidewalls are straight and the subpubic arch curves gently. (Steer CM. Moloy's evaluation of the pelvis in obstetrics. 2nd ed. Philadelphia: WB Saunders, 1959.)

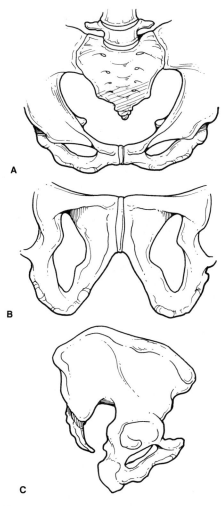

Figure 6-3. Typical android pelvis. (**A**) Inlet view. The inlet is almost heart shaped, and the widest transverse diameter is in the far posterior portion of the pelvic inlet. (**B**) Lateral view. The sacrum curves forward, and therefore the sacrosciatic notch is narrow. (**C**) Subpubic arch view. The bones are heavy. The sidewalls converge, and the subpubic arch is narrower than that seen in Figure 6-2. (Steer CM. Moloy's evaluation of the pelvis in obstetrics. 2nd ed. Philadelphia: WB Saunders, 1959.)

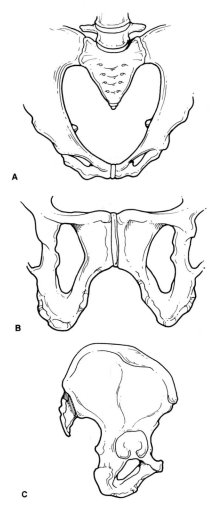

A

B

C

Figure 6-4. Typical anthropoid pelvis. (**A**) Inlet view. Notice that the anteroposterior diameter of the inlet, unlike the other pelvic types, is larger than the widest transverse diameter. (**B**) Lateral view. The sacrosciatic notch is wide. (**C**) subpubic arch view. Although the sidewalls are straight, there is some narrowing of the subpubic arch. (Steer CM. Moloy's evaluation of the pelvis in obstetrics. 2nd ed. Philadelphia: WB Saunders, 1959.)

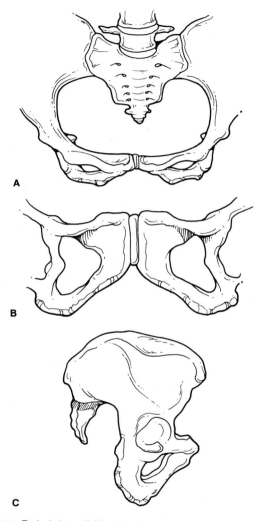

Figure 6-5. Typical platypelloid pelvis. (**A**) Inlet view. The anteroposterior diameter is short, and the transverse diameter is wide. (**B**) Lateral view. The sacrum is inclined anteriorly, decreasing the anteroposterior dimensions. (**C**) Subpubic arch view. The arch is shallow and wide. (Steer CM. Moloy's evaluation of the pelvis in obstetrics. 2nd ed. Philadelphia: WB Saunders, 1959.)

✧ *X-ray pelvimetry*
More precise than clinical examination
Utility is limited
Some risk associated with radiography
CT pelvimetry associated with less radiation exposure
Indications
- pelvic deformity
- abnormal fetal presentation
Standard values (Table 6-4)
- determined in patients with arrest of labor or abnormal presentation

✧ *Soft tissue obstruction*
Ovarian tumors
Uterine leiomyomata
Cervical carcinoma
Vaginal septa
- usually yields to forces of labor or can be incised

◆ The Passenger

✧ *Nomenclature*
Fetal attitude: relationship of fetal parts to one another independent of mother

---

TABLE 6-4. Pelvic Diameters Determined by X-ray Pelvimetry

Pelvic Diameters	Measurement (cm)	
	Mean	SD
Anteroposterior of inlet (obstetric conjugate)	12.2	1.2
Transverse of inlet	13.1	1.0
Transverse of midpelvis (interspinous)	10.2	0.8

Varner MW, Cruikshank DP, Laube DW. X-ray pelvimetry in clinical obstetrics. Obstet Gynecol 1980:56:296.

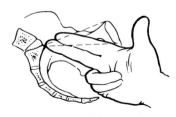

Figure 6-6. Measurement of the diagonal conjugate. (Steer CM. Moloy's evaluation of the pelvis in obstetrics. 2nd ed. Philadelphia: WB Saunders, 1959.)

Fetal presentation: portion of fetus that overlies pelvic inlet
- cephalic in 95% of term labors

Fetal position: orientation of fetal presenting part to maternal bony pelvis

✧ *Clinical evaluation*

Determined by abdominal examination, vaginal examination, ultrasound as needed

Malpresentations in cephalic lie (Fig. 6-7)
- complete extension of head; face presentation
- military attitude: deflexed vertex presentation
- sinciput; brow presentation
  - cannot deliver vaginally

Position determined by palpation of skull sutures (Fig. 6-8)

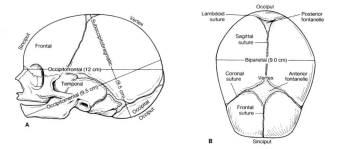

Figure 6-7. The relation among the bones, sutures, and fontanelles of the fetal head.

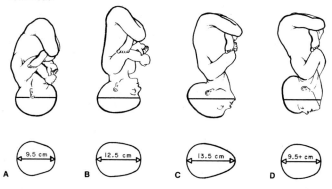

Figure 6-8. Types of cephalic presentations according to the degree of flexion or extension. (**A**) Vertex. (**B**) Sinciput or deflexed vertex. (**C**) Brow. (**D**) Face. The dimensions refer to the presenting diameters of the term-size fetus.

MECHANISM OF LABOR

Five cardinal movements (Fig. 6-9)
1. engagement
2. descent
3. flexion
4. internal rotation
5. extension

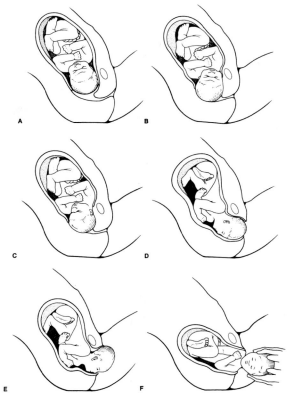

Figure 6-9. Typical mechanism of labor in the gynecoid pelvis. (**A**) The vertex engages in the transverse position. (**B**) With further descent, resistance of the pelvic floor results in increased flexion. (**C**) In the midpelvis, internal rotation occurs. (**D,E**) With further descent, birth of the head results from extension of the head. (**F**) After delivery of the head, external rotation of the vertex returns the body to its former transverse position. (Birth Atlas. 5th ed. New York: Maternity Center Association, 1960.)

◆ **Pearls**

1. BPD is the narrowest presenting diameter of the fetal head. In most labors it is necessary for this narrowest portion of the fetal oval to be accommodated to the narrowest portion of the maternal pelvis

2. The occiput tends to rotate to the widest (most ample) portion at any level in the maternal pelvis

◆ **Engagement**

Occiput usually engages in gynecoid pelvis in transverse position (see #1 above)

Engagement inferred when leading bony point has reached the level of the ischial spine (zero station)

Sacrum should be partially filled by head as descent occurs

◆ **Descent**

Station +1, +2, +3 refer to centimeters above or below the plane of the ischial spine

Extreme molding can confuse the actual station (Fig. 6-10)

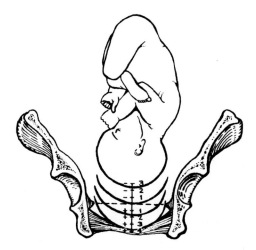

Figure 6-10. Stations of fetal head. At the 0 station, the fetal head has descended to the level of the ischial spines. The levels above this are designated as −1, −2, and −3, referring to the distance in centimeters between the head and the ischial spines. With further descent, the stations are designated by positive integers, such as +1, +2, and +3.

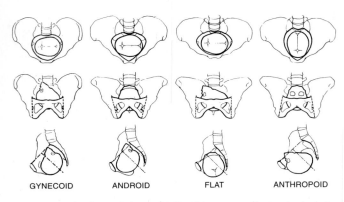

GYNECOID   ANDROID   FLAT   ANTHROPOID

Figure 6-11. Influence of characteristic pelvic types on the mechanism of labor. (Danforth DN, Ellis AH. Midforceps delivery—a vanishing art? Am J Obstet Gynecol 1963;86:29.)

◆ Flexion

Increased resistance to fetal descent results in flexion of head on neck

◆ Internal rotation

Occurs at level of spines
Smallest diameter of fetal head (BPD) passes through mid-pelvis and AP diameter

◆ Extension

Further descent allows delivery by extension of head
External rotation after delivery of head

✧ *Pelvic types*

Mechanism of labor influenced by type of bony pelvis (Fig. 6-11)
- anthropoid
  - roomy posterior pelvis so internal rotation to posterior position common
- android
  - narrow fore-pelvis directs head posteriorly
- platypelloid
  - descent occurs in transverse position
  - delivery may occur as transverse (if at all) or late rotation or perineum

✧ *Breech and face presentation*

Breech delivery entails three movements of internal rotation
Negotiates mid-pelvis as sacrum transverse

- breech delivered by lateral flexion
- fetal back moves anteriorly
- fetal shoulders enter pelvis in transverse diameter
- further rotation of back to sacrum transverse
- shoulders pass AP through mid-pelvis
- back rotates anteriorly again
- fetal head passes through mid-pelvis in AP orientation

Face presentation
- delivery occurs by flexion of chin under pubic symphysis
  - mentum posterior position will not deliver vaginally
  - usually rotates anteriorly

CLINICAL CONDUCT OF LABOR AND DELIVERY

◆ Patient Instruction

Education is critical regarding specific events
- bleeding
- SROM
- change in normal fetal activity

Nullipara patients usually told to remain home until contractions every five minutes for 1 hour

Multipara patients told to come in as soon as they perceive labor beginning

◆ Admission

Initial assessment very important

History
- EDC
- fetal well-being
- contractions
- membrane condition
- pregnancy complications

Examination
- vital signs
- fetal lie/presentation
- estimated fetal weight
- cervical examination
  - if term and no bleeding, perform examination
  - defer if ruptured membranes and preterm gestation
  - dilation and effacement as well as cervical position (anterior, posterior) and consistency should be noted

Fetal condition
- electronic fetal heart rate (FHR) monitoring
  - initial evaluation for 20 to 30 minutes
  - if abnormal, institute continuous FHR monitoring
- continuous monitoring in low-risk patient is not therapeutic
  - physician and others must be skilled in interpretation
- intermittent auscultation

- low-risk patient
- initially reassuring FHR tracing
- occasional 15- to 30-minute session of continuous FHR
- reinstitute continuous EFM for changes in fetal status
  - abnormal labor
  - meconium
  - bleeding
  - blood pressure elevation in mother
  - decelerations

◆ Laboratory Evaluations

Depends on circumstances
Usually type and screen, hematocrit, and urine for protein

◆ Routine Procedures

No longer perform extensive shaving or routine enema
Individualized care to each patient
Oral intake limited
Ambulation or various positions in chair or bed encouraged

◆ Subsequent Care

Temperature every four hours
Pulse and blood pressure every hour
Fetal heart rate (if not on continuous monitoring)
- every 30 minutes in latent phase
- every 15 minutes in active phase
- every 5 minutes in second stage
Vaginal examinations
- performed based on individual labors
- usually hourly in active phase labor
Amniotomy
- allows for internal FHR monitoring
- commits latent phase patients to delivery
- shorten active phase labor/check for meconium
- can lead to cord prolapse with high stations

◆ Meconium

Related to gestational age (Table 6-5)
Usually a soft indication of fetal distress
- meconium is common; asphyxia is not
Meconium aspiration
- may be related to increased pulmonary vascular resistance secondary to in utero hypoxia
- airway management at delivery may be less important than originally thought but still a critical component of neonatal resuscitation

TABLE 6-5. Prevalence of Meconium Staining Related to Gestational Age

Weeks of Gestation	Meconium-Stained Amniotic Fluid (%)
≤36	8
37	10
38	11
39	13
40	17
41	21
42	28
≥43	34

Data from University of Iowa Hospitals—10,244 births, 1982-1986.

SECOND STAGE OF LABOR

Critical time for the fetus
Cord compression may become more severe

◆ Location and Maternal Position

Birthing room/labor-delivery-recovery room births now more common
  • wall coverings do not matter; observation of FHR, sufficient light and access to instruments does matter
Position
  • usually dorsal lithotomy
  • semi-sitting
  • left lateral
    • rare in the United States
Delivery of head
  • gentle counter-pressure
  • perineum usually washed with antiseptic solution

◆ Episiotomy

Neither routinely required nor routinely avoided
  • may be preferred to uncontrolled laceration
Midline or mediolateral
  • midline usually preferred but extension into rectum is more common

◆ Delivery of Head/Body

After head is delivered, suction nose and mouth with bulb
  • DeLee suction trap used if meconium present
    • intubation after umbilical cord is cut
Shoulders delivered with gentle downward pressure
Body of fetus then delivered in controlled fashion

Cord clamped and cut
Staff prepared for need of resuscitation (based on Apgar scores)
Section of cord can be clamped and cut for cord gas assessment
   (Table 6-6)

THIRD STAGE OF LABOR

No attempt at removal of placenta until signs of separation
- uterus rises in abdomen
- shape changes from discoid to globular
- cord lengthens
- gush of blood

Gentle traction on cord with support of uterus (Fig. 6-12)
Oxytocin usually given after delivery of placenta
- 4 U intravenous bolus
- 20 to 30 U/liter intravenous fluid
- 10 U IM
- Indications for manual removal
- heavy bleeding
- third stage greater than 30 minutes
- narcotic, neuroleptic, general anesthesia required

Failure of removal may be indication of placenta accreta
- hysterectomy may be required if hemorrhage occurs

FOURTH STAGE OF LABOR

Evaluation of vagina, cervix, and placenta
Cervical laceration
- repair if extended greater than half way up to vaginal fornix

Vaginal laceration/episiotomy
- repaired to provide anatomic reapproximation

TABLE 6-6. Cord Blood Gas Values for Term Vaginally Delivered, Vertex Presenting Newborns

Source	Mean	SD
Arterial Blood		
pH	7.26	.07
P	45.98	8.21
P	16.86	6.73
Base excess	−6.06	3.34
Venous Blood		
pH	7.34	.06
P	35.66	5.23
P	28.49	6.73
Base excess	−5.03	2.53

Courtesy of EW Kandel, M.D., University of Iowa, IA.

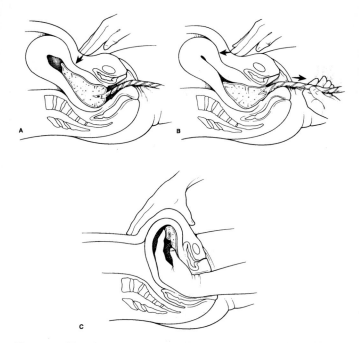

Figure 6-12. Technique of placental delivery. (**A**) Tractiion should not be applied to the umbilical cord until signs of placental separation are noted. (**B**) At this point, gentle traction on the cord coupled with elevation of the uterine corpus with the operator's other hand results in placental delivery. (Adapted from Wilson JR, Atlas of Obstetric technique. St Louis: CV Mosby, 1961.) (**C**) Manual removal of the placenta may be necessary. (Adapted from Davis ME, Rubin R, eds. DeLee's obstetrics for nurses. 17th ed. Philadfelphia: WB Saunders, 1962.)

Postpartum hemorrhage
- 90% result of uterine atony
    - massage uterus
    - oxytocin
    - methylergonovine (0.2 mg) IM
    - 15 methylprostaglandin F_2a (0.25 mg IM)
        - contraindicated in patient with history of asthma
    - maternal hypertension may be worsened with both of the last two agents

INDUCTION OF LABOR

◆ Elective induction

Only when risk approaches zero
Iatrogenic prematurity was previously greatest risk
Requirements
- parous patient
- favorable cervix (greater than 2 cm dilated)
- singleton, vertex
- 39-week gestation
- eager patient

◆ Indicated Induction

Can be one of the most difficult obstetric decisions
Oxytocin usually required
- relative contraindication
  - cephalopelvic disproportion
  - nonvertex presentation
  - scarred uterus
  - very-distended uterus
  - advanced maternal age or parity

Dosing
- 0.5 to 1.0 mU/min increased by 1 to 2 mU/min every 30 to 40 minutes

Prostaglandin E_2 gel
- may be useful in cases of unfavorable cervix in planned induction

7

◆ Obstetric Anesthesia and Analgesia

PAIN OF PARTURITION

Pain of contraction
Conducted via paracervical and inferior hypogastric plexuses to
    sympathetic nerve chain at L2-L3
* enter spinal cord through nerve roots of T10, T11, T12 (Fig. 7-1)
Transmitted through small-diameter myelinated delta A fibers
    and unmyelinated C fibers (Fig. 7-2)
Several ascending pathways
Modulated by input from several nuclei

◆ Intensity

Related to physical factors
* strength, duration of contraction
* degree of distention of vagina, perineal tissues
* use of oxytocin
Psychologic factors
* fear
* exhaustion
* nausea, vomiting

SYSTEMIC ANALGESIA AND SEDATION

◆ Systemic Narcotics

✧ *Meperidine (Demerol)*
Less emesis than morphine, decreased fetal CNS effects
* maximal fetal depression 2 to 4 hours after administration
Usual dose 25 to 50 mg IM or IV
Elimination half-life of 22.7 hours in neonatal blood

✧ *Morphine*
Pharmacologically more potent than meperidine by factor of 10
Alleged to cause more neonatal depression than meperidine

✧ *Fentanyl*
100 times the potency of morphine

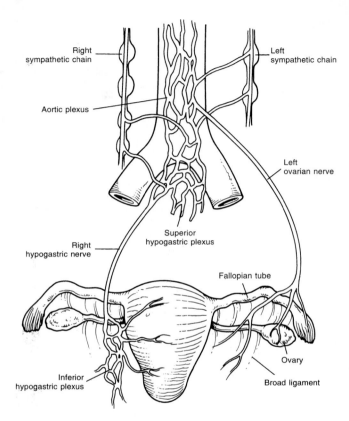

Figure 7-1. Sympathetic nerve supply of the uterus from the pelvic and abdominal distribution. The uterine nerves arise from the upper part of the uterus (i.e., upper uterine segment), the contraction of which contributes to pain; the lower part of the uterus (i.e., lower uterine segment), the contraction of which contributes to pain; and the cervix, the dilation of which contributes to pain. The ovarian nerve supplies the ovary, fallopian tube, broad ligament, round ligament, and the side of the uterus, and it communicates with the uterine plexus. The sympathetic efferent and afferent fibers are shown together. (Abouleish E. Pain control in obstetrics. Philadelphia; JB Lippincott, 1977.)

Short duration (20 to 30 minutes) with rapid onset
Brief reduction in fetal heart rate reactivity may occur
Probably underused in management of pain during labor in the
United States

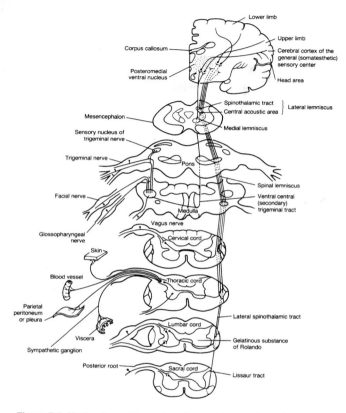

Figure 7-2. Nociceptive pathways from the periphery to the brain. (Bonica JJ. Labor pain mechanisms and pathways. In Marx GF, Bassel GM eds. Obstetric analgesia and anesthesia. New York: Elsevier, 1980:173-195.)

✧ *Nalbuphine (Nubian)*
Narcotic agonist-antagonist
No significant advantage over Meperidine
Possible transient depressive effect on fetal CNS

✧ *Butorphanol (Stadol)*
Synthetic agonist-antagonist
- Five times more potent than morphine; 40 times more potent than meperidine

Moderately popular in the United States

Usual dose 1 to 2 mg IV

✧ *Patient-Controlled Systemic Analgesia (PCA)*

Episodic and increasing nature of labor pain reduces efficacy of PCA

Not widely used for management of labor

May be beneficial management of postcesarean pain

✧ *Narcotic Antagonists*

Naloxone (Narcan) reverses opioid-induced respiratory depression

- maternal dose, 0.4 mg IV bolus
- neonatal dose, 0.01 mg/kg (IV or IM)

◆ Nonnarcotic Drugs

✧ *Benzodiazepines*

Used as seizure prophylaxis in other parts of the world

Amnestic properties present in Midazolam

- used in cesarean section induction for general anesthetic

✧ *Barbiturates*

No longer widely used

◆ Use of Systemic Medications

✧ *Maternal effects*

Nausea

Vomiting

Sedation

Decreased gastric motility

Respiratory depression

✧ *Neonatal effects*

CNS depression

Respiratory depression

Altered neuroadaptive behavior

Decreased temperature regulation

REGIONAL ANALGESIA

◆ Local Anesthetic Agents (Table 7-1)

Block exchange of sodium and potassium ions across cell membrane

Manufactured as chloride salts

Ester configuration (chloroprocaine)

- rapid onset of action
- short duration
- low toxicity

Amide configuration (lidocaine, bupivacaine)

- slow onset

TABLE 7-1. Characteristics, Concentrations, and Properties of Local Anesthetics

Characteristics	Chloroprocaine (Nesacaine)	Tetracaine (Pontocaine)	Lidocaine (Xylocaine)	Bupivacaine (Marcaine)
Type	Ester	Ester	Amide	Amide
Potency	Moderate	High	Moderate	High
Duration	Short	Long	Intermediate	Long
Physiochemical Properties				
Molecular weight	302	300	234	325
Plasma protein binding (%)		75	64	95
Concentratons				
Infiltration (%)	1–2		0.5–1	0.125
Field block (%)	1		0.50–1	0.125–0.25
Pudendal, paracervical (%)	1.5		1	0.25–0.50
Spinal (mg)		4–12	20100	5–15
Epidural block				
Labor (%)	1.5–2	1–1.5	0.25–0.5	
Surgery (%)	3	2	0.50	
Maximal initial dose (mg/kg)	20	1.5	7	2–3

Akamatsu TA, Bonica JJ. Spinal and extradural analgesia: anesthesia for parturition. Clin Obstet Gynecol 1974;17:183.

- long duration of action
- usually greater toxicity

◆ Side Effects of Local Anesthetic Drugs

✧ *Systemic toxicity*
Normal safe doses
- lidocaine, 7 mg/kg (300 mg)
- bupivacaine, 2 to 3 mg/kg (175 mg)
- chloroprocaine, 20 mg/kg (800 to 1000 mg)

Signs and symptoms of toxicity
- relaxed feeling
- drowsiness
- lightheadedness
- tinnitus
- metallic taste
- slurred speech
- blurred vision
- unconsciousness
- convulsions
- cardiac dysrhythmias and arrest

Management of toxicity
- avoidance
- systemic support
- oxygen
- IV fluids
- airway management if required

◆ Use of Local Anesthesia

✧ *Local infiltration of perineum*
Usually 10 to 20 mL of solution
Preferred drugs lidocaine (1%), chloroprocaine (2%)

✧ *Pudendal block*
Easily performed
- inject laterally, posteriorly to iliac spine
- inject through sacrospinous ligament into pudendal canal
- always aspirate before injecting

Good local block
Complications
- infection
- abscess

✧ *Paracervical block*
May result in brachycardia
- probably from uterine artery vasoconstriction

Use has decreased greatly since onset of monitoring

LUMBAR EPIDURAL ANALGESIA

Most common agents
- 2-chloroprocaine (1% to 2%)
- bupivacaine (0.0625% to 0.5%)
- lidocaine (1% to 2%)

Technique
- insertion of 17- or 18-gauge Tuohy needle through the ligamentum flavum into epidural space
- performed at L4-L5, L4-L3, or L2-L3 interspace
- fine catheter placed in cephalad direction

◆ Epidural Opioids

- Combination with local anesthetics has become popular
- Fentanyl and Bupivacaine
- Sufentanil and Bupivacaine
- Alfentanil and Bupivacaine

◆ Effects of Epidural Analgesia on Labor

May slow progression if administered before active phase or in absence of oxytocin

Definitely prolongs second stage

May increase cesarean section rate for dystocia in nulliparous patient

◆ Effects of Epidural Analgesia on Uterine Blood Flow

- negligible effect if patient has been adequately hydrated

◆ Advantages-Disadvantages

✧ *Three principle advantages*
1. patient awake and cooperative
2. incidence of complications low
3. can be used for vaginal or cesarean delivery

✧ *Disadvantages*
May yield poor perineal block

"Hot spots" or "windows" can develop

Technical failure in 4%

Hypotension is common
- treat with position changes, IV fluid, oxygen, ephedrine 5 to 10 mg if needed

◆ Indications-Contraindications

✧ *Indications*
Pain in labor

Certain cardiac disorders

Breech delivery

Multiple gestation

✧ *Contraindications*

Patient refusal
Infection at puncture site
Preexisting CNS disease
Hypovolemia, severe anemia
Lack of experience by anesthetist
Thrombocytopenia (less than 50,000)

CAUDAL ANALGESIA

Complications are rare
Virtually replaced by lumbar epidural analgesia

SUBARACHNOID ANALGESIA (SPINAL ANALGESIA)

Popular for cesarean delivery
Uses low doses of local anesthetic
Rapid onset
Hypotension is common

◆ Postsubarachnoid Block Headache (spinal headache)

Incidence 50% with large gauge epidural needle
Decrease in CSF volume causes tractions on vessels and supporting structures in brain
Treatment
- IV fluid
- bedrest
- IV caffeine
- analgesia
- epidural blood patch or Gelfoam patch (blood patch most effective)

◆ Neurologic Complications

Rare 19/10,000
Most related to intraoperative positioning problems (peroneal nerve palsy)
Epidural hematoma very rare

PSYCHOLOGIC METHODS OF PAIN RELIEF

◆ Prepared Childbirth

Specific education provided
Relaxation methods
Breathing patterns

ANESTHESIA FOR CESAREAN SECTION DELIVERY

◆ Epidural Analgesia

Accounts for one third of all anesthetics used for cesarean
Requires level to T6 dermatome
Epidural opioids may be useful for visceral pain
Several advantages with few disadvantages

◆ Subarachnoid Block

Excellent analgesia for cesarean section
Used in one third of cases
Usually for elective or urgent cesarean
Prehydration important as for epidural
  • hypotension common
Block usually occurs within 20 seconds of placement

◆ General Anesthesia

Use for emergency cesarean section
Failed intubation with aspiration can occur
Prior to induction of anesthesia, oral antacid along with H2
  blocker should be administered
Preoxygenate
Induction agent
  • sodium pentothal
  • propofol

✧ *Failed intubation*

After three attempts
Regional block or awake blind oral or nasal intubation
Anticipation of difficult intubation is key

◆ Analgesia After Cesarean Section

Postoperative epidural analgesia has proved to be safe
Appropriate monitoring should be performed
  • risk of maternal respiratory depression is real

8

◆ The Neonate and Resuscitation

PHYSIOLOGY OF THE FETUS

◆ Lung Development and Alveolar Differentiation

Pseudoglandular phase completed by 16 weeks gestation
Canalicular phase completed by 16th to 24th week
Terminal sac phase completed by 24th week and beyond
- appearance of structural characteristics for extrauterine life
  - increased number of air spaces
  - tissues remodeled into mature parenchyma
  - decreased connective tissue
  - epithelium thinner
    - more efficient air-blood interface

✧ *Fetal lung fluid*

Production of fetal lung fluid essential for air space development
- tracheal drainage—hypoplastic lungs
- tracheal occlusion—hyperinflated lungs

✧ *Fetal breathing*

Appears as early as 11 weeks
Increases with gestational age
- 40% to 60% of the time during the final 10 weeks of pregnancy
May decrease prior to labor

✧ *Surface tension and lung function*

Surfactant is surface tension-reducing substance
- reduces work required for lung expansion

◆ Circulation

Fetal, neonatal, and adult circulations differ (Fig. 8-1)
Acute asphyxiation results in increased pulmonary resistance
- reduces pulmonary flow and maintains fetal circulatory pattern

◆ Thermoregulation

Placenta is principal fetal heat exchanger

Maternal temperature greater than 41.5C may result in adverse fetal effects

◆ Respiratory Gas Exchange Across the Placenta

Gradients across the placenta for H+ and CO_2 are small
- fetus is neither acidotic nor hypercapnic

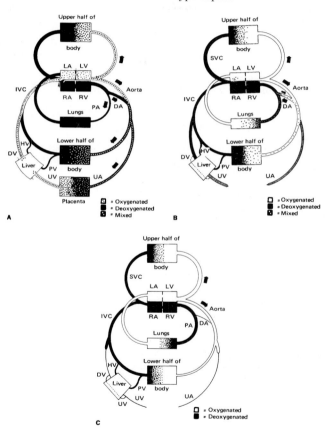

Figure 8-1. Schematic representations of (**A**) fetal, (**B**) neonatal, and (**C**) adult circulations. Arrows indicate the direction of blood flow. (DA, ductus arteriosus; DV, ductus venosus; HV, hepatic vein; IVC, inferior vena cava; LA, left atrium; LV, left ventricle; PA, pulmonary artery; PV, portal vein; RA, right atrium; RV, right ventricle; SVC, superior vena cava; UA, umbilical artery; UV, umbilical vein.)

Oxygen tension low but adequate, tissue oxygen maintained in umbilical vein by O_2 saturation of 80% and high cardiac output

PHYSIOLOGY OF THE NEWBORN

◆ Birth Asphyxia

Oxygen levels in umbilical arterial blood range from 0% to 70% saturation
- average CO_2 58 mm Hg
- average pH 7.28

Relates to the disturbance of the functional relationship between fetus and mother
- not an adaptation to a hypoxic environment

◆ Breathing at Birth

Fluid in lung must be replaced by air
- alveoli require 20 to 25 cm H_2O to expand

5 minutes after delivery the lungs should sound clear

◆ Recovery From Birth Asphyxia

After delivery arterial O_2 increases, arterial CO_2 tension decreases
- as a result of pulmonary elimination of CO_2

Inhibition of recovery
- neurologic impairment
- chemical impairment (analgesia, anesthetics)
- increased metabolic rate (exposure to cold air)

TRANSITION PERIOD AT BIRTH

◆ Changes in the Circulation at Birth

Marked fall in pulmonary vascular resistance with lung expansion and increase in oxygen tension
Pressure rises systemically from increased systemic resistance
Pressure rises in left ventricle and atrium
- change in pressure between atria closes foramen ovale

Ductus arteriosus slowly constricts over 16 hours
Circulatory instability continues until the ductus is firmly closed

◆ Failure to Breathe

Maternal medication
Birth asphyxia
Obstruction of the respiratory tract (rare)
Cerebral trauma
Prematurity is seldom the sole etiology

◆ Thermoregulation

Excessive heat loss occurs after delivery

Oxygen consumption is a function of temperature gradient between body surface and environment

Heat production comes from skeletal muscle and brown adipose tissue

RESUSCITATION

◆ Initial Treatment and Appraisal of the Infant

Initial appraisal should start at time of delivery

Scoring system introduced by Virginia Apgar in 1952 (Table 8-1)

- determines resuscitation required

  7 to10: no resuscitation needed

  4 to 6: some resuscitation needed

  0 to 3: aggressive resuscitation needed

◆ Treatment of the Moderately Depressed Infant

If no response to initial resuscitory within 1.5 minutes, administer oropharyngeal oxygen at 16 to 20 cm H_2O for 1 to 2 seconds

- no response → intubation (Fig. 8-2)

◆ Treatment of the Severely Depressed Infant

Immediate intubation

Cardiac massage

- rate 100 to 200/minute
- middle/lower one third of sternum
- compressions with index and middle finger
- interrupt every 5 seconds for ventilation

TABLE 8-1. Clinical Evaluation of the Newborn Infant in the Delivery Room by the Apgar Scoring Method

Sign	0	1	2
Heart rate	None	Below 100	Over 100
Respiratory effort	None	Weak cry; hypoventilation	Good; strong cry
Muscle tone	Limp	Some flexion of extremities	Active motion; extremities well flexed
Reflex irritability (i.e. response to stimulation of sole of foot)	No response	Grimace	Cry
Color	Pale	Blue	Completely pink

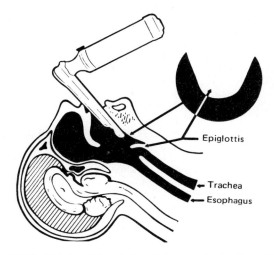

Figure 8-2. Sagittal view of the mouth and pharynx, showing the relation of the laryngoscope blade to the epiglottis.

Epinephrine
- 1 : 10,000 (0.1 to 0.3 mL/kg) IV or endotracheal (ET)
- administer for heart rate <80 after 30 seconds of CPR

Volume expanders
- administer 10 mL/kg over 10 minutes for signs of hypovolemia
- normal saline
- Ringer lactate
- 5% albumin
- whole blood

Correction of pH
- administration of alkali can have adverse effects
- correct slowly
- effective ventilation must precede administration
- initial dose 2 mL/kg of 4.2% solution (0.5 mEq/mL) IV over 2 minutes

Analeptics and drug antagonists
- Narcan useful to correct depression from transplacental opioids
- 0.1 mg/kg of body weight IV or ET

◆ Meconium Aspiration

Infant may be critically ill at delivery
- increased sensitivity of pulmonary arterioles to decreased oxygen

Oxygenation is crucial

Infant is unstable and difficult to manage
- over-ventilation can damage lungs

Most severe complications can be avoided by aggressive pulmonary care

◆ Duration of Resuscitation Efforts

Severe asphyxia
- heart rate does not return after good lung expansion, CPR, epinephrine, volume expansion, and alkali administration
  - consider halting efforts as severe neurologic damage is likely

PHYSICAL EXAMINATION IN THE DELIVERY ROOM

◆ Transitional Period

Respiratory rate 60 to 80/min
Heart rate 20 to 40 beats per minute >intrauterine rate
Autonomic reactivity
- passage of meconium
Initial period of activity followed by period of unresponsiveness followed by second period of activity

◆ Skin

Color should be pink
- extremities may be cyanotic
  - persistence of differential cyanosis
    - failure of ductal closure
    - increased pulmonary vascular resistance
    - preductal coarctation of the aorta
Vernix and lanugo are often present
Petechiae can be seen
Rashes are rare

◆ Head and Neck

Molding is often present
Cephalohematoma, forceps, and vacuum marks can occur
- examine for nerve injuries
Anterior fontanelle open, posterior fontanelle closed
Eyes may be open
Ear size, shape, and texture should be noted
Palate, nasal patency should be assured

◆ Thorax

By 5 minutes of age, adventitious sounds should be heard only in the precordial area
By 20 minutes chest should be cleared
Warning signs
- persistence of advential sounds
- sternal or intercostal retractions
- prolonged expiration with or without grunting

- unilateral diminished or absent breath sounds

Palpation of clavicles and ribs

Cardiac auscultation
- rate 160 to 170
- pansystolic crescendo murmur in 15% of all infants during first 2 hours
  - probably from ductus arteriosus, shunting, or regurgitation through mitral or tricuspid valves

◆ Abdomen

Oropharyngeal catheter should be tested to pass into stomach
- failure to pass must raise suspicion of esophageal atresia or tracheoesophageal fistula

Inspection of liver, kidneys, bladder, and anus should be performed

◆ Genitalia

Female examination limited to inspection of labia and clitoris

Male examination should include location of testes

◆ Back and Extremities

Sacrum examined for pigmentation and abnormal hair
- can be associated with occult spina bifida

Observe limb position and movement

◆ Nervous System

Testing of grasp and Moro reflexes

In depressed infant evaluate anterior fontanelles for signs of brain swelling (suture separation)

Examine for retinal hemorrhages

◆ Weight and Gestational Age

Infants <2500 g may be small for gestational age (Fig. 8-3)

Features useful in distinguishing preterm infant from SGA infant
- consistency of scalp hair
- pliability of ear lobes
- pigmentation of breasts
- presence of upper breast mound
- presence of sole creases
- presence of scrotal rugae

◆ Placenta and Membranes

Examination should be routine (see Chapter 9)

◆ Laboratory Procedures

Cord blood for Coombs typing in cases of blood incompatibility

Blood gases as indicated
Sepsis evaluation as indicated

◆ Respiratory Distress Syndrome

Failure of the cardiopulmonary system to adapt to extrauterine
conditions

Most common in preterm infants

Mildly affected infants may recover gradually with warmth and
oxygen

More severely affected infants may require prompt evaluation
and support

Use of artificial surfactant (eg: Exosurf) has decreased morbidity and mortality associated with RDS

Prevention by administration of antenatal steroids has been documented in several studies

- no adverse neonatal effects demonstrable

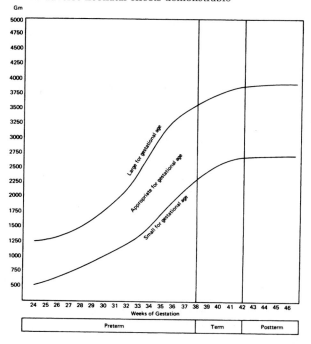

Figure 8-3. Classification of newborns by birth weight and gestational age.
(Lubchenko LO, Hansmann C, Boyd E. Intrauterine growth in length and
head circumference as estimated from live births at gestational ages from
26 to 42 weeks. Pediatrics 1966;37:403.)

9

◆ The Normal and Abnormal Puerperium

DEVELOPMENTAL CHANGES

◆ Genital Tract

◇ *Uterine changes*
At level of umbilicus immediately after delivery
Midway between symphysis and umbilicus by 1 week postpartum
Pelvic organ by 2 weeks postpartum
Nonpregnant size by 6 weeks postpartum

◇ *Lochia*
Blood, necrotic membrane remnants and decidua shed from uterine cavity

◇ *Cervix*
Original form regained within hours after delivery
Slit like external os retained as permanent feature

◇ *Vagina*
Normally well-healed by 6 weeks
Can be pale without rugae in breast-feeding patient because of hypoestrogenic state

◆ Breasts

Engorgement usually occurs by day 3

◆ Cardiovascular System

Reversal of pregnancy changes over 2 to 3 weeks
Cardiac output increases in immediate puerperium
• increased venous return
High-risk period for patients with cardiac defects

◆ Other Systems

Leukocytosis persists
Weight loss
• 5 to 6 kg lost at delivery
• 3 to 5 kg lost during first week postpartum

MANAGEMENT

◆ Observation

Most serious complications are postpartum hemorrhage and infection
* complicate 1% to 5% of all pregnancies
Careful vital signs and observation of bleeding needed
Maternal temperature should be observed closely

◆ Analgesia

Usually for perineal discomfort only
Afterpains occur especially with breast-feeding
Drugs of choice for pain control
* aspirin
* acetaminophen
* NSAIDS

◆ Immunizations

Puerperium is an ideal time for rubella vaccine
Breastfeeding is not contraindication
Rh-negative women with Rh-positive babies should receive Rh
immune globulin

◆ Contraception

Plans should be made prior to discharge
Oral contraceptives
Foam and condoms
Diaphragm (wait until 6 week visit for fitting)

◆ Instructions

Early discharge common in the United States
May limit patient education
Support services should be in place prior to discharge

COMPLICATIONS

◆ Hemorrhage

Average blood loss is 500 mL at vaginal delivery
Bleeding greater than 1000 mL represents a postpartum hemorrhage

◇ *Etiology*

Uterine atony (Fig. 9-1)
* treat by bimanual compression
* oxytoxic agents
Retained placental fragments
Lacerations

Uterine rupture
Uterine inversion
Coagulation defects
Vulvovaginal hematomas (Fig. 9-2)

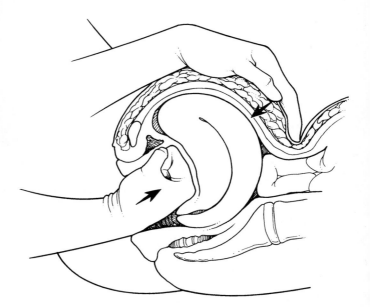

Figure 9-1. Bimanual compression of the uterus can halt persistent uterine bleeding until the administered oxytocics cause myometrial contraction.

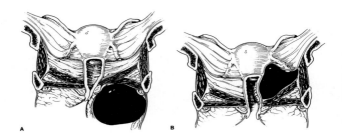

Figure 9-2. (**A**) Vulvar hematoma. (**B**) Paravaginal hematoma.

◆ Infection

Endomyometritis most common cause of infection of early puerperium

Polymicrobial

✧ *Risk factors*

PROM

Long labor with multiple exams

Cesarean delivery

✱ *Signs of infection*

Fever

Uterine tenderness

✧ *Treatment*

IV antibiotics

Single agent therapy

- extended spectrum cephalosporins or penicillins

Combination therapy

- gentamicin, clindamycin
- add ampicillin if severely ill

Switch to oral antibiotics if 24 to 48 hours afebrile

Oral antibiotics have not been proven to be necessary after IV antibiotic therapy

Failure to respond

- consider abscess
- appendicitis
- necrotizing fascitis

◆ Other Complications

✧ *Puerperal ovarian vein thromboebitis*

Usually presents as right lower quadrant pain in first week of puerperium

Heparin is treatment of choice

Ultrasound and CT are valuable tools for making this diagnosis

Septic pelvic vein thrombephlebitis occurs late in the course of a recognized puerperal infection

✧ *Postpartum hemolytic uremic syndrome*

Rare

Poor prognosis

✧ *Episiotomy breakdown*

Local wound care with early repair may be possible

✧ *Postpartum blues*

Transient, mild depression

✧ *Postpartum depression*

Frankly psychotic state

History of depression should alert obstetrician to this possibility

Evaluate for hypothyroidism as well

BREAST-FEEDING

◆ Trends

60% of newborns were breast fed in 1982, rate fell to 50% by 1989

Human breast milk is superior for human nutrition

Obstetrician should be strong advocate for breast-feeding

◆ Lactation Physiology

Mammary gland has 15 to 25 lobes

Extensive development of terminal ducts alveoli occur in pregnancy

- requires estrogen, progesterone, prolactin, and placental lactogen

Lactogenesis results from withdrawal of estradiol and progesterone in human placental lactogen

Tactile stimuli results in release of prolactin and oxytocin

Composition of the milk changes with time

- colostrum
  - thin yellow product of first week
- transitional milk (week 2)
- mature milk
  - more protein
  - less fat and lactose
  - more cells
  - more immunoglobulins

Human milk vs. cow's milk

- human contains whey proteins (lactalbumin and lactoferrin) and cow's milk contains curd protein (casein)

◆ Advantages

Avoidance of unsafe waters in developing countries

Immunoprotective element

Allergic reactions to cow milk can occur

Psychologic benefits regarding mother-infant interactions

◆ Principles and Techniques

Age, heredity and pregnancy have greater effects on breast shape than breast-feeding

Flat nipples can be helped to evert during third trimester, using a rigid plastic nipple shell

Attempt to breast feed in first hour after delivery

Rigid time limits are inappropriate

- five minutes per side is reasonable at the beginning
- increase to 10 to 15 minutes per side as lactation is established

Maternal nutrition

Increase 500 kcal/day for nonpregnant state

◆ Problems

◇ *Engorgement*

Manual expression prior to nursing may help newborn grasp nipple

◇ *Painful or cracked nipples*

Sore or cracked nipples may benefit from exposure to air or dry heat

Ointments may make matters worse

Mechanical pump may be used until nipple heals

◇ *Inadequate supply*

Increase frequency of feeding

Consider oxytocin nasal spray if letdown is a problem

◇ *Plugged duct*

Tender lump

Massage the involved area and manually express milk

◇ *Mastitis*

Usually later than 2 to 3 days postpartum

Unilateral pain and erythema

Treat with antibiotics that have staphylococci coverage

Development of breast abscess is rare

◆ Contraception

Breast-feeding women usually amenorrheic for several months

Ovulation suppressed for three months if infant exclusively breast-fed

Barrier methods appropriate

Oral contraceptions should be deferred for several weeks as they affect milk production

◆ Drug Use

Transfer to breast milk is variable

Specific contraindications exist (Table 9-1)

◆ Maternal Contraindications

Carcinoma of the breast

Severely ill mother

HIV-infected mother

Untreated active TB

Active herpatic lesion on the breast

Hepatitis B surface antigen positive mother (may breast-feed if the neonate has received HBIG and HBV)

**TABLE 9-1. Drugs That Are Contraindicated During
Breast-Feeding**

Drug	Reported Sign or Symptom in Infant or Effect on Lactation
Bromocriptine	Suppresses lactation
Cocaine	Cocaine intoxication
Cyclophosphamide	Possible immunosuppression; unknown effect on growth or association with carcinogenesis; neutropenia
Cyclosporine	Possible immunosuppression; unknown effect on growth or association with carcinogenesis
Doxorubicin*	Possible immunosuppression; unknown effect on growth or association with carcinogenesis
Ergotamine	Vomiting, diarrhea; convulsions at doses used in migraine medications
Lithium	33% to 50% of the therapeutic blood concentration found in infants
Methotrexate	Possible immunosuppression; unknown effect on growth or association with carcinogenesis; neutropenia
Phencyclidine (PCP)	Potent hallucinogen
Phenindione	Anticoagulant; increased prothrombin and partial thromboplastin time in one infant (not used in United States)

*Drug is concentrated in human milk.
(The Committee on Drugs, American Academy of Pediatrics. Transfer of drugs
and other chemicals into human milk. Pediatrics 1989;84:924.)

◆ Lactation Suppression

Bromocriptine no longer indicated for lactation suppression
  based on manufacturer's recommendations
Tight bra or binder with ice packs and analgesics can be very
  effective

10

◆ Early Pregnancy Loss

INTRODUCTION

"Abortion" gradually being replaced by the term "miscarriage"
- both terms traditionally refer to first trimester pregnancy losses
  - this represents an arbitrary time limit

A more clinically relevant classification is based on whether or not a live fetus was ever present

EPIDEMIOLOGY AND ETIOLOGY

◆ Background

Miscarriage is the most common complication of pregnancy
- 15% incidence among clinically recognized pregnancies
- 30% to 45% incidence detected with sensitive β-hCG assays
  - prevalence increases with maternal age
    - 12% in <20-year-old woman
    - >50% in >45-year-old woman

◆ Embryonic Factors

Most sporadic abortions are caused by intrinsic defects
- abnormal germ cells
  - 95% of morphologic/cytogenetic errors eliminated
- defective implantation of normal trophoblast
- injury to developing embryo

✧ *Chromosomal abnormalities*

Present in 60% of first-trimester losses, decreases to 7% at 24 weeks

Frequency (in decreasing incidence)
- autosomal trisomies (16, 21, 22 most common)
  - monosomy X (45 XO)—most common single karyotype
  - triploidy
  - tetraploidy
  - translocations
  - mosaics

Parental factors
- most often normal parental karyotypes,
- rarely a balanced translocation

CLINICAL FEATURES AND TREATMENT

◆ Threatened Abortion

As many as 25% of pregnancies complicated by first-trimester bleeding
- 50% of these eventually abort

Cervix closed and uneffaced

No convincing evidence that any treatments influence outcome
- sympathetic physician attitude probably the most helpful

Fetal cardiac activity is reassuring
- 95% of pregnancies continue beyond first trimester once cardiac activity visualized by ultrasound

Poor outcome predicted by:
- falling β-hCG titers
- gestational sac without fetal pole
- progressive bleeding/cramping

◆ Inevitable and Incomplete Abortion

Inevitable: bleeding or SROM with pain and cervical dilation
Incomplete: partial passage of products of conception (POC)
Aim of therapy
- evacuate uterus to prevent further hemorrhage or infection

Technique
- paracervical block ± IV sedation
- IV hydration
- suction curettage until "gritty" texture appreciated
- observe 4 to 6 hours after procedure
- Rh negative patients should receive Rh immune globulin (RhoGAM)
  - 50 μg or 300 μg dose
- always check pathology (presence of POC, rule out mole, ectopic, etc.)

◆ Complete Abortion

Pain and bleeding ceases after passage of tissue
Cervical os closed; uterus small and nontender
Usually no other therapy needed
Submit POC to pathology
Administer Rh immune globulin as above

◆ Missed Abortion

Expulsion does not occur for prolonged period after fetal death
May be associated with septate uterus

DIC rare in first half of pregnancy

Treatment of choice is suction curettage in first trimester
- may result in hemorrhage above anticipated amount
- perform in hospital setting with IV access and blood available

Second-trimester terminations have greater morbidity
- dilation and evacuation (D&E) especially 13 to 16 weeks
  - use laminaria preoperatively to reduce cervical trauma
- prostaglandin E$_2$ (PGE$_2$) suppositories
  - 20 mg suppository in vaginal fornix every 4 hours
  - 2.5 to 5 mg diphenoxylate (Lomotil) for diarrhea
  - Prochlorperazine (Compazine), 10 mg IM for nausea

◆ Septic Abortion

Previously a significant source of maternal morbidity and mortality
- now much less frequent since Roe vs. Wade

Signs and symptoms: fever, abdominal pain, uterine tenderness
- prompt evaluation crucial (Table 10-1)

Polymicrobial infection (Table 10-2)

Can progress to septic shock

RECURRENT SPONTANEOUS ABORTION (RSA)

◆ Background

Usually defined as three or more consecutive first-trimester losses (Table 10-3)

2% of couples experience this problem

Primary: no previous successful pregnancies

Secondary: repetitive losses after live birth

No classification of women with multiple losses interspersed with normal pregnancies

---

TABLE 10-1. Initial Evaluation of Patient with Septic Abortion

---

Physical and pelvic examination
Complete blood count, electrolytes, renal panel
Type and screen or crossmatch
Smears from cervix for Gram stain
Aerobic and anaerobic cultures from blood, cervix, POC
Foley catheter
IV fluid replacement through large-bore angiocatheter
Administer tetanus prophylaxis
  - immunized patient: 0.5 mL toxoid SC
  - nonimmunized: 250 U tetanus immune globulin IM
Supine and upright abdominal X-rays
  - detect free air or foreign bodies

TABLE 10-2. Antibiotic Regimens for Septic Abortion

A. Gram-positive anaerobe and aerobic coverage*
   1. Aqueous penicillin G, 4-5 million units IV q 4-6 h (20-30 million U / 24 hr); or
   2. Ampicillin 2 g IV q 6 hr; or
   3. Clindamycin 600 mg IV q 6 hr or 900 mg q 8 hr; or
   4. Cephalothin (or other cephalosporin) 2 g IV q 4-6 hr
      (for penicillin-allergic patients there is 10% cross allergy); or
   5. Imipenem-cilastin 250-500 mg q 6 hr (dose reduce for patients < 70 kg or renal compromise)
B. Resistant gram-negative aerobic organism coverage
   1. Gentamycin 1-1.5 mg/kg IV q 8 hr (adjust dose based on blood levels, renal compromise); or
   2. Aztreonam 1-2 g IV q 8-12 hr or q 6 hr in cases of serious infection
      (good alternative to gentamycin in face of toxicity or renal compromise); or
   3. Imipenem-cilastin (see previous dose schedule)
C. Gram-negative anaerobic organism coverage
   1. Clindamycin 600 mg IV q 6 hr or 900 q 8 hr; or
   2. Metronidazole 1 g IV loading dose followed by 500 mg q 6 hr; or
   3. Imipenem (cilastatin) (see previous dose schedule)

*The usual approach is to start one drug from each group; nonessential antibiotics are discontinued when the results of cultures and sensitivities are known. Recommended regimens are based on clinical effectiveness and may change as new antibiotics become available.

TABLE 10-3. Suggested Routine Evaluation for Patient with Recurrent Miscarriage

History

Determine pattern and trimester of pregnancy losses and whether a live fetus was present; clues suggestive of autoimmune disease; unusual exposure to environmental toxins, drugs, infections; previous gynecologic disorders or surgery including dilation and curettage; and previous diagnostic tests and treatments*

Physical

Abnormalities on pelvic examination, including findings suggestive of abnormal cervix, DES exposure, or uterine anomalies.

Tests

Hysterosalpingogram
Luteal-phase endometrial biopsy
Parental chromosome analysis
Screening test for lupus anticoagulant and anticardiolipin
Other laboratory tests if suggested by history and physical examination

*Ultrasound examination at 6 weeks of gestation in the next pregnancy and chromosome analysis of the POC from any subsequent spontaneous abortion.

◆ Etiology

See Figure 10-1

◆ Evaluation

Table 10-3

◆ Specific Clinical Causes

◇ *Structural uterine defects*

Several types

- Müllerian anomalies (asymmetric fusion defects have worst prognosis)
- DES exposure
- submucous myomas
- intrauterine synechiae

Diagnostic tests: hysterosalpingogram, hysteroscopy, laparoscopy

Therapy: hysteroscopic resection of septum, adhesions, or myomas

Outcome: live birth rate often >80%

◇ *Luteal phase deficiency*

Controversial entity

Presumed etiology is inadequate production or response to progesterone

- decreased GnRH secretion
- decreases FSH secretion
- inadequate LH secretion
- inadequate ovarian steroidogenesis
- endometrial receptor defect

Diagnosis

- endometrial biopsy in late luteal phase
- lag of >2 to 3 days is suspect
- confirm by repeat biopsy

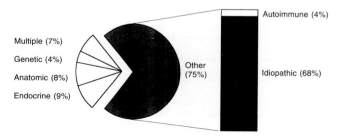

Figure 10-1. Factors considered responsible for recurrent pregnancy loss in more than 400 patients evaluated at the University of Utah.

Therapy (no controlled studies)
- progesterone 25 mg vaginal suppositories BID
- begin at ovulation, continue to 8 to 10 weeks gestation

✧ *Chromosomal abnormalities*
Found in 5% of couples with RSA
Most abnormalities are balanced translocations
- two thirds reciprocal (50% loss rate)
- one third Robertsonian (25% loss rate)
Homologous Robertsonian translocation **precludes** successful
  pregnancy
Future research may reveal molecular basis of RSA

✧ *Autoimmunity*
Association with antiphospholipid antibodies first described in
  1980s
5% of patients have lupus anticoagulant or anticardiolipin
Previous reproductive history crucial
Mechanism of action unclear (Fig. 10-2)

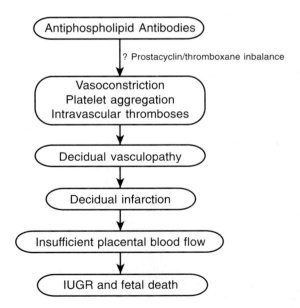

Figure 10-2. Possible mechanism of antiphospholipids and adverse pregnancy outcome.

Treatment
- initial studies used prednisone (40 mg/day) and aspirin (80 mg/day)
  - 60% to 80% live birth rate
- more recently subcutaneous heparin therapy shown to be helpful
  - 7500 U q BID
  - ± aspirin 80 mg/day
  - live birth rate equivalent to corticosteroid group
- steroids should **not** be used with heparin
  - not more effective
  - substantial risk of severe osteoporosis

◆ Idiopathic Causes

Alloimmune factors long suspected
- no practical tests available
- diagnosis is by exclusion

Several types of immunotherapy advocated
- paternal leukocyte transfusion
  - based on transplant studies using pretransplant blood transfusions
- immunization with third party donor cells or trophoblast membrane
- IV immune globulin

Success rates similar for all (50% to 80%)
- however, success rates are 40% to 60% without therapy

Value of immunotherapy remains controversial

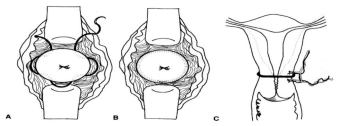

Figure 10-3. Incompetent cervix can be treated by three procedures. **(A)** In the McDonald cerclage procedure, a multiple-bite suture using large, monofilament nylon is placed around the cervix and tied securely to reduce the diameter of the cervical canal to a few millimeters. **(B)** In the Shirodkar procedure, Mersaline tape encircling the cervix is passed under the mucosa and anchored to the cervix anteriorly and posteriorly with interrupted sutures. **(C)** With transabdominal cervicoisthmic cerclage, a Mersaline band is placed in an avascular space medial to the uterine vessels at the level of the cervicouterine junction.

◆ Cervical Incompetence

Premature cervical dilation in second trimester
- painless and gradual with eventual expulsion of previable fetus

Etiology obscure
- previous cervical trauma
- congenital structural defects in cervical connective tissue
- DES exposure

Diagnosis
- absolute: membranes bulging through partially dilated cervix
- presumptive: obstetric history with previous losses

Treatment
- surgical approach most accepted (Fig. 10-3)
  - usually vaginal under regional anesthesia
  - prophylactic placement at end of first trimester
  - placement after cervical change less effective

Exclusion criteria
- diagnosis uncertain
- SROM
- vaginal bleeding or cramping

No evidence that postoperative antibiotics, progesterone, or tocolytics are useful

Management
- remove cerclage at time of SROM or labor
- elective removal after 37 weeks

Success rates 80% to 90%
- little difference between McDonald and Shirodkar techniques

11

◆ Ectopic Pregnancy

INTRODUCTION

Ectopic pregnancy defined as an implantation outside the endometrial cavity

Expectant management (60% mortality) was recommended until 1884 when Lawton Tait proposed surgical intervention

Most common cause of maternal death in first half of pregnancy but mortality is decreasing

- five deaths/10,000 pregnancies in 1987 vs. 35/10,000 in 1972

Factors responsible for increased incidence (diagnosis) of ectopic pregnancy

- pelvic inflammatory disease
- improved diagnostic methods
- sensitive and specific hCG assays
- high resolution ultrasound
- diagnostic laparoscopy
- increased awareness

ETIOLOGY

◆ Tubal Factors

Damage to fallopian tube may increase ectopic rates as high as 27%

History of salpingitis in 30% to 50% of women operated on for ectopic pregnancy

Histologic evidence of chronic salpingitis in 50%

Salpingitis isthmica nodosa may be related to tubal dysfunction

Other risk factors

- prior tubal surgery (15%)
- prior ectopic pregnancy (20% recurrence risk)

◆ Contraceptive Failure

Risk of ectopic pregnancy may approach 60% in pregnancies after elective sterilization

IUD more effective at preventing intrauterine rather than ectopic pregnancies
- 4% to 9% of pregnancies with IUDs in place are ectopic

◆ Hormonal Effects

Alteration of tubal motility
Tenfold increase in ectopic pregnancy with "morning after pill" failures
Fivefold increase in users of progestin-only mini pill
7% in IVF patients
May be result of preexisting tubal disease

ANATOMIC CONSIDERATIONS

◆ Frequency and Implantation Site (Fig. 11-1)

Most frequent location is tubal (97%)
- 86% in distal half of tube
Isthmic ectopics present earlier
- decreased distensibility of the region
Intraluminal vs. extraluminal growth
- 70% of ruptured tubes have tubal wall invasion vs. 14% of unruptured

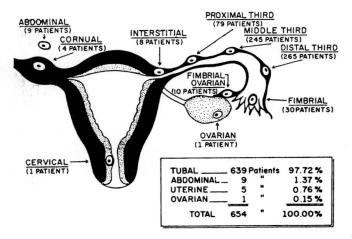

Figure 11-1. Incidence of ectopic pregnancy by anatomic site. (Breen JL. A 21-year survey of 654 ectopic pregnancies. Am J Obstet Gynecol 1970;106:1004.)

UNUSUAL LOCATIONS

◆ Abdominal Pregnancy

9.2/1000 ectopics (10.8/100,000 births)
Mortality rate much higher
• Ninetyfold higher than for intrauterine pregnancy
Perinatal survival 5% to 25%
Deliver by laparotomy
• hemodynamic monitoring
• placenta left intact
  • usually absorbs without complication

◆ Ovarian Pregnancy

Spiegelberg criteria
• intact fallopian tubes
• pregnancy attached to uterus by uteroovarian vasculature
• tissue specimen includes ovarian tissue
• location normally occupied by ovary
Blood transfusion necessary in as many as 35% of patients
Perform ovarian wedge resection or oophorectomy

◆ Cervical Pregnancy

Implantation within endocervical canal
Very rare (1/1000 to 1/95,000 pregnancies)
Newer conservative methods effective
• methotrexate

◆ Heterotopic Pregnancy

Implantation at different sites
Higher incidence with increased use of Assisted Reproductive
   Technology
Surgical or direct medical management with methotrexate

SIGNS AND SYMPTOMS

◆ Differential Diagnosis

Threatened or incomplete abortion
Ruptured corpus luteum
Dysfunctional bleeding
Appendicitis
Adnexal torsion
Endometrioma
Pelvic Inflammatory Disease
Degenerating fibroid

TABLE 11-1. Symptoms of Ectopic Pregnancy

Symptoms	Patients With Symptoms (%)
Abdominal pain	90-100
Amenorrhea	75-95
Vaginal bleeding	50-80
Dizziness, fainting	20-35
Pregnancy symptoms	10-25
Urge to defecate	5-15
Passage of tissue	5-10

Weckstein LN. Current perspective on ectopic pregnancy. Obstet Gynecol Surv 1985;40:259.

TABLE 11-2. Signs of Ectopic Pregnancy

Sign	Patients With Sign (%)
Adnexal tenderness	75-90
Abdominal tenderness	80-95
Adnexal mass*	50
Uterine enlargement	20-30
Orthostatic changes	10-15
Fever	5-10

*20% percent of masses occur on the side opposite the ectopic pregnancy.
Weckstein LN. Current perspective on ectopic pregnancy. Obstet Gynecol Surv 1985;40:259.

DIAGNOSTIC STRATEGIES

◆ Human Chorionic Gonadotropin Assay and Adjunctive Methods

Development of sensitive radioimmunoassay has resulted in early diagnosis of ectopic pregnancy
- Serum hCG usually lower than normal
- Serial values also very helpful, rate of rise slower in ectopic pregnancy
  - doubling time for normal pregnancy 1.4 to 2.2 days
    - 15% of normal pregnancies fail to show normal rise
    - 13% of ectopic show normal increase

◆ Progesterone Determination

Progesterone level greater than 25ng/mL suggests normal IUP
Level less than 5 ng/mL suggests ectopic or abnormal IUP
Concentration, 5 to 25 ng/mL indeterminate

◆ Ultrasound

Greatly aided ability to detect early ectopic pregnancies
"Gold standard" in combination with serum hCG

Correlation of ultrasound and hCG dependent on hCG standards of different labs

◆ Laboratory Standards

Many initially used the second international standard (2nd IS) to quantify hCG

Later replaced by the International Reference Preparation (IRP)
- uses purified hCG
- avoids the use of large amounts of free alpha and beta subunits

2nd IS is now replaced by 3rd IS (equal potency to IRP)
- $2 \times$ 2nd IS = IRP

Discriminatory zone 1000 to 2000 IU/L (IRP)

Fetal pole 9050 to 21,000 IU/L

Gestational sac
- 1cm → see yolk sac
- 2cm → see fetal pole
- 3cm → see cardiac activity

◆ Culdocentesis

Needle puncture into posterior cul-de-sac

Positive result is the finding of nonclotted blood with hematocrit >15%

Positive predicted value of 70% to 97%

Negative culdocentesis does not exclude a nonbleeding ectopic

Positive result not specific for ectopic

With increased resolution of ultrasound fewer indications for culdocentesis

◆ Dilation and Curettage

Can be useful for abnormally rising hCG level or serum progesterone less than 5 ng/mL (Fig. 11-2)

◆ Laparoscopy

Often diagnosis made by direct visualization

Can be performed too early
- if unable to detect laparoscopically, consider medical treatment to avoid second surgery

TREATMENT

◆ Expectant Management

More successful in patients with small early ectopic pregnancies

Future fertility consequences unclear

◆ Surgical Management

Salpingostomy has replaced salpingectomy except in cases of irreparable tubal rupture tumor and hemorrhage

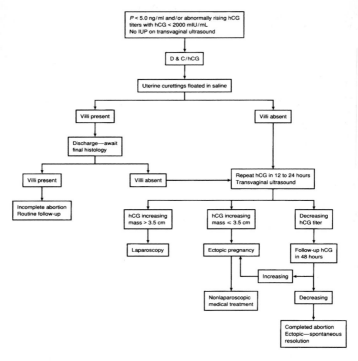

Figure 11-2. Treatment algorithm for patients with abnormally rising human chorionic gonadotropin (hCG) titers or low serum progesterone concentrations, or both. (Stovall TG, Ling FW. Some new approaches to ectopic pregnancy. Contemp Obstet Gynecol 1992;37:37.)

Laparoscopic treatment preferred method in many institutions
- **must** follow hCG levels postoperative if salpingostomy is performed

◆ Medical Treatment

Obvious benefits
Methotrexate first studied for use in gestational trophoblastic neoplasia
- inexpensive
- easy to obtain
- well tolerated

Means of action
- folate antagonist

- inhibits dihydrofolate reductase
- tissues with rapid cell growth most effected

Single-dose therapy 50 mg/m^2 IM

✧ *Inclusion criteria*
- Hemodynamically stable
- Tubal diameter less than 3 to 4 cm
- Unruptured tube
- No fetal cardiac activity
- hCG less than 15,000 IU/L (failure rates higher with increasing hCG levels)

✧ *Exclusion*
- Sensitivity to methotrexate
- Hepatic, renal failure
- Evidence of bone marrow suppression

◆ Reproductive Outcome

One Previous Ectopic Pregnancy
- 52% pregnant
- 87% IUP
- 13% ectopic

Two or More Ectopic Pregnancies
- 65% pregnant
- 25% IUP
- 40% ectopic

Three Ectopic Pregnancies
- 42% pregnancy
- 16% term IUP
- 26% repeat ectopics

Operative method had no significant difference in outcome
Medical management produces similar rates

COMPLICATIONS AND CAVEATS

◆ Persistent Ectopic Pregnancy

Recognized complication of conservative surgical treatment
Incidence may be as high as 7%
Methotrexate may be useful in management

◆ Rh Disease

Despite widespread underuse of Rh$_o$GAM, no sensitization from an early ectopic pregnancy has been reported
Mini dose (50 µg) sufficient in first trimester

◆ Diagnostic Pitfalls

Serum hCG is not necessarily proportional to size of ectopic pregnancy

Tubal rupture can occur with falling levels of hCG
Rarely ectopics detected with undetected hCG levels
Delay of diagnosis
- up to 50% missed at first visit
- early recognition is paramount to allow early intervention

12

◆ Genetics and Prenatal Diagnosis

INTRODUCTION

More than 20 million Americans have a diagnosed genetic disease
Newborns
- 1% have recognized Mendelian disorder
- 0.5% have a chromosomal syndrome
- 2% have a polygenic, multifactorial disorder

Identification of genetic disorders can have a great impact on a
patient's reproductive health

PATTERNS OF INHERITANCE

◆ Types of Birth Defects

Deformation   Any abnormal form, shape, or pattern caused by
mechanical forces

Malformation   A morphologic defect resulting from abnormal
development

Disruption   A morphologic defect resulting from an extensive
breakdown or interference with normal development

Anomaly   Structural features that depart from normal form

Syndrome   A recognizable pattern of structural defects that often has a predictable natural history that allows diagnosis

Association   A group of anomalies that frequently occur together but are not syndromes

Sequence   Pattern of defects that results from a single effect
early in pregnancy

◆ Definitions

✧ *Autosomal dominant*
Disease expressed in heterozygous individuals
Typically have <100% penetrance

Male and female offspring affected with equal frequency and
severity

Usually lethal in homozygous individuals

✧ *Autosomal recessive*
Expressed only in persons with both alleles abnormal

Male and female offspring affected with equal severity and frequency

Offspring of two carriers
- 25% affected
- 50% carrier
- 25% neither carrier nor affected

Horizontal pedigree pattern
- most carriers mate with unaffected individuals

✧ *X-linked*
A trait carried on the X chromosome

Higher male incidence

Never transmitted from father to son

All daughters of an affected male are carriers

X-linked dominant disorders are much rarer
- all daughters have the disorder
- female offspring twice as likely to be affected
- no sons are affected (if father is affected)

✧ *Y-linked*
No known genetic diseases are transmitted in this fashion

✧ *Mitochondrial*
Inherited exclusively through oocyte cytoplasm

**TABLE 12-1. Types of Chromosomal Abnormalities in
Spontaneous Abortuses**

Abnormality	Frequenty (%)
Trisomy 14	3.7
Trisomy 15	4.2
Trisomy 16	16.4
Trisomy 18	3.0
Trisomy 21	4.7
Trisomy 22	5.7
Other trisomies	14.3
45.X	18
Triploid	17
Tetraploid	6
Unbalanced translocations	3
Other	4

Carr DH, Gedeon M. Population cytogenetics of human abortuses. The
frequency of chromosome abnormalities in consecutive newborn studies: results
by sex and by severity of phenotypic involvement. In Hook EB, Porter IH, eds.
Population cytogenetics. New York: Academic Press, 1977:1.

◆ Polygenic, Multifactorial Disorders

Most common form of inheritance
* most congenital anomalies show multifactorial inheritance
* Prediction of recurrence rates may require assistance from medical geneticist

Works according to threshold model
* many different factors must collaborate

Race, sex bias can be present

◆ Cytogenetic Disorders

Involve loss or duplication of a large number of genes

Diagnostic clues range from subtle dysmorphic features to major structural malformations

Usually associated with mental retardation and IUGR

Increased perinatal loss and spontaneous abortion (Table 12-1)

Cytogenetic studies used clinically for approximately 35 years
* modern banding technology developed in 1970

Specific descriptive terminology regarding karyotype analysis

TABLE 12-2. Risk of Karotypic Abnormalities Related to Maternal Age at Delivery

Maternal (y)	Incidence of Trisomy 21		Incidence of Any Abnormality	
	Live Birth	Amnio-centesis	Live Birth	Amnio-centesis
20	1/1734 ·	1/1231	1/526	
25	1/1250	1/887	1/476	
30	1/965	· 1/685	1/385	
31	1/915	1/650	1/385	
32	1/794	1/563	1/322	
33	1/639	1/452	1/286	
34	1/496	1/352	1/238	1/83
35	1/386	1/274	1/192	1/76
37	1/234	1/166	1/127	1/67
38	1/182	1/129	1/102	1/58
39	1/141	1/100	1/83	1/49
40	1/100	1/78	1/66	1/40
41	1/86	1/61	1/53	1/32
42	1/66	1/47	1/42	1/26
43	1/52	1/37	1/33	1/21
44	1/40	1/29	1/26	1/19
45	1/31	1/22	1/21	1/15
46	1/24	1/17	1/16	1/12
47	1/19	1/13	1/13	1/20
48	1/15	1/10	1/10	1/18
49	1/11	1/8	1/8	1/16

Hook EB, Cross PK, Schreinemachers DM. Chromosomal abnormality rates at amniocentesis and in live-born infants. JAMA 1983;249:2034.

Indication for obtaining a fetal karyotype includes
- advanced maternal age (Table 12-2)
- fetal anomalies on ultrasound

GENETIC EVALUATION

◆ Genetic History and Physical Examination

Adequate counseling should be presented as well as further evaluation

History remains one of the most important tools
- a few well-considered questions may be all that is needed (Fig. 12-1)

◆ Pregnancy Termination

Emphasize fetal diagnosis and prognosis

Encourage patient to take advantage of support services

Reinforce the fact that patient did not cause the genetic defect

◆ Laboratory Screening

Population screening is appropriate when defining subset is at risk and an accurate and inexpensive heterozygote test is available (Table 12-3)

Goal of screening programs
- early diagnosis
- identification of at-risk matings

PRENATAL DIAGNOSIS

◆ Maternal Serum Screening

◇ *High maternal serum α-fetoprotein (MSAFP)*

Screening introduced in the 1980s

Testing for neural tube defects (NTD)

Risk for neural tube defects varies
- 1% in Ireland, Wales, Alexandria, and the Punjab
- 1/1000 to 1/2000 in the United States
- recurrence risk 2% to 3% after one affected child
  - 6.4% after two
  - 25% after three

Cut-off of 2.5 multiples of the median
- 98% detection rate
- 0.8% false positive rate
  - usually inaccurate gestational dating

Must correct for weight, race, and diabetes

◇ *Low MSAFP*

1/5 to 1/3 of Down fetuses exhibit low AFP (median 0.7)

Detection rate may be improved by addition of urinary estriol and hCG

PRENATAL GENETICS SCREENING FORM

Last Name _____ First Name _____ Date _____

1. Will you be 35 yers or older when the baby is due?   Yes ☐   No ☐

Genetic Diseases Common to Certain Ethnic Groups
1. Are you or the baby's father of African descent?   Yes ☐   No ☐
   If yes, have either of you been screened for sickle cell trait?   Yes ☐   No ☐
2. Are you or the baby's father of Eastern European Jewish
   descent (Ashkenazi)?   Yes ☐   No ☐
   If yes, have either of you been screened for Tay-Sachs
   disease?   Yes ☐   No ☐
3. Do you or your partner have any close relatives from Italy,
   Greece, or other Mediterranean countries?   Yes ☐   No ☐
   If yes, have either of you been screened for β-thalassemia?   Yes ☐   No ☐
4. Do you or your partner have any close relatives from the
   Philippines or Southeast Asia?   Yes ☐   No ☐
   If yes, have either of you been screened for α-thalassemia?   Yes ☐   No ☐

Personal and Family Genetic History
1. Have you, the baby's father, or any member of your respective families ever had
   any of the following disorders:
   Down syndrome (mongolism)?   Yes ☐   No ☐
   Other chromosomal abnormalities?   Yes ☐   No ☐
   Congenital heart defect?   Yes ☐   No ☐
   Hemophilia?   Yes ☐   No ☐
   Muscular dystrophy?   Yes ☐   No ☐
   Cystic fibrosis?   Yes ☐   No ☐
   Spina bifida (open spine), hydrocephaly (water on the brain)
      or anencephaly (absent brain)?   Yes ☐   No ☐
   A genetic disorder or birth defect not listed above?   Yes ☐   No ☐
   If yes, please list. _____
   If a relative had any of the above, please indicate their relationship to you.
   _____
2. Do you or the baby's father have a birth defect?   Yes ☐   No ☐
   If yes, please describe. _____
3. Have you ever had a baby who died in the womb or a baby
   with a birth defect?   Yes ☐   No ☐
4. Have you had three or more first-trimester (first 12 weeks of
   pregnancy) miscarriages?   Yes ☐   No ☐
5. Do you or the father of your baby have any relatives with
   mental retardation?   Yes ☐   No ☐
6. Excluding iron or prenatal vitamins, have you taken any
   medications during pregnancy?   Yes ☐   No ☐
   If yes, please list. _____
7. Have you used any recreational drugs (e.g., alcohol, cocaine,
   speed) during pregnancy?   Yes ☐   No ☐
   If yes, please list. _____
8. Is there any reason you are especially concerned about having
   a baby with a birth defect or problems with your pregnancy?   Yes ☐   No ☐

Figure 12-1. Genetic screening questionnaires.

TABLE 12-3. Population Screening: Incidence Estimates for Selected Autosomal Recessive Disorders in Defined Ethnic Groups

Disease	Ethnic Group	Carrier Frequency	Disease Incidence in Newborns	At-Risk Couple Frequency*	Screening Test
Sickle cell anemia	Blacks	0.08	1/600	1/150	Presence of sickle cell hemoglobin; confirmation hemoglobin electrophoresis
Tay-Sachs disease	Ashkenazi Jews	0.032	1/3600	1/900	Decreased serum hexosaminidase A
β-Thalassemia	Greeks, Italians	0.032	1/3600	1/900	Mean corpuscular volume <80%; confirmatory hemoglobin electrophoresis
α-Thalassemia	Southeast Asians and Chinese	0.04	1/2500	1/625	Mean corpuscular volume <80%; confirmatory hemoglobin electrophoresis
Cystic fibrosis	Northern Europeans	0.04	1/2500	1/625	Reverse dot blot for common mutations
Phenylketonuria	Europeans	0.016	1/16,000	1/4000	Newborn phenylalanine level

*Likelihood that both members of a couple are carriers, assuming nonconsanguinity and that both are of the at-risk ethnic group.

◆ Fetal Imaging

High-resolution ultrasound has revolutionized fetal imaging
More advanced techniques, CT/MRI (have limited applications)
Direct visualization rarely indicated

◆ Fetal Sampling for Prenatal Diagnosis

◇ *Amniocentesis*

Performed at approximately 15 weeks gestation
- 30 mL of fluid removed under ultrasound guidance
  - α-fetoprotein levels routinely obtained
  - fetal cells grown for karyotype

Administer Rh$_0$GAM for patients at risk
Fetal loss usually reported less than 1/200

◇ *Chorionic villus sampling*

Introduced to United States in 1980s
Small sample of chorionic villi taken for chromosomal analysis
Performed either transcervically or transabdominally
Results
- 0.8% procedure-related loss rate
- 2% of first-trimester CVS samples reveal cytogenic discrepancy between fetus and placenta
  - further testing required (usually amniocentesis)
- small incidence of limb reduction defects

◇ *Fetal blood sampling and fetal biopsy*

Improvements in ultrasound greatly simplified cordocentesis
- not performed until greater than 17 weeks
- procedure-related loss rate approximately 1%
- useful assay for
  - fetal hematocrit in isoimmunization
  - fetal platelet count
  - fetal karyotype
- fetal biopsy rarely indicated
  - rarely performed under fetoscopy
  - can be done with ultrasound guidance

◇ *Early amniocentesis*

Similar to traditional amniocentesis except that it is performed at 10 to 12 weeks
Fetal loss rate and safety not yet well defined
May result in higher losses

13

◆ Teratology and Drug Use During Pregnancy

PRINCIPLES OF TERATOLOGY

Drugs ingested during pregnancy can affect the fetus
- should be used only when necessary
- risk-benefit ratio should justify the use of any drug

Passage of drugs influenced by several factors
- lipid-soluble substances passed readily across the placenta
- water-soluble substances pass less well
- protein bound fraction
  - only free drug can cross placenta

Developmental defects
- drug exposure responsible for 2% to 3%
- genetic defects 25%
- unknown etiology in most cases

Major malformation 2% to 3% of all deliveries
Minor malformation 7% to 10%
Marked species specificity exists in drug teratogenicity

◆ FDA Categories

✧ Category A
Controlled studies in women fail to demonstrate a risk to the fetus in the first trimester, and the possibility of fetal harm appears remote

✧ Category B
Animal studies do not indicate a risk to the fetus, and there are no controlled human studies or animal studies to show an adverse effect on the fetus, but well-controlled studies in pregnant women have failed to demonstrate a risk to the fetus

✧ Category C
Studies have shown the drug to have animal teratogenic or embryocidal effects, but there are no controlled studies of women or no available studies of animals or women

◇ *Category D*

Positive evidence of human fetal risk exists, but benefits in certain situations (e.g. life-threatening situations or serious diseases) may make use of the drug acceptable despite its risks

◇ *Category X*

Studies in animals or humans have demonstrated fetal abnormalities, or there is evidence of fetal risk based on human experience, or both, and the risk clearly outweighs any possible benefit

◆ **Timing of Teratogenesis**

Classic teratogenic period is from day 31 to day 71 (Fig. 13-1)
- critical period of organogenesis means that early exposure usually results in all-or-none effect

Later exposure can result in problems
- DES exposure in second trimester
- alcohol use in later stages of pregnancy

Breast milk secretion of drugs often pharmacologically insignificant

EFFECTS OF THERAPEUTIC DRUGS

◆ **Vitamin A Derivatives**

◇ *Isotretinoin (Accutane)*

A significant human teratogen (Category X)

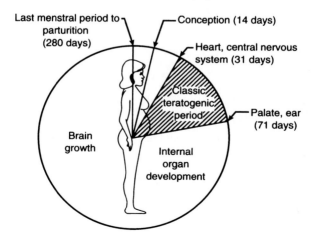

Figure 13-1. The gestational clock shows the classic teratogenic period. (Niebyl JR. Drug use in pregnancy. 2nd ed. Philadelphia: Lea & Febiger, 1988:2)

Risk of anomalies about 25%, mental retardation present in 25%
Malformations
- CNS
- craniofacial
- cardiac
- thymic

Topical use not associated with teratogenic risk

✧ *Etretinate (Tegison)*
May be similar risk to isotretinoin
Half-life of several months
- should avoid pregnancy within six months of use

✧ *Vitamin A*
No evidence for teratogenicity
Large doses (greater than 25,000 IU/day should be discouraged)
- cases of birth defects have been reported for these doses

◆ **Antineoplastic Drugs and Immunosuppressants**

✧ *Methotrexate*
First-trimester teratogen

✧ *Azothioprine (Imuran)*
No documented increase in anomalies

✧ *Cyclosporin A*
No documented increase in anomalies

✧ *Cyclophosphamide (Cytoxan)*
First-trimester exposure may have some risk

✧ *Chloroquine*
Safe in doses for malarial prophylaxis
Large antiinflammatory doses (250 to 500 mg/day) may increase
  risk of anomalies

◆ **Anticonvulsants**

Infants of epileptic mothers
- 5% risk of major malformations
- 2% to 3% risk of epilepsy (5 times general population risk)

✧ *Phenytoin*
Decreases folate absorption
- increased risk for neural tube defects
Fetal hydantoin syndrome (5% to 10%)
- microcephaly
- growth deficiency
- developmental delay
Genetic predisposition to phenytoin-induced defects
- epoxide hydrolase activity levels

✧ *Carbamazepine*
Similar syndrome to hydantoin
1% of risk of neural tube defect
- α-fetoprotein (AFP) surveillance recommended

✧ *Valproic acid*
1% risk of neural tube defect
AFP screening recommended

◆ Anticoagulants

✧ *Warfarin (Coumadin)*
Associated with chondrodysplasia punctata
Presumably a result of microhemorrhages during development

✧ *Heparin*
Does not cross placenta
Full anticoagulation
- not justified in patient with only a history of thrombosis
- recommended in patients with cardiac valve prostheses

◆ Lithium

11% rate of anomalies if used in first trimester
- high rate of cardiovascular anomalies
  - Ebstein anomaly
    - additional studies suggest lower risk
- offer ultrasound and fetal echocardiogram
- monitor serum lithium level
- usually recommended that drug therapy be changed from lithium to another drug during pregnancy
  - may result in relapse of affective disorder

◆ Thyroid and Antithyroid Drugs

Propylthiouracil (PTU) and methimazole (Tapazole) can cross placenta
- may cause fetal goiter
  - fetal hypothyroidism cannot be corrected by maternal ingestion of thyroid hormone
- PTU is drug of choice
Radioactive iodine
- not concentrated by fetal thyroid until after 12 weeks
- inadvertent exposure probably causes insignificant risk
Thyroxine
- safe in pregnancy
- dose normally needs to be increased

◆ Tranquilizers

Prospective studies have failed to demonstrate teratogenicity in first trimester

Regular use associated with a syndrome
- CNS dysfunction
- growth retardation
- dysmorphism

In most cases risk/benefit ratio does not justify their use in pregnancy

◆ Antiemetics

Bendectin
10 mg of doxylamine, 10 mg of pyridoxine (vitamin B6)
Teratogenicity not confirmed in large, controlled studies
Vitamin B6 alone may be effective as single agent
Since withdrawal of bendectin from the market, a similar mixture can be created:
- Unisom (25 mg)
- vitamin B6 (25 mg)
- full 25 mg dose of each at bedtime and half dose in morning and afternoon

◇ *Meclizine (Bonine, Antivert)*
No teratogenic evidence
May be effective antiemedic

◇ *Dimenhydrinate (Dramamine)*
No teratogenicity
29% failure rate

◇ *Diphenhydramine (Benadryl)*
No teratogenicity

◇ *Trimethobenzamide*
Small number of patients
Conflicting data regarding teratogenicity

◇ *Phenothiazines*
Compazine and promethazine (Phenergan) effective and safe
Thorazine may be associated with increased risk of malformations

◆ Antihistamines and Decongestants

Use for trivial indications should be discouraged
Use single therapy, not combination
No risk of anomalies demonstrated from most of the commonly used antihistamines
Little date available on terfenadine (seldane)

◆ Analgesics

◇ *Aspirin*
No first-trimester teratogenic effects
Low dose use may be useful in preventing hypertensive disorders in high-risk patients
Prolongs bleeding time

✧ *Acetaminophen*
No evidence of teratogenicity
No effect on bleeding time

✧ *Propoxyphene (Darvon)*
No human teratogenicity
Potential for narcotic addiction

✧ *Codeine*
No increased risk of malformations
Can cause addiction

◆ Antibiotics and Antiinfective Agents
✧ *Penicillins*
Safe in pregnancy
Erythromycin and cephalosporins also safe

✧ *Sulfonamides*
Can place premature infants at risk for hyperbilirubinemia
- not first choice in third trimester especially if patient is at risk for preterm labor

No risk of malformations noted with use of Septra (sulfamethoxazole-trimethoprim)

✧ *Sulfasalazine*
Used in ulcerative colitis and Crohn's disease
Does cross the placenta
No fetal or neonatal effects documented

✧ *Tetracyclines*
Not recommended in pregnancy
- use after 26 weeks can affect enamel of decidual teeth
- may inhibit bone growth

✧ *Nitrofurantoin*
No risk of birth defects
Can induce hemolytic anemia in G6PD deficiency patients
- theoretically could affect newborn
- no reported cases

✧ *Aminoglycosides and other antituberculosis drugs*
Streptomycin
- no first-trimester teratogenicity
- 3% to 11% incidence of ototoxicity in newborns of mothers on prolonged therapy

Other safe antituberculan agents
- isoniazid
- paraminosalicylate
- rifampin
- ethambutol
- ethionamide may be associated with CNS anomalies

◇ *Metronidazole*
No risk documented
Defer use until after first trimester
- controversy developed out of results of Ames test results (mutagenic risk)

◇ *Lindane (Kwell)*
Use during pregnancy limited to two doses
Mother can absorb through hands while washing children's hair
- alternative treatments usually recommended
- pyrethrins with piperonyl butoxide

◆ Antiasthmatics

◇ *Theophylline and aminophylline*
Safe in pregnancy

◇ *Epinephrine*
Slight increase in minor malformations after first trimester exposure but not statistically significant

◇ *Terbutaline*
Safe
Increased risked of glucose intolerance

◇ *Cromolyn sodium*
Safe

◇ *Isoproterenol and metaproterenol*
Inhaled doses safe
Oral or IV doses may alter uterine blood flow
- use with caution

◇ *Corticosteroids*
All cross the placenta to some degree
Prednisone, prednisolone inactivated by placenta
No evidence for teratogenicity

◇ *Iodide*
Contained in some cough medicines
Can cross placenta and cause fetal goiter

◆ Cardiovascular Drugs

◇ *Digoxin*
No teratogenic effects
May not easily cross placenta in hydropic fetus

◇ *Aldomet and hydralazine*
No teratogenic effects

◇ *Angiotensin-converting enzyme inhibitors*
Not recommended for pregnancy
Can result in fetal renal failure

- oligohydramnios
- limb contractures
- craniofacial deformities
- hypoplastic lung development
- fetal skull ossification defects can occur as well

✧ ***Sympathetic blocking agents***
Propranolol (Inderal)
- no teratogenic effect
- may adversely affect fetal growth
- close surveillance recommended
Atenolol
- may result in improved outcome

◆ **Ovulation Induction**

No teratogenic risk for clomiphene or bromocriptine

INADVERTENT EXPOSURE TO MEDICATIONS

◆ **Estrogens and Progestins**

Little to no risk associated with these agents in first trimester
Given medical-legal climate, a pregnancy test is warranted before prescribing these agents

◆ **Androgens**

May maculinize a developing female fetus
- most often synthetic testosterone derivatives
Danazol has been implicated at doses of 800 mg/day in first trimester

◆ **Spermicides**

Not associated with increased malformations

SOCIAL DRUG EXPOSURE

◆ **Smoking**

Associated with poor outcomes
- decreased birth weight
- increased prematurity
- increased spontaneous abortion
- increased risk of abruption, PROM
Discontinuation or reduction of smoking can improve outcome

◆ **Alcohol**

Fetal alcohol syndrome (FAS) has strict criteria
One characteristic of each category must be present

1. gross retardation before or after birth
2. facial anomalies
   - small palpebral fissures
   - indistinct/absent philtrum
   - epicanthric folds
   - flattened nasal bridge
   - short length of nose
   - thin upper lip
   - low set, unparalleled ears
   - retarded midfacial development
3. CNS dysfunction
   - microcephaly
   - mental retardation
   - other abnormal neurobehavioral development
   - attention deficit disorder with hyperactivity

Confirmatory evidence is history of heavy drinking in pregnancy
Alcoholics have poor perinatal outcomes
43% to 71% of infants abnormal
No degree of drinking is known to be safe in pregnancy

◆ Caffeine

No evidence of teratogenicity
May increase rate of anemia
Studies must control for associated tobacco and alcohol use

◆ Aspartame (NutraSweet)

Metabolized into three products
- aspartic acid
- methanol
- phenylalanine
Levels of these three are not significant
Unlikely that aspartame causes problems

◆ Narcotics

Methadone maintenance goal is 20 to 40 mg/daily
Manipulation of dose should be avoided in third trimester
Withdrawal should be avoided during pregnancy

◆ Marijuana

No teratogenic effect documented
May stimulate uterine activity

◆ Cocaine

Studies suggest increased risk of urinary anomalies with first-trimester use
May also result in fetal disruption
- bowel infarction

- limb reduction defects
- CNS bleeding

DRUGS IN BREAST MILK

Rate of transfer depends on lipid solubility, molecular weight, protein binding, ionization

Dose to infant is usually 1% to 2% maternal dose

Secretion into colostrum is minimal

Generally medications should be taken after breast feeding, and long-acting preparations should be avoided

◆ Drugs Contraindicated During Breast Feeding

✧ *Drugs of abuse*
Cocaine, heroine, marijuana, etc.

✧ *Cytotoxic agents*
Cyclophosphamide, cyclosporine, doxorubicin may cause immunosuppression

✧ *Bromocriptine*
Inhibitory effect on lactation

✧ *Ergotamine*
Doses used for migraine may be associated with vomiting, diarrhea, and convulsions in infant

Dosing for postpartum uterine contractility does not contraindicate nursing

✧ *Lithium*
Milk levels average 40% of maternal serum concentration

✧ *Radiopharmaceuticals*
Interrupt feeding for variable time to avoid radioactivity present in milk

- gallium 67, 2 weeks
- iodine 131, 2 to 14 days
- radioactive sodium, 4 days
- technetium 99, 24 hours to 1 to 3 days

◆ Drugs With Unknown Effects

Psychiatric agents
- antianxiety
- antidepressants
- antipsychotics

Metronidazole
- single-dose therapy preferred

◆ Drugs Compatible With Breast Feeding

✧ *Narcotics, sedatives, and anticonvulsants*
No evidence for adverse effects
Dose in breast milk 1% to 2% of maternal dose
Accumulation can occur in barbiturates or benzodiazepine use

✧ *Analgesics*
Aspirin transferred in small amounts
• risk only at dose >16 (300 mg) tablets per day
Acetaminophen safe
Propoxyphene could result in poor muscle tone in infant at maximal maternal dose

✧ *Antihistamines and phenothiazines*
No harmful effects noted or observed
Avoid decongestants in women having trouble producing adequate milk

✧ *Aminophylline*
Nursing infant receives less than 1% of maternal dose
No adverse effects noted
Recommend breast feeding immediately before taking medication

✧ *Amphetamines*
No evidence of stimulation in infants

✧ *Antihypertensives*
Total infant dose usually less than 1% of therapeutic dose

✧ *Anticoagulants*
Heparin does not cross
Warfarin
• difficult to detect in breast milk
• safe with careful monitoring
• watch for evidence of drug accumulation

✧ *Corticosteroids*
Negligible amounts passed on to the infant
Safe in breast feeding

✧ *Digoxin*
No adverse effects noted
Infant receives 1% of maternal dose

✧ *Antibiotics*
Penicillins, cephalosporins safe
Tetracycline injection by mother has not resulted in problems in breast-fed infants
Sulfonamides appear in small amount
• best avoided during first 5 days of life or in premature infants when hyperbilirubinemia may be a problem
Isoniazid, acyclovir are safe

⬥ *Oral contraceptives*
  Combination pills with 50 μg of estrogen dose have been associated with decreased milk production
  Recommend starting low dose pills three weeks postpartum
  • no risk to infant
  Progestin-only pills do not alter breast milk composition or volume
  • ideal for breast-feeding mothers

⬥ *Alcohol*
  Levels in milk similar to maternal blood
  Can effect odor of the milk and decrease consumption

⬥ *Lithium*
  Breast milk levels are one half of maternal serum levels
  • much lower than during pregnancy
  • risk/benefit ratio should be considered

⬥ *Propylthiouracil*
  Found in breast milk in small amounts
  Safe with close supervision of infants

⬥ *Caffeine*
  No adverse effects
  Can accumulate in cases of excessive maternal consumption

⬥ *Smoking*
  No significant risk from fetal ingestion
  Passive smoking may cause respiratory problems in infants

RADIATION

◆ **Diagnostic**

  Not teratogenic at current levels
  Doses <5 to 10 cGy incapable of producing any effects
  Usual doses received by the fetus
    Chest x-ray: 0.008 cGy
    IVP: 0.4 cGy
    CT: 0.250 cGy/slice
    Upper GI: 0.550 cGy
    Barium enema: 1 cGy
    Technetium 99 scan: 1 to 3 cGy
    Thallium 201 scan: 0.5 to 1.0 cGy
  Exposure to as little as 2 cGy may increase risk of childhood leukemia (1.3- to 1.8-fold increase)

◆ **Therapeutic**

  Levels to treat malignancy are teratogenic
  CNS, eyes, hemtopoietic system sensitive throughout pregnancy

◆ Video Display Terminals

No increased risk of spontaneous abortion or birth defects
X-ray absorbed by glass screen
Nonionizing radiation not significantly increased

◆ Hyperthermia

Prospective studies have not confirmed associating with birth
defects
Recommend that pregnant women using hot tub at 40°C stay in
for less than 10 minutes

14

◆ Ultrasound During Pregnancy

INTRODUCTION

◆ Techniques

Two-dimensional and M-mode ultrasound produced by electrical stimulation of a piezoelectric crystal

As frequency of transducer increases, resolution increases but penetration of tissue decreases

✧ *Two dimensional ultrasound*

Produces images
- useful for fetal measurement, anatomic survey, and assessment of fetal condition

✧ *M-mode*

High resolution information about one series of points over time
- useful for cardiac evaluation

✧ *Doppler*

Measure velocity of flow

Color Doppler and pulsed Doppler assessment

◆ Instrumentation

Major types of transducers
- linear array
- sector
- curvilinear
- vaginal

◆ Applications

Measure the fetus

Assess anatomy

Establish viability or well-being

NIH consensus report recommends limiting ultrasound studies to specific indications (Table 14-1)

High-risk groups should also be included (Table 14-2)

TABLE 14-1. Indications for Use of Diagnostic Ultrasound

Estimation of gestational age for patients with uncertain clinical dates
Evaluation of fetal growth
Vaginal bleeding of undetermined cause in pregnancy
Determination of fetal presentation
Suspected multiple gestation
Adjunct to amniocentesis
Significant uterine size-date discrepancy
Pelvic mass
Suspected hydatidiform mole
Suspected polyhydramnios or oligohydramnios
Suspected abruptio placentae
External version
Estimation of fetal weight with premature rupture of membranes or
    premature labor
Abnormal serum α-fetoprotein
Follow-up an identified fetal anomaly
Follow-up placental location with identified placenta previa
History of congenital anomaly
Serial evaluation of fetal growth in multiple gestation
Adjunct to cerclage
Suspected ectopic pregnancy
Special procedures
Suspected fetal death
Suspected uterine abnormality
Intrauterine device localization
Ovarian follicle development surveillance
Biophysical evolution after 28 wk
Observation of intrapartum events
Evaluation of fetal condition in late registrants for prenatal care

National Institute of Child Health and Development. Diagnostic ultrasound
imaging in pregnancy. Report of the Consensus Development Conference. NIH
Publ. No. 84-667. Washington, DC: Government Printing Office, 1984.

◆ Information Obtained from the Anatomic Survey

Depends on the trimester (Table 14-3)
Certain essential features of an ultrasound survey (Table 14-4)

◆ Measurement Scans

Based on measurements of crown rump length, head, abdomen,
    or femur
Accuracy dependent on several factors (Table 14-5)

◇ *Crown rump length (Table 14-6)*
  • measure from fetal head to fetal rump
  • accurate within 4 to 7 days
    · one of the most precise predictors of age

TABLE 14-2. High-Risk Groups

History of Anomalies
Growth retardation
Premature labor

Maternal Conditions Predisposing to Anomalies
Diabetes, insulin dependent
Connective tissue disease
Isoimmunization
Phenylketonuria
Age

Maternal Conditions Predisposing to Growth Retardation
Hypertension
Vascular disease
Cyanosis

Exposure to Drugs
Diphenylhydantoin
Lithium
Isotretinoin
Alcohol

Exposure to Viruses
Rubella
Toxoplasmosis
Cytomegalovirus
Parvovirus

Abnormal Pregnancy Progression
Abnormal growth
Abnormal amniotic fluid volume
Multiple gestation
Abnormal ultrasound
Anomalies
Hydrops
Premature labor
Bleeding
Persistent malpresentation
Decreased fetal movement
Fetal arrhythmia

TABLE 14-3. Data Obtained From Ultrasound Examination

First Trimester	Second Trimester	Third Trimester
Pregnancy location	Fetal size for dates	Fetal size for growth
Size of fetus and sac	Detailed fetal anatomy	Fetal anatomy
Pregnancy viability		Biophysical behavior
Gross anatomy		
Limits: Fetal size (small)	Limits: fetal size (small); fetal age (early)	Limits: fetal size (large); fetal position

---

TABLE 14-4. Essentials of Second- or Third-Trimester Ultrasound

Number of fetuses
Position
Placental location
Amniotic fluid volume
Pelvic masses
Measurements
    Biparietal diamenter (BPD)
        Occipitofrontal diamenter (OFD)
        Head circumference (HC)
    Abdominal diameter of circumference (AC)
    Femur length (FL)
    Ratios and calculations
        BPD/OFD (cephalic index)
        HC/AC
        BPD/FL
        Fetal weight
Anatomy
    Neural tube; ventricles, spine
    Heart: four-chamber view
    Abdomen
        Wall
        Stomach
        Kidneys

TABLE 14-5. Clinical and Ultrasound Estimation of Gestational Age

Criterion	Trimester	Variation
Last menstrual period		3 wk
Pelvic examination	1	2 wk
Crown-rump length	1	5 d
Biparietal diameter	1,2	10 d
Femur length	1,2	10 d
Biparietal diameter	3	2-3 wk
Femur length	3	3 wk
Head circumference	3	2-3 wk
Abdominal circumference	3	2-3 wk

◇ *Biparietal diameter (Table 14-7)*
Measure at level of thalamus, and cavum septi pellucidi
Less reliable with increasing gestational age
Head malformations may be from associated CNS anomalies

◇ *Abdominal circumference (Table 14-8)*
Measure at level of intraabdominal umbilical vein, at branching point, or at ductus venosus
Useful in assessing growth retardation
• after 36 weeks abdominal circumfrence should be greater than head circumfrence

◇ *Femur (Table 14-9)*
Diaphysis is measured, excluding distal epiphyseal cartilage

◆ Anatomy

Major anatomic defects should always be excluded
Detailed scans examine anatomy more extensively (Table 14-10)

◆ Amniotic Fluid

Decreases with advanced gestational age
Definitions of oligo- and polyhydraminios vary

◆ Placenta

Examine for location
Assign grade
Grade I: some irregularity of chorionic plate, scattered areas of echogenicity
Grade II: large indentations, basal echogenicity detected near the uterine wall
Grade III: chorionic plate indentations that reach the uterine wall, extreme calicifications

TABLE 14-6. Gestation Age Based on Crown-Rump Length

Crown-Rump Length (cm)	Gestational Age (wk + d)			Crown-Rump Length (cm)	Gestational age (wk + d)		
	MacGregor et al	Robinson and Fleming*	Drumm et al†		MacGregor et al	Robinson and Fleming*	Drumm et al†
1.0	7 + 5	7 + 0	6 + 6	3.9	10 + 6	10 + 4	10 + 5
1.2	8 + 0	7 + 3	7 + 2	4.1	11 + 0	10 + 5	10 + 6
1.4	8 + 1	7 + 5	7 + 4	4.3	11 + 1	11 + 0	11 + 0
1.6	8 + 3	8 + 0	7 + 6	4.5	11 + 3	11 + 1	11 + 2
1.8	8 + 5	8 + 2	8 + 1	4.7	11 + 4	11 + 2	11 + 3
2.0	8 + 6	8 + 4	8 + 3	4.9	11 + 5	11 + 3	11 + 4
2.2	9 + 1	8 + 6	8 + 5	5.1	12 + 0	11 + 4	11 + 5
2.4	9 + 2	9 + 0	9 + 0	5.3	12 + 1	11 + 5	12 + 0
2.6	9 + 4	9 + 2	9 + 2	5.5	12 + 2	11 + 6	12 + 1
2.8	9 + 5	9 + 3	9 + 3	5.7	12 + 3	12 + 1	12 + 2
3.0	9 + 6	9 + 5	9 + 5	5.9	12 + 4	12 + 2	12 + 3
3.2	10 + 1	9 + 6	10 + 0	6.1	12 + 6	12 + 3	12 + 5
3.4	10 + 2	10 + 1	10 + 1	6.3	13 + 0	12 + 4	12 + 6
3.6	10 + 4	10 + 2	10 + 3	6.5	13 + 1	12 + 5	13 + 0
3.8	10 + 5	10 + 3	10 + 4				

* Robinson HP, Fleming JEE. A critical evaluation of sonar "crown-rump length" measurements. Br J Obstet Gynaecol 1975; 82: 702
† Drumm JE. Clinch J, MacKenzie CT. The ultrasonic measurement of the fetal crown-rump length as a method of assessing gestational age. Br J Obstet Gynaecol 1976; 83:471.
MacGregor SN, Tamura RK, Sabbagha RE. Underestimation of gestational age by conventional crown-rump length dating curves. Obstet Gynecol 1987;70:344.

TABLE 14-7. Correlation of Predicted Menstrual Age Based on Biparietal Diameters

Menstrual Age (wk)	Biparietal Diameter (mm)			
	*Kurtz et al**	*Hadlock et al†*	*Shepard and Filly‡*	*Jeanty and Romero§*
14	26	27	28	28
16	33	33	34	36
18	40	40	40	43
20	46	46	46	49
22	53	53	52	55
24	59	58	57	61
26	64	64	63	67
28	70	70	68	72
30	75	75	73	77
32	79	79	78	82
34	84	84	83	86
36	88	88	88	90
38	92	91	92	
40	95	95	97	

* Kurtz AB et al. J Clin Ultrasound 1980;8:319.
† Hadlock RP, Deter RL, Harrist RB, Park SK. Fetal biparietal diameter: a critical re-evaluation of the relation to menstrual age by means of real-time ultrasound. J Ultrasound Med 1982; 1:97.
‡ Shepard Mr. Filly RA. A standardized plane for biparietal diameter measurement. J Ultrasound Med 1982; 1:145.
§ Jeanty P, Romero R. Obstetrical ultrasound. New York: McGraw-Hill, 1984. Sanders RC, James AE, eds. Ultrasonography in obstetrics and gynecology. 3rd ed. Norwalk, CT: Appleton Century-Crofts, 1985:626.

TABLE 14-8. Predicted Menstrual Age for Abdominal Circumference Values

Abdominal Circumference (cm)	Menstrual Age (wk)	Abdominal Circumference (cm)	Menstrual Age (wk)
10.0	15.6	23.5	27.7
11.0	16.5	24.5	28.7
12.0	17.3	25.5	29.7
13.0	18.2	26.5	30.6
14.0	19.1	27.5	31.6
15.0	20.0	28.5	32.6
16.0	20.8	29.5	33.6
17.0	21.7	30.5	34.6
18.0	22.6	31.5	35.6
19.0	23.6	32.5	36.6
20.0	24.5	33.5	37.6
21.0	25.4	34.5	38.7
22.0	26.3	35.5	39.7
23.0	27.3	36.5	40.8

Menstrual age = 7.6070 + 0.7645 (abdominal circumference) + 0.00393 (abdominal circumference)^2; multiple correlation coefficeint + 97.8%; standard deviation = 1.2 wk.
Hadlock FP, Deter RL, Harrist RB, Park SK. Fetal abdominal circumference as a predictor of menstrual age. AJR AM J Roentgenol 1982; 139:367.

TABLE 14-9. Predicted Femur Lengths at Points in Gestation

Menstrual Age (wk)	Femur Length (mm)			
	Filly et al [*][†]	*Jeanty et al* [‡][§]	*Hadlock et al* [†][‖]	*Hadlock et al* [§][‖]
12		09	14	08
14		15	19	15
16	22	22	23	21
18	28	28	28	27
20	35	33	33	33
22	41	39	38	39
24	47	44	42	44
26	53	49	47	49
28	57	53	52	54
30	63	58	57	58
32		62	61	63
34		65	66	66
36		69	71	70
38		72	76	73
40		75	80	76

[*] Filly RA, Golbus, Ms Carey JC, et al. Short-limbed dwarfism: ultrasonographic diagnosis by mensuration of fetal femoral length. Radiology 1981; 138:653.
[†] Linear Function
[‡] Jeanty P, Kirkpatrick C, Dramaix-Wilmet M, et al. Ultrasonic evaluation of fetal limb growth. Radiology 1981; 140:165
[§] Linear quadratic function
[‖] Hadlock FP, Harrist RB, Deter RL, Park SK. Fetal femur length as a predictor of menstrual age: sonographically measured. AJR Am J Roentgenol 1982; 138:875.
Jeanty P, Romero R. Obstetrical ultrasound. New York: McGraw-Hill, 1984; 327.

TABLE 14-10. Detailed Ultrasound Examinations

Structure	Additonal Detail	Condition or Anomaly
Cerebral ventricles	Thalamus	Hydrocephalus
	Cavum septi pellucidi	Anencephalus
	Atria	Microcephaly
	Cisterna magna	Encephalocele
Face in profile	Palate	Cleft
		Orbits
Neck		Thyroid mass
		Edema
		Cystic hygroma
Spine		Meningomyelocele
Longitudinal		Spina bifida
Transverse		
Coronal		
Thorax		
Lungs		Pleural effusion
		Masses
		Hypoplasia
		Diaphragmatic hernia
Heart	Four chambers	Congenital heart
	Great vessels	disease
	Aortic arch	
	Ductal arch	
Abdomen		
Wall		Gastroschisis
		Omphalocele
Stomach		Tracheoesophageal fistula
Liver		Enlargement
Spleen		Absence, enlargement
Gallbladder		Stones, cyst
Cystic masses		Intestinal atresia
Kidneys		Agenesis
		Hydronephrosis
		Multicystic
		Polycystic
Bladder		Obstruction
Extremities		Skeletal dysplasia
		Amniotic disruption sequence

15

◆ Assessment of Fetal Well-Being

INTRODUCTION

Approach dependent on gestational age

◆ First Trimester

Establish viability
Number of fetuses
Document intrauterine location
Prenatal diagnosis (CVS)

◆ Second Trimester

Gestational age
Anatomic malformations
Prenatal diagnosis (amniocentesis)

◆ Third Trimester

Antepartum fetal testing
Intrapartum fetal monitoring

GESTATIONAL AGE

Key point in assessing fetal risks and benefits for delivery
Documentation of fetal growth dependent on appropriate assignment of gestational age

◆ First-Trimester Examination

Pelvic examination
Ausculation of heart tones
• Doppler, 10 to 12 weeks
• fetoscope, 17 to 20 weeks
Early ultrasound
• most accurate method

◆ Second- and Third-Trimester Evaluation

Ultrasound dating limited by variability of normal fetal growth
Reassignment of gestational age requires careful consideration
of historical information

FETAL LUNG MATURITY

Pulmonary immaturity previously a leading cause of infant
mortality
- iatrogenic etiology as a result of misdating a pregnancy
- now markedly reduced as a result of better evaluation

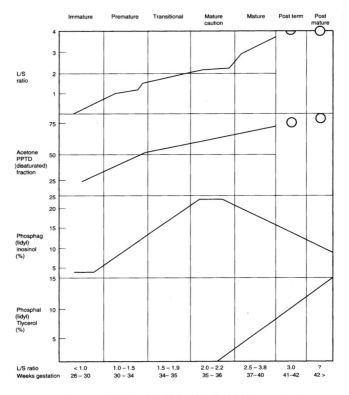

Figure 15-1. Lung profile. (Gluck L, Kulovich MV. Fetal lung maturity. In: Eden RP, Boehm FH, Haire M, eds. Assessment and care of the fetus. Norwalk, CT: Appleton & Lange, 1990:412.)

◆ Amniocentesis

First developed to evaluate fetal condition in Rh incompatibility
Amniotic fluid collected with ultrasound guidance under sterile conditions
  * assessment of lung maturity (Fig. 15-1)
  * fetal squamous cells grown to assess karyotype

◇ *Risk of amniocentesis*

Genetic amniocentesis
  * pregnancy loss of 1/300 normal fetuses above background rate
Lung maturation (third-trimester amniocentesis)
  * loss rate extremely low
  * acute complications can occur
  * emergency cesarean delivery may be required

◆ Surfactant

Mixture of 80% to 90% lipid, 10% to 20% protein
Detergent-like substance
  * secreted by type II fetal pulmonary cells
  * decreases alveoli surface tension
Absence leads to poorly compliant or stiff lungs
Composition of surfactant changes within increasing gestational age

◇ *Lecithin*

Major component of phospholipid portion at term
Increases exponentially after 34 to 36 weeks

◇ *Sphingomyelin*

Lipid component of all membranes
Appears early in gestation
Acts as internal control for assessment of lecithin

◆ L/S Ratio

Increases after 34 weeks
Correlates with gestational age-dependent risk of RDS
  * ratios of 1 : 5 to 2 : 0 are transitional
  * seldom associated with lethal RDS in nondiabetic patient

◇ *Diabetic pregnancies*

Increased risk of RDS for any given L/S ratio in White classes A to C
  * some recommend using ratio of greater than 2 : 5 for diagnosis of pulmonary maturity in these cases
  * others recommend use of different measures (PG)
More rapid pulmonary maturity present in severe diabetics (White D, F, R)
  * primarily related to fetal stress and production of endogenous fetal steroid

◇ *Contamination*
Levels affected by other bodily fluids

Laboratory variation
Usually determined by thin layer of chromatography
Variations and values between laboratories occur
Each laboratory should document correlation with known controls

◆ Phosphatidylglycerol

Acidic phospholipid in surfactant
Increases after 35 weeks
Laboratory methods simpler and less expensive
PG levels greater than 3% associated with low incidence of RDS
(less than 1%)
- not affected by presence of other fluids
- can be tested for in vaginal pool samples

◆ Ultrasound

BPD >9.3 cm
Femoral length >7.4 cm
- incidence of RDS less than 1% (in absence of diabetes)
- these are strict criteria

ANTEPARTUM TESTING

◆ History

Approximately 1% of all third-trimester low-risk pregnancies
end in fetal death in absence of surveillance
- two thirds occur in utero
High-risk pregnancy associated with higher rate
Electronic fetal monitoring
- provides objective data
- allow correlation with fetal acid base status
- extended to antepartum period

◇ *Contractions stress test (CST)*
Labor intensive
Sensitive but nonspecific

◇ *Nonstress test (NST)*
Simpler
Not as predictive as CST

◇ *Biophysical profile (BPP)*
Developed to improve sensitivity and specificity
Sensitive and convenient testing regime for high-risk conditions

ELECTRONIC FETAL MONITORING

Early retrospective studies demonstrated reduction in intrapartum and neonatal mortality in high-risk patients

Became standard practice in 1970s

◆ Anatomy of a Fetal Heart Rate Tracing

Two pen lines on continuous graph paper

Fine vertical lines every 10 seconds

Darker lines mark every minute
- top pen fetal heart rate
- bottom pen uterine activity

Monitor
- internal
  - fetal scalp electrode
    - use during labor
- external (anytime)
  - subject to artifacts (Fig. 15-2)
  - affected by maternal body habitus

Pressure measurements
- external tocodynometer
- internal transducer (IUPC)
  - direct measurement
  - can be used as a therapeutic tool
    - amnioinfusion
- early introduction of IUPC may result in increased amnionitis

◆ Interpreting Fetal Heart Rate Tracings

✧ *Uterine activity*

Frequency

Intensity
- early labor 20 to 30 mm Hg

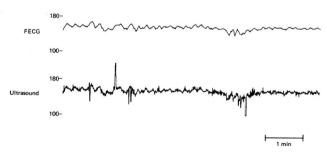

Figure 15-2. Manner in which the fetal heart rate is depicted on the monitor chart when it is recorded by direct (*top*) and indirect (*bottom*) methods. (Courtesy Richard H. Paul.)

- active labor 50 mm Hg
- second stage 70 to 80 mm Hg
  - Montevideo unit
    - average peak pressure minus baseline pressure times the number of contractions over 10 minutes
    - >200 considered adequate

Baseline
  - hypertonus may represent iatrogenic effects or altered normal response

◆ Fetal Heart Rate

Baseline rate
- most prominent for average rate between contraction in absence of decelerations
- should persist for greater than 15 minutes
- normal range 110 to 160 BPM
- less than 120 BPM should have normal variability to be considered normal variant

Fetal tachycardia
- greater than 160 BPM
- fetal immaturity
- maternal fever
- fetal infection
- mild hypoxia
- reflex tachycardia (recovery from bradycardia)
- fetal tachyarrhythmias
- maternal hyperthyroidism
- pharmaceuticals

Periodic changes
- brief accelerations or deceleration followed by return to baseline
- can be reassuring or concerning

✧ *Accelerations*
Usually in response to fetal movement
Reassuring
Reactivity defined by most as two increased greater than 50 BPM above baseline lasting 15 seconds in a 20 minute window

✧ *Decelerations*
Three types: early, late, variable (Fig. 15-3)

✧ *Early deceleration*
Most benign
Probably normal vagal response
Not associated with hypoxia or acidosis

✧ *Variable decelerations*
Most common (50% of all heart rate tracings)
Result from cord compression

Nonuniform shape, duration, depth
Fetal risk depends on severity and persistence of decelerations
May be alleviated by introduction of saline through IUPC (amnio-
  infusion)

✧ *Late deceleration*
Most concerning periodic change
Return to baseline after contraction
Smooth shape
Usually repetitive
70% associated with suboptimal outcome
• especially in the absence of other reassuring components

✧ *Sinusoidal pattern*
Rare but ominous
Seen in association with severe fetal anemia

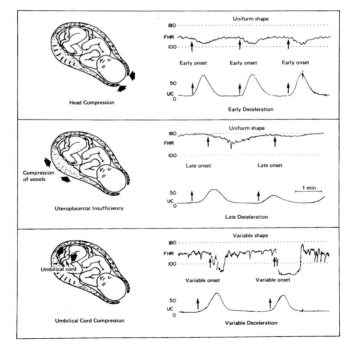

Figure 15-3. Deceleration patterns of the fetal heart rate (FHR) and their implied causative mechanisms. Intrauterine pressure (UC) is measured in millimeters of mercury. (Hon EH. An atlas of fetal heart rate patterns. New Haven, CT: Harty Press, 1968.)

ANTEPARTUM FETAL TESTING

◆ Contraction Stress Test

Based on observation of adverse outcomes in fetus with late decelerations after spontaneous uterine contractions

Low-dose oxytocin infused to stimulate three contractions in 10 minutes

Sensitive test for uteroplacental insufficiency
- time-intensive
- poor specificity
- test often equivocable or uninterpretable

◆ Nonstress Test

Criteria varied between institution

Reactive test usually defined as noted previously
- associated with perinatal mortality 1 to 4/1000 in high-risk patient

Nonreactive nonstress test
- perinatal mortality 20% to 26%

Nervous system maturation limits utility at gestational ages <30 weeks

◆ Fetal Acoustic Stimulation

Performed by placement of an artificial larynx device against abdomen for 1-second sound blast
- has reduced required testing time during NST

Safety seems to be confirmed by longitudinal follow-up studies

◆ Biophysical Profile

Developed by Manning in 1985 as an in utero Apgar score

Maximum score of 10 in 30 minute observation period (Table 15-1)

Low false-positive rate

Low false-negative rate (0.5 to 0.7 per 1000)

Utility during labor is uncertain

◆ Amniotic Fluid Volume and the Modified Biophysical Profile

Postdates pregnancy outcome related to amniotic fluid volume
- use of nonstress test and Amniotic Fluid Index (AFI) may be appropriate testing in some cases
- twice weekly testing reduces perinatal mortality and postdates pregnancy to that of term population

Normal AFI 5 to 20 cm

Polyhydramnios >20 cm

Oligohydramnios <5 cm

TABLE 15-1. Technique and Interpretation of Biophysical Profile Scoring

Biophysical Variable	Normal (Score = 2)	Abnormal (Score = 0)
Fetal breathing movements (FBM)	At least one episode of FBM of at least 30-sec duration in 30-min observation	Absent FBM or no episode of >30 sec in 30 min
Gross body movement	At least three discrete body or limb movements in 30 min (episodes of active continuous movement considered as single movement)	Two or fewer episodes of body or limb movements in 30 min
Fetal tone	At least one episode of active extension with return to flexion of fetal limb(s) or trunk. Opening and closing of hand considered normal tone	Either slow extension with return to partial flexion or movement of limb in full extension, absent fetal movement
Reactive fetal heart rate (FHR)	At least two episodes of FHR acceleration of >15 bpm and of at least 15-sec duration	Fewer than two episodes of acceleration of FHR or acceleration of >15 bpm in 30 min
Qualitative amniotic fluid (AF) volume	At least one pocket of AF that measures at least 1 cm in two perpendicular planes	Either no AF pockets or a pocket <1 cm in two perpendicular planes

bpm, beats per minute
Manning FA, Harman CR. The fetal biophysical profile. In: Eden RD, Boehm FH, Haire M, Jonas HS, eds. Assessment and care of the fetus. Norwalk, CT: Appleton & Lange, 1990:389.)

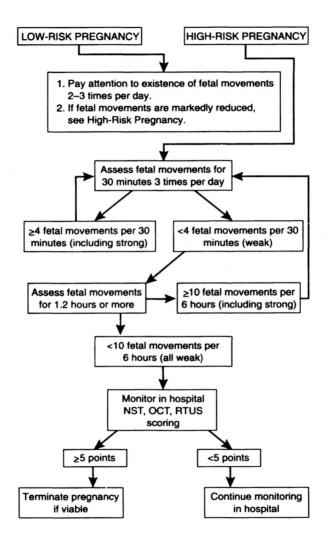

Figure 15-4. Protocol for fetal movement assessment. (Sadovsky E. Fetal movements. In: Contemp Obstet Gynecol 1985:341.)

◆ Fetal Kick Counts

Represents near continuous surveillance
Supported by animal data
Preliminary reports suggests reduction in perinatal mortality
Protocols vary between institutions (Fig 15-4)

◆ Fetal Doppler Studies

Can be used to evaluate relative flow
Prospective studies not yet performed
May not add additional information to BPP

◆ Fetal Scalp Sampling

Usually performed in cases where fetal tracing difficult to inter-
pret
- plastic cone placed in vagina
- scalp cleansed with disinfectant
- superficial scalp incision made
- sample collected in capillary tube

Can be very time consuming

✧ *Evaluating results*

pH <7.20 → fetal acidosis → delivery indicated
7.20-7.25 → concerning, repeat test required within 20 to 30
minutes
7.25-7.35 → normal

◆ Percutaneous Umbilical Blood Sampling

Very useful in certain clinical settings
- Rh disease
- platelet disorders
- genetic assessment

2% complication risk

FETAL DISTRESS

A state that will by best estimates deteriorate to a potentially
lethal condition

◆ Examples of Fetal Distress

Prolonged brachycardia unresponsive to maneuvers
Repetitive late deceleration unresponsive to intrauterine resus-
citation
Ominous nonreactive tracing with minimal variability in
previously normal fetus
Gross distortion in fetal heart rate tracing unresponsive to intra-
uterine resuscitation
Worsening hydrops

Persistent BPP <6
Gross and persistent deterioration of fetal Doppler studies
Worsening cardiac arrhythmia
• with tricuspid regurgitation or cardiac dilation
Documented acidosis

16

◆ Causes and Management of Preterm Labor

INTRODUCTION

7% to 10% of infants are born prematurely
Responsible for 75% of perinatal morbidity and mortality

◆ Definition of Preterm Labor

Gestational age <37 weeks **or** weight <2500 g
• **one third are not premature but growth retarded**
Regular uterine contractions (3 to 4 in 30 minutes)
Cervical change (dilation or effacement)

MECHANISMS FOR THE ONSET OF PARTURITION

◆ Background

Labor represents conversion of uterine environment from containment to expulsion
Preterm labor prevention and treatment has received much attention
• preterm birth rate has not been significantly reduced
Several animal models have been useful with similar findings regarding parturition
• increase in myometrial oxytocin receptors
• development of gap junctions between uterine cells
• increased responsiveness to uterotonic agents
• physical and biochemical changes in the cervix resulting in softening

◆ Progesterone-Estrogen Effects

Withdrawal of progesterone initiates labor in some animal models
• in sheep, changes are initiated in fetal adrenal cells with increased cortisol production
• primate studies do not support this model
• human studies reveal nocturnal shifts in the estrogen and progesterone surges

- forward shift in the timing of the estrogen surge results in several hours of relative unopposed estrogen
- uterine activity increases at this time

RU486 (progesterone receptor antagonist) increases uterine activity

◆ Oxytocin

Precise role difficult to ascertain because of measurement difficulty and pulsatile release

Receptors increase with gestational age and during labor

Locally and centrally produced oxytocin may play a role in the initiation of parturition

◆ Prostaglandins

Release mediated by oxytocin action on decidual receptors

Also released by infection of the membranes

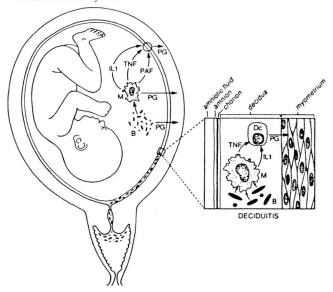

Figure 16-1. Romero's conception of the ascending route of vaginal infection to stimulate contractions either by action of the bacteria or by the resultant host response. (B, bacteria, DC, decidua; IL1, interleukin 1; M, monocyte/macrophage; PAF, platelet-activating factor; PG, prostaglandin; TNF, tumor necrosis factor/cachetin. (Romero R, Auila C, Drekus CA, et al. The role of systemic and intrauterine infection in preterm parturition. In: Garfield RE, ed. Uterine contractility. Norwell, MA: Serono Symposium, 1990:319.)

Labor associated with increased plasma and amniotic fluid prostaglandin concentration

◆ Infection

Bacterial products may stimulate prostaglandin release
- bacterial phospholipase may release arachidonic acid from amnion
- gram-negative organisms may stimulate decidual or membrane production of prostaglandins via endotoxin
- gram-positive organisms may stimulate prostaglandin activity via peptidoglycans

Infection may also influence arachidonic acid metabolism (Fig. 16-1)
- increasing amniotic fluid levels of leukotrienes, cytokines, and other substances

ETIOLOGY OF PRETERM LABOR

◆ Demographics

Increased incidence
- upper and lower extremes of age
  - may be related to confounding factors
- lower socio-economic status
- inadequate prenatal care
- race
  - some studies suggest a twofold increase in blacks

◆ Lifestyle and Employment

Proven to increase incidence
- smoking
- drug use

Possibly increase incidence
- prolonged periods of standing
- fatigue and long hours at work
- heavy work and lifting in patients predisposed to preterm delivery

◆ Reproductive History

Major factor in assigning risk in current pregnancy (Table 16-1)

◆ Uterine Anomalies

Presence of leiomyomata may also increase incidence of preterm labor

Some anomalies have strong association (Table 16-2)

◆ Weight Gain

Low weight or low weight gain may increase risk

TABLE 16-1. Risk of Preterm Birth in Subsequent Pregnancies

First Birth	Second Birth	Subsequent Preterm Birth (%)
Not preterm		4.2
Preterm		14.3
Not preterm	Not preterm	2.6
Preterm	Not preterm	5.7
Not preterm	Preterm	9.0
Preterm	Preterm	28.1

TABLE 16-2. Relation of Uterine Anomalies to Preterm Labor

Anomaly	Number of patients	Patients with preterm labor (%)
Unicornate	8	37
Didelphic	17	35
Bicornuate		
Bicollis	5	80
Unicollis	66	27
Arcuate	33	18
Septate	24	4
Incomplete	36	17

◆ Anemia

At most a weak predictor
Probably related to other risk factors

◆ Uterine Size and Placental Abnormalities

Distended uterus (may increase gap junction formation)
• multiple gestation
• polyhydramnios
Placental abnormalities
• placenta previa
• abruption

◆ Premature Rupture of Membranes (PROM)

A very common cause of preterm labor and delivery
• 50% of patients enter labor within 24 hours
• 75% to 90% enter labor within 7 days
Longer latent period observed in patients more remote from term

◆ Vaginal Bleeding

First-trimester bleeding results in increased risk
Risk increased if bleeding occurs in more than one trimester

◆ Surgery

Abdominal procedures greatly increase risk of preterm labor

◆ Nonuterine Infection

Maternal infections predispose to preterm labor
Asymptomatic bacteriuria strongly associated (twice the risk)
Pyelonephritis (30% incidence if untreated)
Pneumonia (25% risk)
Malaria/typhoid fever (50% risk)

◆ Genital Tract Infection

Many organisms implicated, few proven
- "proven"
  - *Treponema pallidum*
    - 50% prematurity rate in untreated 1° or 2° syphilis
  - *Neisseria gonorrhea*
  - Group B streptococcus
    - found in 20% of women at some time in pregnancy
    - associated with PROM
    - bacteriuria may be major associated factor
  - *Bacteroides* sp.
    - heavy vaginal growth increases relative risk 1.7 to 2.0
  - *G vaginalis* (conflicting data)
  - *Trichomonas vaginalis* (conflicting data)
- "questionable" association
  - *Chlamydia trachomatis*
  - *Ureaplasma urealyticum*
Amniotic fluid infection
- positive cultures by amniocentesis in up to 30% of patients with preterm labor
- most frequent organisms isolated
  - *U urealyticum*
  - *Fusobacterium* sp.
  - *Mycoplasma hominis*

◆ Other Associations

Fetal gender (male fetuses have shorter gestation period)
Coitus/orgasm
- not an apparent risk factor except in patients predisposed to preterm labor
Low magnesium levels
Fetal fibronectin levels in cervical/vaginal secretions

HIGH-RISK POPULATIONS AND SPECIAL PRENATAL CARE

◆ Recognized Risk Factors

Low socioeconomic status
Prior preterm delivery
Multiple gestation
Uterine malformation
Cervical incompetence
Bacterial vaginosis
Unexplained high maternal α-fetoprotein levels
Urinary tract infection

◆ Special Prenatal Care for High-risk Women

Frequent visits for weeks 22 to 32
Cervical GBS and urine culture at 24 weeks
Vaginal examination for pH and cervical examination
Uterine tone and activity palpated
Education on nutrition and preterm labor
Signs and symptoms reinforced
  • increase or change in vaginal discharge
  • uterine contractions
  • vaginal bleeding or leaking fluid
  • pelvic pressure or backache

MANAGEMENT OF PRETERM LABOR

◆ Diagnosis

Regular uterine contractions
Cervical change
Gestational age <37 weeks or EFW by ultrasound <2500 g

◆ Exclusion criteria for Tocolytic Therapy

PROM
Serious maternal or fetal disease
  • abruption
  • chorioamnionitis
  • PIH - HELLP
  • fetal distress
  • major fetal anomalies incompatible with life
Advanced cervical dilation (usually >6 cm)

◆ Bed Rest and Hydration

Increases uterine blood flow
500 to 1000 cc fluid bolus over 30 to 60 minutes
Continuous monitoring
Tocolytic therapy if this fails

◆ Tocolytics

Many agents developed and used
IV alcohol one of the first agents
• blocks posterior pituitary release of vasopressin and oxytocin
Now most frequently used agents are magnesium sulfate and
β-mimetic agents

◆ Magnesium Sulfate

Administration
• 6 g IV bolus in 250 cc over 30 minutes
• constant IV infusion of 2 to 4 g /hour
Blood levels of 6 to 8 mg/dL optimal
Mechanism of action unknown
• probably decreases free $Ca+2$ ion concentration in intracellular compartment of uterine muscle myosin light chain
Disadvantages
• toxic levels can cause cardiac arrest
• need to follow deep tendon reflexes

◆ β-Mimetics

Acts on the β-2 receptors in myometrium
FDA approved use of ritodrine (Yutopar)
Maternal pulse mirrors serum concentration
• decrease infusion if maternal pulse >120
Disadvantages
• risk of pulmonary edema
  • maternal tachycardia >120 beats per minute
  • multiple gestation
  • maternal infection
  • use of IV preparation of drug for >24 hr
• adverse effect on glucose metabolism
• increased incidence of neonatal intraventricular hemorrhage

◆ Oral Tocolytics

Little benefit
Tachyphylactic effect of oral β-mimetics limit utility

◇ *Efficacy*

Early use (cervix <2 cm) associated with improved success
However, difficulty of diagnosis of real preterm labor makes
  evaluation of success problematic
50% success rate with bed rest and hydration alone
Tocolytic agents may add 25% to this value

◆ Maternal Transport

Patients should be transported to level III center after stabilization

Tocolytic therapy may improve outcome by delaying delivery enough to facilitate transport

◆ Fetal Maturation Therapy

Lung maturity
- glucocorticoid therapy
  - singleton fetus
  - 28 to 32 weeks
  - administer Betamethasone 12 mg IM q 24 hr x 2 doses
  - maximum benefit at 48 hours
  - repeat weekly until 32 weeks
- thyrotropin-releasing hormone (TRH)
  - crosses placenta and stimulates fetal thyroid
  - 400 µg IV q 8 hr x 6 doses
  - useful in conjunction with steroids

Prevention of intraventricular hemorrhage
- phenobarbitol may be useful
  - 60 mg q day
  - active multicenter trials using high dose IV phenobarbitol currently in progress

CONTROVERSIES

Risk scoring systems
- variable utility

Home uterine monitoring
- not useful and not endorsed by FDA or ACOG

Oral tocolytics
- no prophylactic advantage

Amniocentesis
- routine use to detect infection not supported by data
- may be useful in assessing lung maturity in some cases

17

◆ Premature Rupture of Membranes

DEFINITION AND CAUSE

Rupture of fetal membranes before the onset of labor
- 10% occur at or near term
  - presumably a normal variant

Cause remains unknown in most cases

Risk factors at preterm gestation
- polyhydramnios
- cerclage
- amniocentesis
- abruption
- infection

More common in twin gestation

Seldom associated with trauma

INCIDENCE

10% of all pregnancies

Accounts for more preterm deliveries than any other identifiable cause

COMPLICATIONS

Premature labor and preterm delivery

Maternal and/or fetal infection

Cord compression

◆ Premature Labor

Delay between PROM and labor is called the latency period
- PROM at earlier gestational age is usually associated with longer latency period
- term: latency period 24 hours in 90% of patients
- 28 to 34 weeks: 50% in labor within 24 hours; 80% to 90% in labor by 1 week
- <24 to 26 weeks: 50% in labor by 1 week

◆ Infection

PROM >24 hours associated with significant increased risk of infection at term
- not true in preterm gestation

Maternal infection
- chorioamnionitis
  - infection of membranes prior to delivery
- endometritis
  - infection spreads from endometrium to myometrium and even parametrium
  - clinical infection persisting >24 hours after delivery
  - associated with chorioamnionitis or may occur independently
  - causative organisms (Table 17-1)

◆ Incidence of Chorioamnionitis

0.5% to 1% of all pregnancies
3% to 5% in cases of prolonged PROM at term
15% to 25% in cases of preterm PROM
Neonatal sepsis more likely in preterm fetus

TABLE 17-1. Organisms Cultured From Amniotic Fluid

Low-Virulence Organisms (Not Commonly Associated with Chorioamnionitis)

Aerobes	**Anerobes**
Lactobacilli	*Eubacterium lentum*
Diphtheroids	*Propionibacterium* sp
Staphylococcus epidermidis	*Gaffkya* sp
Micrococcus sp	*Veillonella* sp
Bacillus sp	*Bifidobacterium* sp
Gardnerella vaginalis	

High-Virulence Organisms (Associated With Chorioamnionitis)

Aerobes	**Anaerobes**
Streptococci	*Peptococcus* sp
Group B	*Peptostreptococcus* sp
Enterococci	*Clostridium* sp
Alpha hemolytic	*Bacteroides* sp
Gamma hemolytic	*Fusobacterium* sp
Straphylococcus aureus	
Escherichia coli	
Klebsiella sp	
Proteus sp	
Citrobacter sp	
Enterobacter sp	

Gibbs RS, Blanco JD, St. Clair PJ, et al. Quantitive bacteriology of amniotic fluid from patients with clinical intra-amniotic infection at term. J Infect Dis 1982;145:1

- term infants normally 1/500; 3% in cases of documented chorioamnionitis
- preterm 5%; 15% to 20% in cases of chorioamnionitis

◆ Fetal Distress

Umbilical prolapse more common in cases of PROM (1.5%)

Preterm PROM in labor have 8.5% incidence of fetal distress vs. 1.5% in preterm labor without PROM

Increased rate of stillbirths in unmonitored patients with preterm PROM managed expectantly

Delivery as an option depends on risk/benefit analysis

- prematurity vs. in utero fetal compromise

EVALUATING THE PATIENT WITH PROM

◆ Making the Diagnosis

Correct diagnosis is essential to future management

- 90% of patients with history suggestive of PROM have confirmed PROM on examination

Appropriate evaluation (Table 17-2)

Ultrasound final confirmatory step in some cases

Other important information from speculum examination

- cervical dilation
- prolapse of fetal part or umbilical cord
- collection of samples for culture

TABLE 17-2. Proper Evaluation With Sterile Speculum

- Visualize pool of fluid in vaginal fornix ("pooling")
- Valsalva may reveal leakage of fluid through cervix
- pH of amniotic fluid 7.1 to 7.3
  - normal vagina 4.5 to 6.0
  - nitrazine paper turns blue at pH>6.5
    - false-positive rate (1% to 17%)
      - blood
      - semen
      - vaginal infection
      - alkaline antiseptics
      - alkaline urine
- If diagnosis still uncertain, check for ferning of fluid on glass slide
  - dry for 5 to 7 minutes
  - examine under microscope
  - false negatives
    - blood
    - meconium
    - lubricants
    - heavy vaginal discharge
    - insufficient fluid
  - false positive: usually cervical mucus

- collection of fluid for lung maturity studies
  - PG most reliable
- DO NOT PERFORM DIGITAL INTRACERVICAL EXAMINA-TION IN NONLABORING PATIENT

◆ Establishing Gestational Age and Fetal Maturity

Accurate diagnosis of fetal age is essential
- history, ultrasound, other dating criteria
Oligohydramnios can affect ultrasound measurements (especially BPD)
- femur length and abdominal circumference most reliable
Fetal lung maturity testing
- may be helpful at 32 to 36 weeks
- vaginal pool PG most reliable
  - if negative, consider amniocentesis

◆ Establishing the Onset of Labor

Patient management dictated by the presence or absence of labor
Perform cervical examination in presence of painful, regular contractions
- if in doubt, repeat speculum examination
Early diagnosis of labor is helpful
- provides for prompt assessment of fetal tolerance of labor
- continuous EFM in labor as fetal heart rate abnormalities are common in preterm PROM

◆ Ruling Out Infection

Diagnosis of chorioamnionitis should be made in timely fashion
- maternal fever (>38°C)
- maternal tachycardia
- leukocytosis
- fetal tachycardia
- tender uterus
- malodorous or purulent vaginal discharge
All of the above features usually present only in advanced or virulent infections
More commonly, clinical diagnosis is made when maternal temperature is >38° in patient with PROM
Testing for evaluation of occult chorioamnionitis has not been shown to improve outcome
- amniocentesis
  - chorioamnionitis occurs in 80% of patients with positive Gram stain
- biophysical profile
  - disappearance of fetal breathing can be predictive
- C-reactive protein
  - nonspecific test similar to maternal leukocyte count

◆ Ruling Out Fetal Distress

Underappreciated cause of adverse outcome
Initial period of extended monitoring (12 to 24 hours)
- subsequent daily prolonged NSTs
- reinstitute continuous monitoring in labor or for suspicious tracings

Variable decelerations dictate more continous monitoring
Loss of variability and accelerations may suggest possible sepsis
Determination of amniotic fluid volume may help identify patients at increased risk for fetal compromise

MANAGING THE PATIENT WITH PROM

Term Patient

Immediate induction has been suggested
- this approach may increase risk of infection and cesarean delivery

Suggested management
- perform single speculum examination
- prolonged heart rate monitoring
- rule out infection
- favorable cervix → pitocin induction
- unfavorable cervix → allow 12 to 24 hours for spontaneous labor

Preterm Patient

Complications of prematurity are 3 times as likely to cause perinatal mortality than infection
Survival rate with PROM after 26 weeks is close to 50%

◆ Tocolytics

No significant prolongation of pregnancy
No improvement in neonatal outcome
No increase in rate of infection

◆ Corticosteroids

Metaanalysis suggests a modest reduction in the incidence of RDS
Confirms a small increased risk of maternal infection
- PROM alone may accelerate lung maturity

◆ Antibiotics

Some evidence that use of ampicillin prolongs latent period
Treatment of patients colonized with group B streptococci clearly reduces neonatal sepsis
Positive amniocentesis results demand antibiotic therapy and delivery

◆ Previable Gestational Age Group

PROM at <23 weeks
Vast majority deliver before 26 to 28 weeks
- 25% survival rate
- high rate of neurologic damage
- risk of pulmonary hypoplasia
- Two options for management
1. termination of pregnancy (usually PG suppositories)
2. expectant management until viability (consider outpatient care)

MANAGING CHORIOAMNIONITIS

◆ Delivery

Vaginal delivery is preferred route from maternal aspect
Cesarean section substantially increases infectious complications
No evidence of increased risk to fetus from delay in delivery to allow trial of labor
Antibiotic therapy crucial
Cesarean section reserved for usual obstetric indications
Fetal tachycardia is the rule not the exception
- should not be considered fetal distress in absence of decelerations
- treatment of maternal fever (Tylenol, cooling blanket, etc.) may normalize fetal heart rate tracing

◆ Antibiotics

Maternal treatment BEFORE delivery clearly decreases neonatal sepsis
Antibiotic therapy should be instituted immediately once diagnosis is made
Specific therapy
- mild to moderate infection: IV ampicillin
- more severe infection (rigors, high temperative): ampicillin and gentamycin (and possibly clindamycin)
Most patients defervesce after delivery
- usually continue antibiotics until afebrile for 24 to 48 hours postpartum

18

◆ Fetal Growth Retardation

INTRODUCTION

Evaluation of fetal growth requires estimates of gestational age and fetal weight

Excessive growth

- macrosomia 4000 g or 4500 g birth weight
  - dystocia
  - birth trauma
- insufficient growth (IUGR)
  - lowest 10% of weight for age
  - high-risk for perinatal mortality and morbidity

CONTROLLING FETAL GROWTH

Fetus and placenta grow at different rates

- placental peak growth at 37 weeks
- surface area of 11 m^2

Fetal growth continuous but slow up to 36 to 37 weeks

- increased fat deposition
- high metabolic activity
  - requires glucose, oxygen, amino acids
  - glucose facilitated diffusion
  - amino acid active transport
  - oxygen simple diffusion

ETIOLOGY OF IUGR

Group according to substrate handling

- maternal: substrate availability
- placenta: substrate transfer
- fetal: substrate utilization

◆ Substrate Availability—Maternal

Most common cause of IUGR

Least serious
- infants are small, but most do not have increased mortality or long-term morbidity

Maternal nutrition
- chronic maternal disease

Hypoxemic state
- asthma
- cardiac disease

Malabsorption syndrome
- inflammatory bowel disease

Drug and alcohol use—smoking

◆ Substrate Transfer—Placenta

Poor uterine blood flow
- maternal vascular disease

Reduced placental surface area
- maternal hypertension

◆ Substrate Utilization—Fetus

Major congenital anomalies
- trisomy 13, 18

Cardiovascular anomalies

Congenital infections—TORCH group

DIAGNOSIS

✧ *Clinical examination*
Measurement of uterine fundal height, plot on graph
Accuracy of 75% in diagnosis of IUGR

✧ *Ultrasound*
Measurement of BPD only, not very helpful because of CNS sparing effects
- measurement of abdomen

Amniotic fluid volume may be also helpful

✧ *Biochemical*
Increased MSAFP in early pregnancy
- placental disruption

Decreased estriol, hPL, SP_1 protein is in maternal circulation (urine)

✧ *Doppler flow*
Abnormal systolic-diastolic ratio (>3.0) suggests increased placental vascular resistance
Ultrasound may be more accurate

◆ Asymmetric IUGR

Short duration of abnormal growth

CNS sparing
- abdomen and liver fail to grow appropriately

◆ Symmetric IUGR

Prolonged IUGR—usually more severe
Can be related to intrinsic fetal defects
- chromosomal abnormality
- congenital infections

COMPLICATIONS

Most are infant-related

◆ Fetal Stress/Distress

30% positive OCT
50% hypoxia or acidosis in labor
Oligohydramnios associated with fetal heart rate abnormalities
  in labor
- also increased risk of in utero demise

◆ Neonatal Problems

Meconium aspiration
Compensatory polycythemia
Hyperviscocity syndrome
- thrombosis
- heart failure
Hyperbilirubinemia
Hypoglycemia
Anomalies
Perinatal mortality six to eight times higher
Long-term development
- physically small during first 10 years
- possible defects in neurologic development

MANAGEMENT

Five general principles
- early detection
- elimination of contributing factors
- increase uterine blood flow
- serial fetal surveillance
- early delivery in perinatal center

◆ Early Detection

Preexisting disease (vasculopathy, hypertension)
Poor nutrition, smoking

◆ Contributing Factors

Diet
- 1000 calories intake per day required
- no proven need for prenatal vitamins in presence of adequate diet

Habits
- smoking
- alcohol consumption
- substance abuse program

◆ Uterine Blood Flow

Reduce maternal activity
Bedrest in left lateral decubitous
Good hydration

◆ Fetal Surveillance

Fetal karyotype and TORCH titers in symmetric IUGR
Begin surveillance at time of detection
- may be as early as 26 weeks

Antenatal FHR monitoring for hypoxia detection
- weekly NST
- consider OCT if nonreactive

Weekly AFI for oligohydramnios detection
- four quadrant assessment (normal greater than six)

Serial ultrasound for growth

◆ Early Delivery

In absence of abnormal testing, optimal delivery around 38 weeks
- in cases with mature L/S delivery indicated for
  - positive OCT
  - loss of amniotic fluid (oligohydramnios)
  - ultrasound documentation of growth failure of head

Monitoring during labor is essential
- elevation of baseline FHR can represent acidosis
  - prompt delivery may be necessary
  - attempt in utero fetal resuscitation
    - oxygen
    - fluid bolus
    - maternal left side position
    - tocolytics

Newborn care
- management of meconium
- appropriate resuscitation
- blood glucose monitoring
  - less than 40 mg/dL requires parenteral glucose

Long-term follow-up

19

◆ Postdate Pregnancy

INTRODUCTION

Defined as a pregnancy of 42 or more weeks gestation
Incidence of 3% to 12%

DATING THE PREGNANCY

Only ovulation detection can accurately date pregnancies
Mean gestation 280 days from last menstrual period (LMP)
- Naegele's rule: subtract 3 months from LMP, add 7 days to give expected date of confinement (EDC)

Precise dating requires physical examination, menstrual history, and other parameters
Ultrasound
- accuracy decreases as pregnancy advances

CAUSES

Most frequent causes is inaccurate dating of the pregnancy
Rarer causes
- fetal anecephaly
- placental sufatase deficiency

Mechanism
- unknown
- lack of cervical prostaglandin production
- refractoriness of cervix to prostaglandins

MATERNAL PROBLEMS

Emotional stress
Inconvenience of increased need for medical care
Potential for delivery trauma

INFANT PROBLEMS

Much more serious than those for the mother

◆ Oligohydramnios

Increased incidence of cord accidents
Abnormalities of fetal heart rate in labor
Thick, undiluted meconium

◆ Macrosomia

Birth trauma, obstructive labor
Diagnosis difficult, ultrasound accurate to ± 10%

◆ Meconium aspiration

25% incidence
Usually thicker in postdate pregnancies with oligohydramnios

◆ Placental insufficiency

Placental function normally peaks at 37 weeks
Fetal compromise can occur

MANAGEMENT

◆ Weekly Vaginal Examinations

Plan induction when cervix is favorable (3+ cm dilated)
Use of prostaglandin gel may assist in converting a cervix from
   unfavorable to favorable

◆ Weekly Real-Time Ultrasound Scans

Gradual reduction of amniotic fluid is normal
• maximum volume at 37 to 38 weeks
• decreases slowly
• AFI (four quadrant assessment) are useful
• greater than 6 cm is normal
• oligohydramnios may be treated in labor with amnioinfusion
   of saline (Fig. 19-1)

✧ *Antepartum fetal heart rate monitoring*

Nonstress test weekly
• simpler and fairly sensitive
• if nonreactive, perform contraction stress test

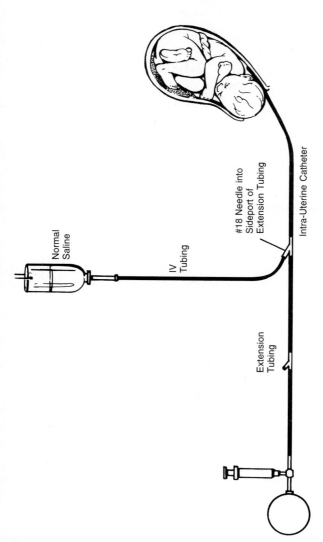

Normal Saline

IV Tubing

#18 Needle into Sideport of Extension Tubing

Intra-Uterine Catheter

Extension Tubing

Figure 19-1. Amniotic infusion setup.

DELIVERY

◆ Labor Dysfunction—Shoulder Dystocia

Consider elective cesarean section if estimated fetal weight is greater than 5000 g

Obstructed labor should alert physician to possible macrosomia

Management requires prompt physician intervention

◆ Meconium Aspiration

Amnioinfusion may help to dilute thick meconium
- prevention of fetal hypoxia in labor may reduce inutero gasping, which pulls the meconium deep into the lungs and damages tissue

Use of DeLee suction trap on the perineum after the delivery of the head will not eliminate all problems

Intubation of neonate with tracheal aspiration of meconium

◆ Fetal Distress

Greatly increased in postdate pregnancies

Emergency cesarean section sometimes required
- faster is better
- in utero resuscitation should be attempted while preparing for surgery
- patient placed on left side
- IV hydration
- arrest of uterine activity (0.25 mg terbutaline, subcutaneously)
- oxygen

20

◆ Multiple Pregnancies

TWIN GESTATION

INTRODUCTION

Represent a high-risk pregnancy
- 1% of all births
  - 12% of all perinatal mortality
    - fetal mortality rate increased fourfold
    - neonatal mortality rate increased sixfold
    - perinatal mortality rate increased tenfold
- <2500 g twin infants have better survival rate than single-tons of the same weight
- >2500 g twins infants have more complications than single-ton of the same weight

ETIOLOGY AND EPIDEMIOLOGY

Monozygotic
- chance occurrence
- 3 to 4/1000
- increased slightly with delayed implantation

Dizygotic
- frequency varies throughout the world
- heredity is important on mother's side
- race-specific rates
  - 7 to 10/1000 in Caucasians
  - 10 to 40/1000 in Africans
  - 3/1000 in Asians
- increased in women greater than 35 years-of-age and in obese women
- fertility drug use associated with dizygotic twinning
  - Clomid 10%
  - Pergonal 30% to 50%

PLACENTATION

Dizygotic—two individual placental units
Monozygotic dependent on timing of division (Fig. 20-1)
- <3 days → diamniotic, dichorionic
- 3 to 8 days → diamniotic, monochorionic
- 8 to 13 days → monochorionic
- >13 days → conjoined twins

Diagnosis
- clinical examination (misses one third of all twins)
  - uterine size greater than dates
  - two fetuses palpated
  - two heart rates auscultated

Biochemical
- increased MSAFP, hCG, hPL, estriol

Biophysical assessment
- ultrasound
- can sometimes underestimate number of fetuses

MATERNAL COMPLICATIONS

◆ Physiologic Changes

Greater increase in blood volume, pulse, cardiac output, and weight gain (40 to 44 pounds)
Increased rate of antepartum, intrapartum, postpartum complications (Table 20-1)

INFANT COMPLICATIONS

◆ Prematurity

Average age of delivery, 37 weeks
Lung maturity often by 31 to 32 weeks

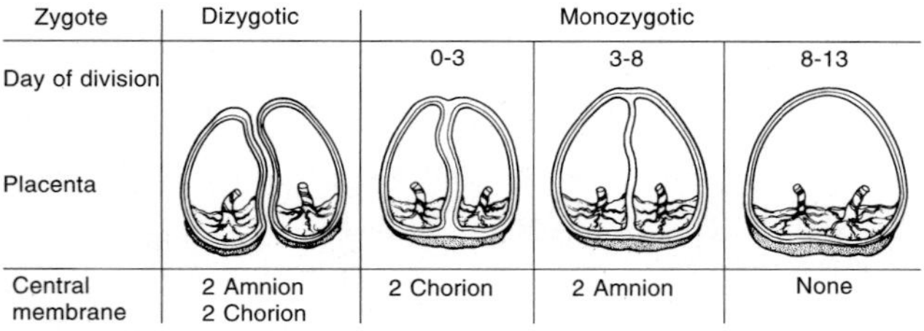

Zygote	Dizygotic	Monozygotic		
Day of division		0-3	3-8	8-13
Placenta				
Central membrane	2 Amnion 2 Chorion	2 Chorion	2 Amnion	None

Figure 20-1. Types of placentation in monozygotic and dizygotic twinning.

TABLE 20-1. Maternal Complications With Twin
            Pregnancies

Problems	Increased Likelihood Over Singleton Pregnancy
Preterm labor	7-10
Hypertension	2-5
Abruption	3
Anemia	2-3
Hydramnios	3-5
Urinary tract infection	1.4
Postpartum hemorrhage	2-4
Cesarean section	2-3

◆ Discordance

Defined as a difference of greater than 20% to 25% in weight
Occurs in 10% of all twins
Etiology
- differences in placental surface area
- twin-twin transfusion syndrome
  - 85% of monochorionic placentas have vascular anastomosis
    - donor twin
      - small
      - pale
      - anemic
      - oligohydramnios
      - neonatal heart failure
    - recipient
      - large
      - plethoric
      - polycythemia
      - polyhydramnios
      - neonatal heart failure, hyperbilirubinemia
Diagnosis
- antepartum difference in BPD of greater than 5 mm or in estimated weight of greater than 25%
- acute polyhydramnios in twin-twin transfusion syndrome
  - poor prognostic sign
  - some benefit in performing repeated therapeutic amniocen-
    tesis

◆ Vanishing Twin

50% of all twin pregnancies in first trimester end up as single-
ton birth
- most show empty gestational sac on early ultrasound
Remnant is whitish plaque on membranes
- no harm to the surviving infant in cases of early loss

◆ Monoamniotic Twin Pregnancy

Result from monozygotic division between day 8 and 13
High-risk pregnancy
- cord entanglement and fetal depth usually before 32 weeks (Fig. 20-2)
  - consider expectant management after 32 weeks as risk decreases significantly

◆ Dead Fetus Syndrome

2% to 7% of twin pregnancies result in fetal death of one twin after 20 weeks
Maternal hypofibrinogenemia (less than 150 mg/mL) rarely occurs
Fetal complications
- dichorionic placenta
  - low risk
- monochorionic placenta
  - high risk for surviving twin
    - acute DIC
    - renal, CNS cysts
      - multicystic encephalomalacia
    - 25% die in utero
      - 50% of survivors have brain damage
  - immediate delivery if viable gestational age at time of fetal demise

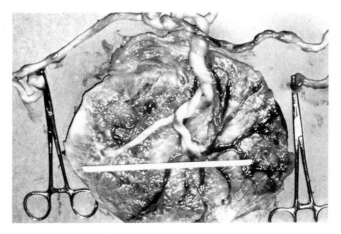

Figure 20-2. In monozygotic twins with no central membrane, cord entanglement can occur with fetal movement, leading to obstruction of blood flow and possible death of the fetuses.

◆ Rare Complications

Locking twins (1/90,000)

Combined pregnancy (heterotopic) pregnancy 1/30,000 pregnancies (intrauterine and ectopic)

Molar pregnancy and fetus

Delayed delivery

- delays of 21 to 143 days reported
- may allow second fetus time to reach viability

MANAGEMENT

◆ Antepartum

Prevention of recognized problems

- preterm labor surveillance
  - regular vaginal examinations
  - bed rest has been advocated after 24 weeks
  - prophylactic tocolytics of no proven value
  - home uterine monitoring
    - may be useful in twin pregnancies compared with singletons
- maternal nutrition
  - anemia more common
  - require 1 mg of folic acid, 60 mg of elemental iron daily
- fetal health
  - determination of type of placentation useful
    - risk for twin-twin transfusion syndrome with monochorionic placentas
  - surveillance for appropriate growth by ultrasound
- prenatal counseling
  - higher risk of congenital anomalies in twins
  - higher risk of chromosomal abnormalities in twins
    - screening recommended at 33 years-of-age for mother if a twin gestation compared with 35 years-of-age for a singleton
    - amniocentesis must check both sacs
      - use glucometer and glucose infusion into fluid to identify each sac
      - avoid the use of dyes
- antenatal fetal testing
  - weekly nonstress test
  - especially in pregnancies complicated by hypertension or other problems

◆ Intrapartum

Delivery

- monitor both fetuses
- after delivery of first twin no optimal interval to delivery of second twin if monitored
- risk of abruption after delivery of first twin

- always be prepared for emergency cesarean section
  - vertex/breech presentation
    - second twin either deliver as breech extraction or perform external cephalic version
- overall cesarean section rate for twins is 50%

◆ Postpartum

Increased risk for atony and hemorrhage
Postpartum depression more common
- assure adequate social support

TRIPLETS

Increasing frequency because of ART
Few large series in literature
- average weight gain 45 to 50 pounds
- usual spontaneous time for delivery is 32 to 34 weeks
  - average weight 1800 to 1900 g
- growth slows after 27 weeks
- 30% rate of growth discordance (10% in twins)
Perinatal mortality similar to twins
Most delivered by cesarean section

QUADRUPLETS OR MORE

Most are a result of ART
Average weight gain 50 to 55 pounds
High risk of preterm labor
- average gestational age of delivery 30 to 31 weeks
- average weight 1200 g to 1500 g
Multifetal reduction has been shown to improve perinatal survival rate

21

◆ Diabetes Mellitus and Pregnancy

CARBOHYDRATE METABOLISM DURING NORMAL PREGNANCY

Blood glucose levels change in pregnancy
- lower fasting
- prolonged elevation of postprandial values
  - probably related to delayed gastric emptying
- pregnancy is an insulin-resistant state

SCREENING FOR DIABETES DURING PREGNANCY

High-risk patient
- screen at the first visit
All patients
- screen by end of second trimester (26 weeks)

◆ Screening Examination

50 g oral glucose load
Plasma glucose checked 1 hour later
Less than 140 mg/dL → normal
Greater than 140 mg/dL → perform oral glucose tolerance test (GTT)
Greater than 200 mg/dL → probably does not need GGT; check fasting glucose first

◆ Glucose Tolerance Test

Begin after 3 days of good diet (250 calories of carbohydrate daily)
- fast for 10 hours prior to test
- 100 g oral glucose solution
- perform blood level tests at fasting 1, 2, and 3 hours after drinking solution
Follow-up
- two or more abnormal values, define gestational diabetes (Table 21-1)
- one abnormal value, repeat GTT in 1 month

TABLE 21-1. Pregnancy Oral Glucose Tolerance Test Using a 100-g Load

Sample	Fasting	1 h	2 h	3 h

Sample	Upper Limits for Normal Glucose Levels (mg/dL)			
	Fasting	1 h	2 h	3 h
Blood	90	165	145	125
Plasma	105	190	165	145

GESTATIONAL DIABETES

Major risk is macrosomic fetus
May manage with diet alone in many cases
• insulin required for elevated fasting levels
Antenatal surveillance with nonstress test after 39 weeks in patient with good control
Postpartum follow-up required to rule out adult onset diabetes

INSULIN-DEPENDENT DIABETES

◆ Maternal problems

✧ *Hypoglycemia*
Usually occurs in first half of pregnancy
Need to adjust insulin dose based on caloric intake

✧ *Hyperglycemia*
Tends to occur in second half of pregnancy
Major increase in insulin is often required between 20 and 30 weeks
• increasing insulin resistance occurs during this period
Sudden drop in insulin requirement may reflect decreasing placental function

✧ *Urinary tract and other infections*
Pregnancy predisposes to urinary tract colonization
Obtain urine cultures at first visit and at 32 weeks or if symptoms develop
Diabetics are at higher risk than other pregnant patients for infectious complications (e.g. wound infection after cesarean)

✧ *Hypertension*
Diabetic women are at higher risk for hypertensive disorders of pregnancy

✧ *Hydramnios*
May occur in 10% to 20% of diabetic pregnancies, especially in poorly controlled patients
Probably result of fetal polyuria resulting from fetal glucosuria

◇ *Retinopathy*
15% of women experience exacerbation of retinopathy
85% of women with proliferative retinopathy experience progression
Close observation and possible laser therapy indicated
Perform opthamologic examination in each trimester

◆ Infant Problems

◇ *Abortion*
Frequency of spontaneous abortion not increased except in patients with poor control

◇ *Congenital anomalies*
Threefold increase overall in anomaly rate
Elevated hemoglobin A_{1c} levels predict anomalies
Preconceptional control is important
Unique diabetic anomaly: sacral agenesis

◇ *Respiratory distress*
Increased fivefold to sixfold for all gestational ages
Related to lung type II pneumocytes production of surfactant
Inverse relationship between amniotic fluid L/S ratios and maternal glucose levels

◇ *Neonatal hypoglycemia*
Common in infant of diabetic mother (IDM)
Monitor infant closely after delivery

◇ *Macrosomia*
Usually defined as infants greater than 4000 or 4500 g
Higher incidence of birth trauma

◇ *Hypocalcemia*
Can present frequently

◇ *Hyperbilirubinemia*
More common in IDM
Often related to increased hematocrit in utero

◇ *Perinatal mortality*
Sudden death often related to hyperglycemia
50% fetal mortality in cases of maternal diabetic ketoacidosis

MANAGEMENT

◆ Glucose Control

◇ *Diet*
35 calories/kg of ideal body weight recommended
- 1.3 g of protein
- 250 g of carbohydrates
Constant dietary intake most important factor in glucose control

✧ *Insulin dose*
First half of gestation: 0.5 units/kg
Second half of gestation: 0.7 units/kg
Split injections may be necessary
- two thirds dose in the morning
  - two thirds NPH, one third regular
- one third dose in the evening
  - one half NPH, one half regular
Inject 30 minutes prior to meals
Dosing in labor is best done with IV insulin drip (begin at one unit per hour)

✧ *Glucose levels*
Home blood glucose monitoring
Maternal glucose values are best index of control
Daily determination required
- fasting (70 to 80 mg/dL target range)
- one hour postprandial (<120 mg/dL target)
- bedtime

✧ *24-hour urine glucose*
Substantial glucosuria indicates poor control
Good guide on blood glucose testing methods (timing, accuracy)

✧ *Hemoglobin A_{1C}*
Reflects glucose control during previous 4 to 5 weeks
Should be monitored monthly during pregnancy

✧ *Amniotic fluid glucose*
Reflects previous 7 days of maternal glucose control
Higher glucose levels have been associated with neonatal depression

✧ *Fetal monitoring*
Antenatal fetal testing most widely used method
NST less sensitive than CST
Biophysical profile data are limited

◆ **Early Delivery**

✧ *Fetal maturity testing*
Lung maturity better documented by PG levels than by L/S ratio
Usually perform amniocentesis 37 to 38 weeks

✧ *Delivery*
Evaluate for macrosomia
Consider elective cesarean delivery if estimated fetal weight is greater than 4500 g
Induction recommended unless obstetric contraindication exists
Delivery should be performed at perinatal center if possible

◆ Postpartum Family Planning

Usually recommend barrier contraception
IUD may also be a good choice in carefully selected patients
Low-dose oral contraceptives may be used but require close surveillance of glycemic control

22

◆ Hypertensive Disorders of Pregnancy

INTRODUCTION

The term "preeclampsia" has replaced the term "toxemia"
Complicates 5% of all pregnancies
20% of nulliparous pregnancies
40% of women with chronic renal disease
Delay of diagnosis and uncertainty of treatment can lead to significant maternal and fetal morbidity and mortality

DIAGNOSIS

Clinical classifications proposed by ACOG
I. Preeclampsia and eclampsia
II. Chronic hypertension of any etiology preceding pregnancy
III. Chronic hypertension with superimposed preeclampsia or eclampsia
IV. Transient hypertension

HYPERTENSION

Defined as blood pressure of at least 140/90 mm Hg or a rise of 30 mm Hg systolic or 15 mm Hg diastolic
Blood pressure usually falls during second trimester
Should use Korotkoff phase V sound
• disappearance of ausculated sound

PREECLAMPSIA

Syndrome of pregnancy-induced hypertension accompanied by proteinuria, edema, and frequently other organ system disturbances
Proteinuria defined as 300 mg of protein over 24 hours
• highly variable and mainly a late symptom

TABLE 22-1. Criteria for Severe Preeclampsia

Blood pressure consistently >160 mm Hg systolic or >110 mm Hg diastolic
New onset of proteinuria >2 g in a 24-h urine collection or >3 + in a randomly collected specimen
Oliguria (<400 mL in 24 h) or increasing serum creatinine levels
Platelet count <100,000/μL, hemolytic anemia, or increase in lactic acid dehydrogenase and direct bilirubin levels
Headache, visual disturbances, or other cerebral signs
Epigastric or right upper quadrant pain
Cardiac decompensation, pulmonary edema, or cyanosis
Fetal growth retardation

Edema usually considered pathologic only if generalized and includes hands, face, and legs
Can range from mild to severe including the HELLP variant (Table 22-1)
- hemolysis (H)
- elevated liver enzymes (EL)
- low platelet count (LP)

ECLAMPSIA

Severe form of preeclampsia with seizure or coma
Convulsions usually preceded by headaches, epigastric pain, hyperreflexia, hemoconcentration
Can occur before labor in 50%, during labor in 25%, and early postpartum in 25%
Late postpartum eclampsia is a controversial entity

CHRONIC HYPERTENSION

Hypertension that antedates pregnancy appears before 20 weeks or presents after delivery
Clinical findings suggestive of chronic hypertension (Table 22-2)
High risk to develop superimposed preeclampsia

TABLE 22-2. Clinical Findings Suggestive of Chronic Hypertension

Multiparity with a history of hypertensive pregnancies
Retinal hemorrhages or exudates
Blood urea nitrogen concentration >20 mg/dL or serum creatinine >1 mg/dL
Radiographic or electrocardiographic evidence of cardiac enlargement
Presence of diabetes mellitus, renal disease, autoimmune or collagen vascular disease, or other predisposing disorders

TRANSIENT HYPERTENSION

No other signs of preeclampsia
Blood pressure normalizes postpartum
May recur in subsequent pregnancies

CAUSES AND PATHOPHYSIOLOGY

Described in 1916 as a "disease of theories"; still true today
• certain predisposing risk factors are recognized (Table 22-3)

IMMUNOGENETIC FACTORS

Exposure to fetal antigens not necessary
• can occur in molar gestation
May be linked to a recessive immune response gene linked to HLA
In general, no solid evidence exists regarding immunogenetic causes

VASCULAR REACTIVITY

Underlying abnormality is a general alteration in increased vascular sensitivity to pressor hormones and eicosanoids
May be the result of prostacyclin, thromboxane imbalance (Fig. 22-1)
Increased pressor response to angiotensin

ORGAN DYSFUNCTION

◆ Renal Problems

Distinct renal lesion associated with preeclampsia
• glomerular capillary endotheliosis
Also associated with decrease glomerular filtration rate and renal plasma flow

---

TABLE 22-3. Risk Factors for Preeclampsia

Primigravid status
Family history of preeclampsia or eclampsia
Previous preeclampsia or eclampsia
New paternity
Extremes of maternal age (younger than 20 y or older than 35 y of age)
Preexisting hypertensive vascular, autoimmune, or renal disease
Diabetes mellitus
Multiple gestation
Nonimmune or alloimmune fetal hydrops
Trisomy 13
Hydatidiform mole

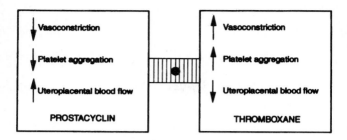

NORMAL PREGNANCY

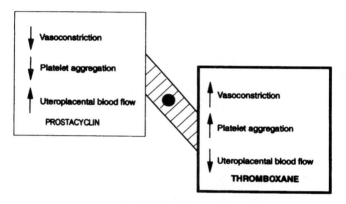

PREECLAMPSIA

Figure 22-1. Physiologic balance of prostacyclin and thromboxane in normal pregnancy and the proposed imbalance resulting in thromboxane dominance in preeclampsia.

◆ Hepatic Problems

Most common and prominent in women with HELLP syndrome
Often presents with atypical clinical picture (Table 22-4)

◆ Placental Problems

Reduction of intervillous perfusion
• main cause of prenatal morbidity and mortality
Increased risk of abruption as well as IUGR

TABLE 22-4. Clinical Features of Six Pregnant Women With HELLP Syndrome*					
RUQ Pain and N&V†	AST (mg/dL)	Bilirubin (mg/dL)	Blood Pressure (mm Hg)	Proteinuria (dipstick)†	Platelets/µL
++++	600	4.6	170/100	++	42,000
++++	240	1.7	150/98	+	15,000
++++	276	2.7	160/100	+	75,000
+++	975	8.3	140/100	+++	27,000
++	428	3.5	140/90	+++	30,000
++++	1450	1.3	190/95	+	29,000

* Women were originally hospitalized for suspected hepatobiliary disease. Diagnoses by various consultants included cholecystitis, hepatitis, pancreatitis, gastroenteritis, appendicitis, and perforated ulcer.
† Pluses indicate severity of symptoms for least (+) to greatest(++++).
AST, aspartate aminotransferase (formerly SGOT); N&V, nausea and vomiting; RUQ, right upper quadrant.

◆ Cardiac and Pulmonary Problems

Hemoconcentration common

Heart failure can occur

Pulmonary edema is more often a complication of the treatment of severe preeclamsia

- only accepted indication (along with CHF) for diuretic therapy in pregnancy

◆ Hematologic Problems

Associated with vasoconstriction and activation of coagulation system

Reduction of platelet count is most common coagulation abnormality; hypofibrogenemia also may occur

◆ Cerebral Problems

Represents a form of hypertensive encephalopathy

Eclamptic women demonstrate white matter hypodensities in up to 50%

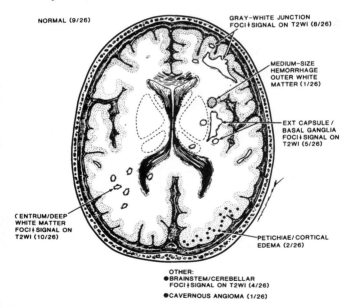

Figure 22-2. Compilation of observed magnetic resonance imaging findings in 26 patients with severe preeclampsia or eclampsia. (Digre KB, Varner MW, Osborn AG, Crawford S. Cranial magnetic resonance imaging in severe pre-eclampsia versus eclampsia. Arch Neurol 1993; 50:399.)

MRI may be more sensitive (Fig. 22-2)
Numerous clinical tests have been proposed but none has proven
  clinically useful

PREVENTION

◆ Aspirin

Binds irreversibly with cyclooxygenase enzymes
- inhibits TxA_2 synthesis
- effects are dose dependent

Low-dose therapy is effective in reducing the risk of preeclampsia
  (Fig. 22-3)
- adverse effects can occur

Limit use to high-risk population
- chronic hypertension
- autoimmune disorders
- anticardiolipin antibody
- multiple gestation
- renal disease
- history of recurring preeclampsia
- transplant recipients

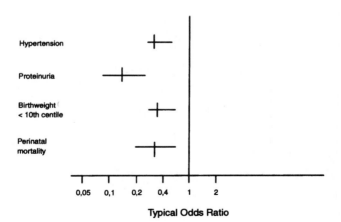

Figure 22-3. Graphic overview of odds ratios and 95% confidence intervals of the effects of low-dose aspirin on the occurrence of hypertension, preeclampsia, and fetal-neonatal sequelae from six randomized, controlled, clinical trials.24-29 In patients at risk, all odds ratios are less than 1 in those who received low-dose aspirin. (Bremer HA, Wallenburg HCS. Aspirin in pregnancy. Fetal Matern Med Rev 1992; 4:37.)

◆ Calcium

Role of calcium in prevention still needs to be addressed

MANAGEMENT

◆ Preeclampsia

Encountered by all obstetricians
Most effective therapy is delivery
Patient remote from term represents a treatment dilemma (Table 22-5)

◆ Mild Preeclampsia

Initial management consists of rest and observation if patient is not a candidate for delivery
• bedrest maximizes uteroplacental flow
If admission is necessary consider close observation as detailed (Table 22-6)
Delivery should be accomplished by 38th week or sooner if cervix is favorable and fetus is mature

TABLE 22-5. Management of Hypertension Complicating Pregnancy

Clinical Condition	Therapy
Preeclampsia or chronic hypertension when the fetus is mature	*Definitive* Prevent convulsions Control blood pressure Deliver fetus
Preeclampsia or chronic hypertension when the fetus is premature, but there is severe preeclampsia or superimposed preeclampsia, fetal growth retardation, or fetal distress	*Definitive* Prevent convulsions Control blood pressure Deliver fetus
Eclampsia, whether the fetus is mature or premature	*Definitive* Treat convulsions Control blood pressure Stabilize mother Deliver fetus
Preeclampsia or chronic hypertension when the fetus is preterm	*Expectant* Ambulatory treatment Hospitalization
Hypertension in the first 20 weeks of gestation	Depends on severity of hypertension

◆ Severe Preeclampsia

Delivery is always the appropriate maternal therapy
Fetal risk must be balanced against maternal risk
- consider conservative management between 25 to 30 weeks
- delivery indicated for severe preeclampsia, IUGR, or fetal distress

◆ Treating Hypertension

Treat for greater than 160/110 mm Hg
Goal is to lower diastolic to 90 to 100 mm Hg
Drug therapy
- hydralazine 5 mg IV, then 5 to 10 mg q 20 minutes
- labetalol 20 to 50 mg IV
Carefully monitor urine output

◆ Preventing Convulsions

Drug of choice is magnesium sulfate
Treat all preeclamptic patients during labor and 24 hours postpartum

◇ *Dosing*

4 g IV load then 2 to 3 g/hour
- keep serum magnesium 4 to 8 mg/dL
IM dosing more painful
- 10 g load IM
- 5 g IM q 4 hours

**TABLE 22-6. Serial Examinations Recommended for
Preeclamptic Hospitalized Patients***

Mother
Blood pressure (four times daily)
Assessment for proteinuria, edema, weight, hyperreflexia, headache, visual disturbance, epigastric pain (daily)
Hematocrit, platelet count (every 2 d)
Serum uric acid and creatinine levels, 24-h urine for total protein and creatinine clearance (twice weelky)
Liver function tests† (weekly)

Fetus
Fetal movement record (daily)
Nonstress test ‡ (twice weekly)
Ultrasound for fetal growth (every 2 wk)

* Recommendations are for hospitalized patients from time of diagnosis to delivery. Frequency of evaluations can be increased or decreased, depending on severity of disease.
† Serum aspartate aminotransferase (formerly SGOT), lactic dehydrogenase, serum bilirubin.
‡ Biophysical profile if nonstress test is nonreactive

TABLE 22-7. Protocol for Treating Eclampsia

1. Turn patient on her side
2. Establish airway and administer oxygen
3. Administer 4-6 g of magnesium sulfate intravenously over 10-15 min, followed by a 2g/h maintenance dose; adjusted dosage later based on patellar reflexes, urine outupt, and serum magnesium levels
4. Obtain arterial blood gas measurement and chest x-ray film
5. If convulsions are controlled and maternal condition is stable, initiate induction or delivery within 3 to 6 h
6. Continue to administer magnesium sulfate for at least 24h after delivery or last convulsion
7. Obtain computed tomographic scan or magnetic resonance imaging if seizures are atypical or coma is prolonged

---

✧ *Toxicity*

Loss of patellar reflexes 8 to 10 mg/dL
Respiratory depression 10 to 15 mg/dL
Defective cardiac conduction >15 mg/dL
Treatment of toxicity
• calcium gluconate 1 g IV over 3 minutes

◆ **Delivery**

Vaginal delivery preferred
Aggressive induction appropriate with clear endpoint (usually 8 to 12 hours from commencement)

◆ **Eclampsia**

Incidence of 0.2%
Protocol for management as noted in Table 22-7
CNS imaging is not necessary in patients with typical presentation of preeclampsia
Maternal stabilization should be obtained prior to induction or cesarean section

◆ **Chronic Hypertension**

Follow closely for worsening blood pressure, worsening renal status
Limit sodium intake
Serial laboratory measurements
• hematocrit, creatinine, uric acid, creatinine clearance, 24-hour urine collection for protein
  • elevation of uric acid greater than 6 mg/dL often early sign of superimposed preeclampsia
Antihypertensive therapy
• aldomet is drug of choice but other drugs can be considered (Table 22-8)
Fetal surveillance is appropriate

◆ Prognosis

Typically resolves following delivery

Discharge usually safe with blood pressure less than 160/100 mm Hg

Oral contraceptive acceptable but wait until blood pressure normalizes

Recurrence rates

- mild disease in primigravidas: rare
- severe preeclampsia: 30% to 50%
- superimposed preeclampsia: 70%

TABLE 22-8. Antihypertensive Therapy for Chronic Hypertension in Pregnant Patients

α_2-Adrenergic Receptor Agonists

Methyldopa is the antihypertensive drug used most extensively during pregnancy. The dosage is 250-500 mg every 6 h. Its safety and efficacy are supported by randomized trials and a 7.5-y follow-up of children born to treated mothers.

α_2-Adrenergic Receptor Agonists and β-Adrenergic Receptor Antagonists

Labetalol appears to be as effective as methyldopa, but no follow-up studies of children born to mothers given labetalol have been conducted, and there is concern about maternal hepatotoxicity.

β-Adrenergic Receptor Agonists

These drugs, especially atenolol and metoprolol, appear to be safe and efficacious in late pregnancy, bet fetal bradycardia can occur. Fetal growth retardation has been reported when treatment was started in early gestation or midgestation.

Angiotensin-Converting Enzyme Inhibitors

Captopril and several converting enzyme inhibitors have been associated with oligohydramnios and neonatal renal failure,[49,50]. They should not be used in pregnancy.

Diuretics

Diuretic therapy begun before conception usually is continued during pregnancy.

Peripheral Vasodilators

Hydralazine commonly is used as adjuvant therapy with methyldopa and β-adrenergic receptor antagonists. Trials with calcium-channel blockers look promising. The experience with minoxidil is limited, and this drug is not recommended.

23

◆ Cardiovascular, Pulmonary, Renal and Hematologic Diseases in Pregnancy

CARDIOVASCULAR DISEASE

◆ Congenital Heart Disease

✧ Left-to-right shunts (uncorrected)

✳ *Atrial septal defect*
Most common congenital lesion seen in pregnancy
Majority of patients tolerate pregnancy well
Major risk
- shunt reversal secondary to systemic hypotension
- obstetrical hemorrhage
- sympathetic blockade
Bacterial endocarditis prophylaxis required

✳ *Ventricular septal defect*
Most patients do well in pregnancy (CHF in 8%)
Bacterial endocarditis prophylaxis required
Major risk
- shunt reversal after delivery

✳ *Patent ductus arteriosus*
Most patients tolerate pregnancy well
Failure can develop
- medical management
- surgical closure in absence of pulmonary hypertension
Antibiotic prophylaxis is necessary
Shunt reversal is major risk

✧ Right-to-left shunts (cyanotic heart disease)

✳ *Tetralogy of fallot*
Most common congenital cyanotic heart disease
- pulmonic stenosis
- VSD
- dextroposition of the aorta (overriding)
- right ventricular hypertrophy
Most patients undergo correction
Partial correction can be performed
- Blalock-Taussig shunt

- Potts repair
- Waterston-Cooley shunt

Pregnancy increases right-to-left shunting
Maternal mortality 5% to 10% in uncorrected lesions
Systemic hypotension is very dangerous
IUGR can occur in presence of cyanotic disease

✳ *Eisenmenger syndrome*
Any right-to-left shunt associated with pulmonary hypertension
Pregnancy is extremely hazardous
- maternal mortality 30% to 50%
- pregnancy worsens right-to-left shunting

Early termination of pregnancy should be offered and sterilization considered
Later termination has same risk as term delivery
Pregnancy management
- hospitalization at 20 weeks
- strict bed rest
- continuous oxygen
- management of congestive heart failure
- antenatal surveillance
- induction with favorable cervix or spontaneous labor is preferable
- Swan-Ganz catheter placement in labor

Avoid cesarean (75% mortality rate)
Avoid Valsalva maneuver
Antibiotic prophylaxis

◇ **Other congenital conditions**

✳ *Coarctation of the aorta*
Usually corrected in childhood
Mortality 3.5% in uncorrected patients
- aortic rupture or dissection
- CVA
- CHF
- bacterial endocarditis

Management
- limitation of activity
- control of hypertension
- repair only for dissection, uncontrollable hypertension
- avoid Valsalva in labor

Perinatal mortality 25%
Fetal surveillance important

✳ *Isolated pulmonic stenosis*
Most patients tolerate pregnancy well
Major risk is right-sided heart failure (5% to 10%)
- usually responds to medical therapy

◇ **Rheumatic heart disease**

✳ *Mitral stenosis*
Rheumatic heart disease in women usually involves mitral valve

90% of RHD seen in pregnancy
Overall mortality is 1%
Higher in more severe cases
Pregnancy aggravates mitral stenosis
- physiologic tachycardia (shortened filling time)
- increased blood volume
- increased cardiac output results in increased left atrial, pulmonary capillary pressure
- decreased serum albumin (risk of pulmonary edema)
- increased incidence of atrial arrhythmias
Early puerperium is dangerous time
Congestive heart failure in 8% of pregnancies
Management
- reduced activity
- atrial fibrillation requires anticoagulation and digitalis treatment
Pulmonary hypertension
- pregnancy is a grave risk (mortality 25%)

✳ *Mitral insufficiency*
Accounts for 6% of cases of RHD in pregnancy
Most patients tolerate pregnancy well
Some risk of atrial fibrillation

✳ *Aortic stenosis*
Seldom encountered (1% of RHD)
Mild cases tolerate pregnancy well
Severe cases can be worrisome
- 17% mortality
Maintain venous return by avoiding hypotension
Antibiotic prophylaxis is recommended

⬦ **Cardiomyopathies**

✳ *Peripartum cardiomyopathy (PPCM)*
Many synonyms
Rare disease (1/1500 to 1/4000 pregnancies)
Three criteria:
1. development of CHF in last month of pregnancy or first 5 months of puerperium
2. lack of any other determining cause
3. lack of any demonstratable evidence of heart disease before last month of pregnancy
Etiology unknown
7% of cases occur after multiple gestation
15% to 30% complicated by preeclampsia
82% begin in first 3 months after delivery
- may present as biventricular failure
- pulmonary embolism 25% to 30%
- arrhythmias (40% with ventricular ectopy, 20% atrial fibrillation)
Prognosis
- dependent on return of heart to normal size

- tends to recur
- oral contraceptives contraindicated

✳ *Hypertrophic cardiomyopathy (IHSS)*
Autosomal dominant disorder
Obstruction of left ventricular outflow tract by muscular hypertrophy
Patients prone to sudden death
Avoid tachycardia
Treatment with ß-blockers may be indicated

✳ *Primary pulmonary hypertension*
Rare disorder
Extremely high mortality (50%)
Pulmonary artery pressures increase because of pulmonary arteriolar fibrosis
Death can occur at any time
First trimester abortion indicated
Hospitalize for bedrest at 20 weeks gestation

✳ *Mitral valve prolapse*
Common disorder (6% to 10% of women)
Midsystolic click and late systolic murmur
Most patients asymptomatic
Antibiotic prophylaxis controversial but most physicians administer antibiotics

✳ *Marfan syndrome*
Autosomal dominant
Maternal mortality 25% to 50%
- aortic root >4 cm is pregnancy contraindication
Restrict activity
ß-blockade to decrease force of myocardial contractions

◆ General Principles

✧ *Bacterial endocarditis prophylaxis*
Regimen 1—Aqueous Pencillin G 2 million units IV or IM, or ampicillin 2 g IV or IM plus Gentamycin 1.5 mg/kg IV or IM
This regimen is given 30 to 60 minutes before delivery and is repeated every 8 hours for 2 additional doses.
Regimen 2—penicillin allergic patients—Vancomycin 1 g IV over 60 minutes plus Gentamycin 1.5 mg/kg IV or IM
This regimen is repeated in 12 hours

◆ Chronic Hypertension

Preexisting hypertension prior to pregnancy
Blood pressure of 140/90mm Hg during first 20 weeks of pregnancy
- pressures may fall in second trimester
- rise in third trimester may be difficult to distinguish from preeclampsia

✧ *Complications*
    IUGR
    Stillbirth
    Abruption
    Fetal distress in labor
    Superimposed preeclampsia (14% to 23%)

✧ *Antepartum care*
    Serial ultrasound for growth
    Baseline renal function studies
    Fetal surveillance
    Drug therapy (blood pressure greater than 105 mm Hg diastolic)
- α-methyldopa 750 mg—2 g/per day
- labetalol 200 mg BID to TID (maximum 2400 mg/day)
- metoprolol and atenolol
- avoid thiazide diuretics and ACE inhibitors

◆ Vascular Disease

✧ *Deep vein thrombosis*
    Clinical diagnosis is not reliable
- 50% of patients with signs have no DVT
- 30% with DVT have no signs

    Diagnosis is best made by impedance plethysmography (IPG) or Doppler ultrasound
    Limited venography also may be useful in third trimester
    Therapy
- anticoagulation
- bedrest with leg elevation (20 cm)
- moist heat
- elastic hose once symptoms subside

✧ *Pulmonary embolism*
    Symptoms: tachycardia, tachypnea, dyspnea
    Most important test is ^{99}Tc perfusion scan coupled with ^{133}Xe ventilation scan
    Matched defects usually the result of other disease processes
    Chest x-ray not very useful
    ABG determinations are nonspecific and insensitive
    EKG may be normal
    Therapy
- anticoagulation
- bedrest (5 to 7 days)
- treat DVT if present
- oxygen therapy is needed

✧ *Anticoagulation in pregnancy*
    Oral agents contraindicated in most cases
    Heparin is anticoagulant of choice
- does not cross placenta

    Initial therapy

- IV heparin for 10 to 14 days
- keep activated PTT 1.5 to 2.0 times pretreatment level
- maintenance dose (Table 23-1)

Labor
- stop with onset of labor
- restart 12 to 24 hours after delivery

✧ *Superficial thrombophlebitis*

Occurs in 1/600 pregnancies, 1/100 women in puerperium

Painful red tender superficial vein

Rule out DVT if any question of diagnosis

Therapy
- bedrest
- limb elevation
- moist heat
- analgesics
- anticoagulation not necessary

✧ *Varicose veins*

Seldom require treatment during pregnancy

Improve or resolve after delivery

Treatment during pregnancy
- 1 hour bedrest every 4 hours
- elevate leg 20 cm
- avoid standing for long periods
- do not sit with crossed legs
- support hose helpful

PULMONARY DISEASE

◆ Asthma

0.4% to 1.3% of all gestations
- effect of pregnancy variable

TABLE 23-1. Anticoagulation With Heparin During Pregnancy

Diagnosis	Acute Event	Duration of Pregnancy	Puerperium
DVT or PE (first 20 wk)	Full dose × 10-14 d	Moderate dose × 3 mo Low dose for duration of pregnancy	Moderate dose × 1-2 wk
DVT or PE (second 20 wk)	Full dose × 10-14 d	Moderate dose for duration of pregnancy	Moderate dose × 1-2 wk
History of DVT or PE		Low dose throughout pregnancy	Low dose × 1-2 wk

DVT, deep vein thrombosis: PE, pulmonary embolism; full dose, heparin intravenously to keep activated partial thromboplastin time at control × 2; moderate dose, 10,000 units subcutaneously b.i.d.; low dose, 5000 units subcutaneously

---

- 80% rate of exacerbations in patients with severe disease
- minimal neonatal effects

Medical management of chronic asthma (same as for nonpregnant state)

- inhaled beta-mimetic (albuterol)
- inhaled cromolyn sodium
- inhaled glucocoritcoids (severe symptoms)
- oral theophylline (many have abandoned this drug)
- oral steroids

Acute attack

- inhaled beta-mimetics (hand-held nebulizer)
- intravenous steroids
- subcutaneous epinephrine/terbutaline
- arterial blood gas
- impending respiratory failure (ICU care needed)
  - pH less than 7.35
  - PO_2 less than 60 mm Hg
  - PCO_2 greater than 35 mm Hg
  - maternal alkalosis (pH greater than 7.6 has adverse fetal effects)

◆ Tuberculosis

Natural history unaffected by pregnancy
Treatment indicated to avoid neonatal exposure
PPD valid throughout pregnancy
Positive test → chest x-ray
At least three morning sputum collections
Treatment

- INH and ethambutol
  - recent PPD converter (within past year)
  - treat after first trimester with INH for one year

Mothers with acute TB

- separate from infant until bacteriologically negative and appropriate neonatal prophylaxis begun

◆ Cystic Fibrosis

More than 140 pregnancies reported
Patients with less severe disease are those who get pregnant
Maternal mortality high but not greater than nonpregnant CF patients
Perinatal mortality 11%
Pregnancy does not seem to affect progression of disease
Cor pulmonale and pulmonary hypertension are contraindications to pregnancy

RENALDISEASE

◆ Urinary Tract Infections

Common medical complication of pregnancy (10% to 15%)
Most common organisms
- *E coli* (75% to 90%)
- *Klebsiella* species (10% to 15%)
- *Proteus* species (5%)
- group B streptococci
  - vaginal culture recommended as well

◆ Asymptomatic Bacteriuria

4% to 10% of all sexually active women
- twice as high in women with sickle trait

✧ *Usual definition*
100,000 organisms/mm3 in asymptomatic patient
- pure culture of gram negative rods with >1000 organisms/mm3 is significant
- >10,000 gram negatives with one other organism is also significant

Increased risk of pyelonephritis
- 25% to 30% if untreated

✧ *Screening*
All pregnant women
Nitrate test on dipstick (low-risk patient)
Culture (high-risk patient)
- history of urinary tract infection
- sickle trait
- diabetes
- chronic renal disease
- hypertension

Perform at initial visit then every 6 to 12 weeks
Clean catch specimen
- 90% accurate
- 4% to 5% infection rate with catheterization

✧ *Treatment*
Ampicillin
Nitrofurantoin
Sulfamethoxazole-trimethoprim
- avoid in first trimester and near term

Repeat culture one week after therapy and every 4 to 6 weeks

◆ Cystitis

Obtain culture before therapy
Pyuria requires >50 leukocytes per high-power fluid on spun specimen

◆ Acute Pyelonephritis

Complicates 1% to 2.5% of pregnancies
Fever, costovertebral angle tenderness, pyuria, and bacteriuria
Frequently associated with preterm labor

✧ *Treatment*

Hospitalization
IV antibiotics
• cefoxitin or first generation cephalosporin 1 to 2 g every six
  hours
Adequate hydration
• 200 mL/hour
Switch to oral antibiotics when afebrile 24 hours
Discharge after 24 hours on oral antibiotics, complete 10 day
  course
Lack of improvement after 48 hours
• change antibiotics based on sensitivities
If no sensitivities available add gentamicin
Still febrile 4 to 5 days later consider perinephric abscess
• renal ultrasound
• IV pyelogram

✧ *Recurrence rate and suppressive therapy*

Recurrence rate 10% to 18%
• reduced to 2.7% with suppression
Similar result with no suppression but close follow-up
Suppressive therapy 100 mg of nitrofurantoin at bedtime
• 1 double strength co-trimoxazole (Septra) at bedtime

◆ Urinary Calculi

Incidence 0.5% to 3.5%
20% to 45% infection rate with stones
• check urine cultures
• consider chronic suppressive therapy
Treatment
• most stones passed spontaneously
• treat with analgesics, hydration, antibiotics as indicated
85% to 90% of stones in pregnancy are radiopaque
Consider evaluation for hyperparathyroidism

◆ Chronic Renal Disease

Risk for development of hypertension (23%)
Natural course of the underlying disease probably not affected
  by pregnancy
Fetal mortality increased in all series
Follow baseline renal functions
Document appropriate fetal growth
Antenatal surveillance is indicated, especially in hypertensive
  patients

◆ Acute Renal Failure

Incidence has been falling as improvements in care have taken place
- fewer septic abortions
- early delivery for preeclampsia

Most cases involve acute tubular necrosis
- 21% bilateral cortical necrosis
- usually related to abruptio placentae

Hemodialysis
- acute and chronic renal failure
- high-risk for preterm labor
  - possible result of decrease in progesterone levels
  - some obstetricians have recommended treatment with 1000 mg progesterone in oil during dialysis

HEMATOLOGIC DISEASE

◆ Red Blood Cell Disorders

✧ *Iron-deficiency anemia*

Anemia refers to hematocrit <30% or hemoglobin <10 g/dL
Complicates 15% to 25% of all pregnancies
- iron-deficient anemia most common (75%)

✳ *Absorption of iron*

Absorbed from duodenum in ferrous state
- 10% of maternal iron absorbed in nonpregnant state
  - 1 to 1.5 mg of iron per day
- 20% absorbed in pregnancy

✳ *Requirements in pregnancy*

1000 mg total requirement
500 mg to increase maternal red blood cell mass
300 mg transported to fetus and placenta
200 mg daily losses
Increased during second half of pregnancy
Supplementation
- important in all pregnant women
- 60 mg of elemental iron
- equivalent to 300 mg ferrous sulfate (Table 23-2)

✳ *Evaluation (Table 23-3)*

RBC indices
Visualization of peripheral smear
Serum iron, ferritin, iron-binding capacity

✳ *Treatment*

Ferrous sulfate 300 mg, BID to TID
Parenteral iron dextran
- deliver by IM IV push or IV infusion
- 0.2 to 0.3% anaphylactic reaction
  - test dose of 0.5 mL, 1 hour prior to treatment

TABLE 23-2. Iron Preparations

Preparations	Elemental Iron Content (%)	Dose Containing 60 mg Elemental Iron
Ferrous (fumarate) Ferostat (Forest) Ferro-Sequels (Lederle)	30	200
Ferrous gluconate Generic Fergon (Winthrop-Breon) Ferralet (Mission)	11	550
Ferrous sulfate Generic Feosol (SmithKline) Iberet (Abbott) Ferro-Gradumet (Abbott)	20	300

TABLE 23-3. Indices of Iron Homeostasis

	Normal Nonpregnant	Normal Pregnant	Iron-Deficiency Anemia in Pregnancy
Hemoglobin (g/dL)	12.5-14.0	11.5-12.5	<10
Hematocrit (%)	37-45	33-38	<30
Mean corpuscular hemoglobin concentration	32-36	32-36	<30
Mean corpuscular volume (cubic microns)	80-100	70-90	
Mean corpuscular hemoglobin (pg/cell)	27-34	23-31	
Serum iron (ug/dL)	50-110	35-100	<30
Unsaturated iron-binding capacity (ug/dL)	250-300	280-400	>400
Transferrin saturation (%)	25-35	16-30	<16
Serum ferritin (ug/L)	75-100	55-70	<10

◇ *Folate-deficiency anemia*
Complicates up to 1% of pregnancies
More common in multiple gestation
Folate found in dietary sources (legumes)

✳ *Daily requirements of folate*
Nonpregnant 50 to 100µg
Pregnancy 150 to 400 µg

✳ *Diagnosis*
Fasting folate less than 3 mg/mL
Anemic patient with macrocytic changes of peripheral smear
  with hypersegmented neutrophils

Supplementation
0.5 to 1 mg daily (contained in most prenatal vitamins)

✥ *Vitamin B$_{12}$ deficiency (pernicious anemia)*
Exceedingly rare (1/8000)
Megaloblastic anemia
  • neurologic symptoms
Vitamin B$_{12}$ levels less than 50 pg/mL suggestive of pernicious anemia
Treatment
  • vitamin B$_{12}$ injections, 1 mg IM weekly for 6 weeks

HEMOGLOBINOPATHIES

Normal adult hemoglobin
  • two alpha, two beta globin chains
Hemoglobin A$_2$
  • two alpha, two delta chains
Fetal hemoglobin
  • two alpha and two gamma chains

◆ Sickle Hemoglobinopathies

Hemoglobin S and C
Single amino acid substitution on beta chain
  • hemoglobin S: valine for glutamic acid at position 6
  • hemoglobin C: lysine for glutamic acid at position 6
Range of disease present (Table 23-4)
Hemoglobin S has altered physiochemical properties
  • forms sickle-shaped cells in deoxygenated state

◆ Sickle Cell Anemia

Homozygous for HbS
Compensated hemolytic anemia
  • hematocrit 20% to 30%

TABLE 23-4. Hemoglobin Electrophoresis Findings in Various Hemoglobinopathies

Condition	HbA (%)	HbA$_2$ (%)	HbS (%)	HbF (%)	HbC (%)
Sickle cell trait	55-60	2-3	40-45	1	
Sickle cell disease	0	2-3	85-95	5-15	
Sickle cell/β-thalassemia	10-20	3-5	60-80	10-20	
Hemoglobin SC disease	0	2-3	45-50	1	45-50
Beta-thalassemia trait (β-thalassemia minor)	82-94	4-8		2-3	
Normal	96-97	2-3		1	

- reticulocyte counts 10% to 25%

Four severe vasoocclusive crises per year on average
Pregnancy associated with worsening of most parameters
- anemia more severe, crises more common

Previously poor outcomes
Now improved with more aggressive care

⟡ *Prenatal care*
Frequent visits
- screen for bacteriuria
- folate supplementation
- iron supplementation
  - if indices indicate iron deficiency anemia

Early hospitalization for crises
- oxygen, IV fluid (0.5% saline)
- fetal surveillance
- transfusion indications
  - severe maternal anemia (less than 15%)
  - prophylaxis
    - controversial
    - usually every 6 to 8 weeks
    - partial exchange transfusion
    - goal hematocrit 30%, hemoglobin A 40% to 50%

◆ Hemoglobin SC Disease

Pregnancy causes marked increase in symptoms
Manage pregnancy in similar fashion to sickle cell disease

◆ Sickle Cell-ß-Thalassemia

Intermediate course between HbSS, HbSC and HbAS, HbAA
Management as for sickle cell anemia

◆ Sickle Trait

Only significant risk in pregnancy is UTIs

◆ Genetic Counseling

Important for all women with sickle hemoglobinopathies
Prenatal diagnosis available
Based on restriction fragment length polymorphism (RFLP) of
    DNA

◆ Thalassemia

Homozygous α-thalassemia
- incompatible with life

Heterozygous α-thalassemia (a-thalassemia minor)
- hypochromic microcytic RBC but no anemia

Homozygous β-thalassemia (Cooley's anemia)

- devastating transfusion-dependent disease

Heterozygous β-thalassemia (β-thalassemia minor)
- mild hypochromic microcytic anemia
  - hematocrit 32% to 33%
  - hemoglobin A_2 4% to 8% (distinguishes it from iron-deficiency anemia)
  - patients tolerate pregnancy well
  - folate supplementation only

COAGULATION DEFECTS

◆ Von Willebrand Disease

1 in 10,000 people, usually inherited as autosomal dominant
Hemorrhagic disorder with near undetectable levels of Factor VIII:C and VIII:R
- factor VIII:C and VIII:R increase during pregnancy
- may normalize by term
- no replacement needed if values greater than 50% of normal unless cesarean delivery needed (85% normal levels required)

Normal platelet count
Therapy
- cryoprecipitate
- fresh frozen plasma

◆ Hemophilia A (Factor VIII Deficiency)

Inherited hemorrhagic disorder (X-linked recessive)
Low to absent factor VIII:C and factor VIII:R
Gene has been sequenced
Probes available for prenatal diagnosis

◆ Hemophilia B (Christmas Disease; Factor IX Deficiency)

X-linked deficiency of factor IX
Carrier women have levels that average 33% of normal level
Clinically indistinguishable from hemophilia A
Gene has been cloned
Probes available for prenatal diagnosis
Some carrier mothers may be at risk for hemorrhage
Treat with FFP or factor IX concentrate

24

◆ Immunologic Disorders in Pregnancy

FUNDAMENTAL IMMUNOBIOLOGY

Immune system is primary function
- protect against foreign antigens and pathogens
- distinguish biologic self from nonself

Highly regulated, nonrandom process (Fig. 24-1)

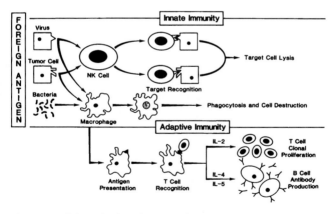

Figure 24-1. Schematic view of innate and adaptive immune systems. Foreign antigen is recognized by phagocytic cells of the innate immune system. The foreign antigen can be microbial pathogens, viral antigens, or tumor antigen. Innate immune responses result in direct cytotoxicity or destruction of the pathogen. Activation of the adaptive immune system depends on interaction with processed antigen provided by cells of the innate immune system. T-cell and B-cell activation results in T-cell clonal proliferation and B-cell antibody production, respectively. IL, interleukin; NK, natural killers. (Dudley DJ. The immune system in health and disease. Ballieres Clin Obstet Gynaecol 1992;6:393.)

MATERNAL FETAL IMMUNOLOGY

Pregnancy is not a state of generalized immune suppression
Differentiated fetal trophoblastic cells are in direct/continuous
    contact with maternal uterine tissue/blood
- do not express classic HLA class I or HLA class II
- resist cellular or Ab mediated immunologic activity
- extravillous cytotrophoblast express nonclassic MHC (HLA-G)

RH IMMUNIZATION

Caused by incompatibility between fetal and maternal blood
- Rh-negative mother becomes sensitized
- Rh-positive fetus at risk for hemolytic anemia
Incidence dramatically reduced since introduction of Rh immu-
    noglobulin (RhIgG)

◆ Pathophysiology

Nomenclature
- genetic locus on chromosome 1
- small protein 7000 to 10,000 molecular weight
- multiple antigenic determinants
- Fisher-Race nomenclature most widely used
  - 3 genetic loci (C, D, E)

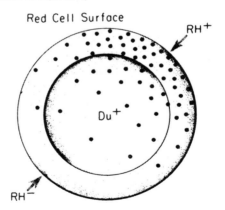

Figure 24-2. Mechanism for the determination of D and Du positivity. One theory suggests that the density of the D antigen on the surface of the red cell determines the results of red cell typing. Patients with no antigen are typed Rh–, patients with low densities of the antigen are typed Du+, and patients with high densities of the antigen are typed Rh+. (Kochenour NK, Scott JR. Rh isoimmunization in pregnancy. In: Scott JR, Rote NS, eds. Immunology in obstetrics and gynecology. Norwalk, CT: Appleton-Century-Crofts, 1984;143.)

- 2 possible alleles of each
- Cc, Dd, Ee
- "d" represents absence of discernible allelic product
- genotypes indicated as pairs of gene products (e.g., CDe/cde)
- several variations of D antigen expression (Fig. 24-2)
  - Du variants are considered Rh positive
  - their erythrocytes can generate anti-D immune response

Fetomaternal hemorrhage
- fetal blood often enters maternal circulation
  - 6.7% first trimester
  - 15.9% second trimester
  - 28.9% third trimester
- minimal amount needed to sensitize Rh-negative volunteers (0.1 mL)
- several factors increase risk of transplacental transfer (Table 24-1)

◆ Immunology

Rh-negative women develop anti-D only when exposed to Rh-positive red blood cells
- 30% of Rh-negative people never respond to exposure

IgM response first

Slow IgG response (6 weeks to 6 months)
- differences in transplacental transfer and heterogeneity of IgG subclasses

IgG coated red blood cells hemolyzed extravascularly
- not a complement fixing reaction

TABLE 24-1. Factors That Influence Whether a Patient Will Become Rh-Immunized

---

Conditions Associated With Increased Risk of Fetomaternal Hemorrhage

Amniocentesis
Threatened abortion, placenta previa, placental abruption
Abdominal trauma
External version
Fetal death
Sinusoidal fetal heart tracing
Multiple pregnancy
Cesarean section
Anemic infant

Factors That Influence Rh Immunization

Incidence and size of fetomaternal hemorrhage
ABO compatibility between mother and fetus
Rh phenotype of fetal red cells
Gender of the baby
Genetic predisposition (responder)

◆ Clinical Manifestations

Fetal anemia
Extramedullary hematopoiesis
Erythroblastosis fetalis (immune hydrops)
- heart failure, ascites, pericardial effusions
Neonatal complications
- anemia
- hyperbilirubinemia
  - low level of glucuronyl transferase
  - bilirubin deposition in basal ganglia (kernicterus)

◆ Prevention with Rh Immunoglobulin

Mechanisms
- antigen blocking (competitive inhibition)
- clearance and antigen deviation
- central inhibition
Clinical use of RhIgG
- more than 350,000 women receive it annually
- no evidence of any HIV risk
- 300 μg anti-D = 30 mL fetal Rh-positive blood (15 mL packed fetal red blood cells)
- 100% effective immunologically if given before sensitization
  - failures usually arise from
    - error in blood typing
    - failure to administer RhIgG
    - unrecognized fetomaternal hemorrhage during delivery
    - inadequate Rh dose
    - patient refusal

◆ Appropriate Management

◇ *First-trimester abortion*

D antigen identified as early as day 38 of gestation
Risk of sensitization 3% to 5%
All Rh-negative women with any type of abortal episode should receive 50 μg RhIgG
- adequate for first trimester
- protects against 5 mL fetal blood
Ectopic pregnancy does not represent sensitization risk
Hydatidiform mole
- no fetal red blood cells or vessels
Most research indicates no Rh antigen on trophoblastic cells

◇ *Amniocentesis*

All Rh-negative women should receive 300 μg RhIgG
If delivery is anticipated within 72 hr, physician could defer RhIgG until fetal blood type is determined

◇ *Antepartum bleeding*

Risk of sensitization with threatened abortion is unknown

Fetomaternal bleeding may be more common in this setting
- can test for fetal blood in maternal circulation
  - if positive, administer RhIgG
    - subsequent abortion: defer RhIgG, previous dose is adequate
    - term pregnancy: RhIgG at 28 weeks

Check K-B in other high-risk situations
- previa
- abruption
- abdominal trauma
- hydrops
- sinusoidal fetal heart rates
- unexplained fetal demise

✧ *Antepartum prophylaxis*
Postpartum administation fails in 1% to 2%
- failure rate reduced to 0.1% with routine prophylaxis at 28 weeks

Indirect Coombs may still be positive at delivery
- if infant is Rh positive, do not withhold RhIgG

✧ *Postpartum management*
300 µg RhIgG IM within 72 hr of delivery
- still indicated at >72 hours

0.4% of patients require >300 µg
- large maternofetal bleed

Occasionally conflicting data
- Rh negative, Du positive
  - either actually Du positive → no RhIgG
  - or large number of fetal erythocytes in blood
    - check K-B

◆ Management

Goal is to time delivery to minimize fetal morbidity/mortality
Protocols for treatment/assessment must be individualized

✧ *Maternal antibody titer*
First sensitized gestation
- risk of fetal involvement is low (anemia/hydrops <10%)
- follow with monthly titer, serial ultrasounds
  - if titers remain low → little risk of anemia

After first affected pregnancy, titers are less predictive
- usually if >1:16 perform amniocentesis
- pattern is that of equal or greater fetal involvement in subsequent pregnancies

✧ *Amniocentesis and amniotic fluid assessment*
Timing of initial amniocentesis requires judgement
Ultrasound guided
Check ∆OD 450, plot on Liley curve (Fig. 24-3)
- Zone I: Rh negative or mildly affected
- Zone II: moderately affected

- Zone III: high risk for IUFD

Can now perform PCR on amniocytes to determine fetal Rh status

✧ *Fetal management*

✳ *Mild to moderate disease*

Sonogram for gestational age at 14 to 16 weeks

Amniotic fluid analysis (see Liley curve, Fig. 24-3), serial sonograms (unless titer is low)

First amniocentesis at 26 to 28 weeks if this is the first sensitized pregnancy or if there is a previous history of mildly affected infant

- management based on ΔOD450
  - zone II and falling → deliver when mature
  - zone II and rising → deliver before maturity

Common error is underestimating the severity of the disease

Delivery optimally at center able to handle neonatal complications

✳ *Severe disease*

First ultrasound at 14 to 16 weeks

Serial scans every 1 to 2 weeks

Hydropic changes indicate Hct <15%

If severe anemia is suspected, perform percutaneous umbilical blood sampling (PUBS) and possibly transfuse in utero

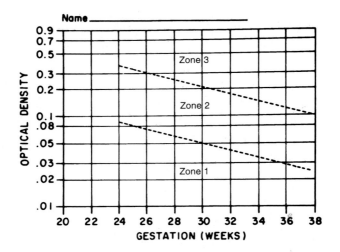

Figure 24-3. The modified Liley graph is divided into three zones to predict severity of isoimmunization and assist in clinical decision making.

ABO INCOMPATIBILITY

ABO incompatibility between fetus/mother in 20% to 25%
Only 10% result in clinically recognized hemolytic process
ABO hemolytic problems almost exclusively A or B infants of O
  mothers
Kernicterus/anemia are rare

IMMUNE THROMBOCYTOPENIA

Two diseases with similar fetal but different maternal consequences
Autoimmune (formerly idiopathic thrombocytopenic purpura)
Alloimmune (formerly isoimmune thrombocytopenia)
Mean antepartum platelet count 246,000/mm^3
- <150,000/mm^3 in 7.6%
- <100,000 /mm^3 in 1%
Differential diagnosis
- HELLP
- SLE
- antiphospholipid syndrome
- AIDS
- TTP
- transfusion reaction
- medication
- pseudothrombocytopenia

AUTOIMMUNE THROMBOCYTOPENIA

Most common autoimmune bleeding disorder encountered during pregnancy
IgG antibodies directed against maternal and fetal platelets
- produced mainly in spleen
Fetal thrombocytopenia can occur

◆ Diagnosis

History of easy bruising
Platelets <100,000 with or without megakaryocytes on smear
Bone marrow biopsy normal or with increased megakaryocytes
Exclusion of other causes
90% have platelet-associated IgG
- levels not predictive of fetal thrombocytopenia

◆ Treatment

Maintain platelets >20,000 for delivery

◇ *Glucocorticoids*

Prednisone 1 to 2 mg/kg/day
Response seen in 75%, complete remission in 25%
Taper prednisone dose by 10% to 20% every 2 weeks

◇ *Splenectomy*

Useful in patients unresponsive to steroids
Complete remission in 80%, often by 1 to 2 weeks
May be performed during second trimester

✧ *Immunoglobulin*

High doses (400 mg/kg/day for 5 days)
Peak platelet count within 7 to 9 days
>80% will be increased to >50,000
Only 2 to 3 days of treatment may be needed in responders
• 800 mg to 1 g/kg doses may suffice as single or double infusion

✧ *Platelet transfusion*

Useful in cases of maternal hemorrhage
6 to 10 units to temporarily control bleeding

◆ **Obstetric Management**

Fetal platelets >50,000 in 80%
Options
• cesarean delivery
• fetal scalp sampling in labor to determine delivery route
• PUBS to determine delivery route (risk not well established)
If planning vaginal delivery
• avoid scalp electrode
• avoid injectible anesthetic or operative delivery
Pediatric follow-up is critical
• platelet counts usually fall after delivery

ALLOIMMUNE THROMBOCYTOPENIA

Suspected when thrombocytopenic infant delivered by normal
  mother
Process analogous to Rh incompatibility
• PL^{A1} platelet-specific alloantigen
• inherited as a codominant trait
  • 69% of people are homozygous PL^{A1} positive
  • 28% heterozygous
  • 2% PL^{A1} negative
Occurs in only 1 to 2/10,000 neonates
Unknown factors prevent sensitization
• more common in certain HLA phenotypes (HLA-DR3)
Often occurs in primiparous patients
75% recurrance rate

◆ **Obstetric Management**

May have more severe neonatal complications than autoimmune
• mortality 10% to 15%
• neurologic impairment (from intracranial hemorrhage) 25%
  • sonographic evidence of IC bleed in utero in 10%
Options
• glucocorticoids
• IV IgG
• transfusion (PUBS)

- sampling of fetal blood near term
  - deliver by cesarean if thrombocytopenic

Disease is self-limited following delivery

SYSTEMIC LUPUS ERYTHEMATOSIS

Chronic multisystem inflammatory disease
>250,000 cases; 50,000 new cases each year
Development of antibodies to autologous DNA and other cellular components
- deposition of antibody-antigen complexes

Genetic factors implicated
10 year survival >90%

◆ Diagnosis

May begin with vague symptoms
Most frequent laboratory abnormalities
- thrombocytopenia
- leukopenia
- presence of autoantibodies
  - 98% have positive ANA
  - high titers of antibody to double-stranded DNA and Smith (Sm) antigen also specific for SLE

◆ SLE and Pregnancy

Clinical course not adversely influenced by pregnancy
Maternal complications correlate with disease activity, renal, and cardiac involvement
- >50% fetal loss rate with initial creatinine >1.5 mg/dL
- >80% if also associated with proteinuria and decreased creatinine clearance

Difficult to distinguish lupus flare from superimposed PIH
- 20% to 30% develop preeclampsia

30% to 50% preterm birth
80% to 90% live birth rate in cases of mild to moderate renal disease in remission

◆ Pregnancy Management

Postpone conception for 1 to 2 years after diagnosis and stabilization of disease
- contraceptive method of choice: barrier (and sterilization)

Mainstay of therapy is use of corticosteroids
- initial dose 60 to 100 mg prednisone daily
- taper over several weeks to 10 to 15 mg/day
- stress doses given in labor 100 mg hydrocortisone IV q 8 hours

Close surveillance during pregnancy (see Table 24-2)
Route of delivery determined by obstetric indications

ANTIPHOSPHOLIPID SYNDROME

Autoimmune disorder characterized by production of high levels
of antiphospholipid antibodies (aPL) (Table 24-3)

Can occur in patients with other autoimmune disorders such as
SLE (secondary APS)

May present in patient with no recognizable autoimmune disease (primary APS)

**TABLE 24-2. Management of Systemic Lupus
Erythematosus During Pregnancy**

Testing Parameter	First Trimester	Second Trimester	Third Trimester
Blood count with platelets	X	X	X
Microscopic urinalysis	X	X	X
24-h urine for protein, creatinine clearance	X	X	X
Urine culture	X		
Lupus anticoagulant	X		
Anticardiolipin	X		
Anti-Ro and anti-LA antibodies	X		
SMA	X		
Clinic visits	Biweekly	Biweekly	Weekly
Sonographic examination	Once	Monthly	Monthly
Fetal heart rate testing			Weekly

**TABLE 24-3. Clinical and Laboratory Criteria for
Antiphospholipid Syndrome**

Clinical Features

Pregnancy loss
Recurrent pregnancy loss
Fetal death
Thrombosis
Venous
Arterial, including stroke
Autoimmune thrombocytopenia
Other
Coombs'-positive hemolytic anemia
Livedo reticularis

Laboratory Features

Lupus anticoagulant
Anticardiolipin antibodies
IgG, medium- or high-positive
IgM, medium- or high-positive and lupus anticoagulant

Patients with antiphospholipid syndrome should have at least one clinical and
one laboratory feature at some time in the course of their disease. Laboratory
test results should be positive on at least two occasions more than 8 weeks
apart.

◆ Laboratory Determination and Interpretation

Three aPL with well-established assays
- biologic false-positive test for syphilis (RPR, VDRL)
- lupus anticoagulant (LA)
- anticardiolipin antibodies (aCL)

Low-positive and isolated IgM aCL results are of questionable clinical value

Results calibrated against standards from APL Standardization Lab in Lexington, Kentucky

LA detected using phospholipid-dependent clotting assays
- activated partial thromboplastin time
- dilute Russell viper venom test
- Kaolin clotting time

Prolongation of clotting time is nonspecific
- need to rule out factor deficiencies

◆ Prevalence

aPL antibody levels in pregnancy do not differ from nonpregnant
- <2% of normal pregnant women have IgG aCL
- >80% of positive values are low positive
  - only 0.2% of IgG, 0.7% IgM results are in clinically significant range

aPL screening in general population not recommended
- useful in patients with recurrent pregnancy loss (5% to 10% positive)

30% to 40% of SLE patients are aPL antibody positive
- fetal loss rate much higher than in isolated aPL (73% vs. 17%)

◆ Clinical Manifestations

Small subset of patients have no clinical evidence

90% of patients with aPL as cause of pregnancy loss have at least one midtrimester fetal death
- prognosis worse in cases of multiple losses

30% to 50% have history of thrombotic events
- 80% related to pregnancy or oral contraceptive use

◆ Pathogenesis

Mechanism has not been elucidated

Nonspecific decidual vasculopathy

Original hypothesis of prostacyclin/thromboxane imbalance not confirmed

◆ Pregnancy Management

Need well-documented history of previous adverse pregnancy outcome or underlying autoimmune disease prior to considering therapy

Glucocorticoids
- associated with numerous adverse effects

Low dose ASA (80 mg/day)

Subcutaneous heparin

No randomized controlled trials but pregnancy outcome improved in all but one series

✧ *University of Utah regimen*

One baby aspirin (80 mg) q day

Heparin instituted after ultrasonography documentation of viability in first trimester

Begin at 15,000 units q day in divided doses
- adjust to therapeutic levels in second trimester

✳ *Risks*

Bleeding from trauma

Heparin-induced osteopenia

Idiopathic thrombocytopenia

Note: Heparin and steroids should NOT be combined

Greatly increased risk of severe osteopenia with no therapeutic benefit

◆ Outcomes

Treatment does not eliminate risk of complicated pregnancy

Careful antepartum surveillance needed
- serial ultrasound examinations
- antepartum testing

High rate of preeclampsia
- often with serious sequelae

Preterm delivery often indicated for maternal or fetal compromise

Fetal/neonatal death prior to 22 weeks may occur

Several cases of puerperal complications resembling autoimmune flare
- treat with glucocorticoids, supportive measures

TRANSPLANTATION

◆ Kidney Transplantation

Experience with pregnancy is greatest in patients with living donor or cadaveric renal transplant

More than 3000 documented pregnancies

GFR usually decreases in third trimester
- usually a reversible defect

UTI common, twofold increase in pyelonephritis

Hypertension and preeclampsia common (30%)

Preterm delivery (45%)

IUGR (20%)

Rarely rejection and even maternal death

◆ Other Transplants

Bone marrow
- limited exposure (at least 11 normal children)

Liver (29 pregnancies reported)
- complications similar to renal

Heart, heart/lung
- five episodes of rejection, three late maternal deaths
- frequent complications hypertension (48%), preeclampsia (24%), preterm labor (28%)

Fetal effects
- all agents cross the placenta
- no statistical increase in rate of congenital anomalies in humans

◆ Prepregnancy Evaluation

Preconception counseling desirable
Ideal timing likely 2 to 5 years posttransplant
Rate of spontaneous abortion not increased
Infection can be a serious problem
Rejection can occur but likely not related to pregnancy
Frank/tactful discussion of long-term survival is appropriate

◆ Prenatal Care

Serial ultrasound for growth
Close surveillance for allograft failure
Treatment of cervical dysplasia
Consider prophylactic ASA use given the risk of PIH
Aggressive treatment of infections

◆ Labor and Delivery

No contraindication to induction, labor, or vaginal delivery
Minimize interventions in attempt to decrease rate of infectious complications
Cesarean, based on obstetric indications
Consider lower midline incision in transplant patients to avoid graft disruption

◆ Neonatal Problems

Most offspring have uncomplicated neonatal course
Mothers advised against breast feeding
Long-term follow-up recommended

25

◆ General Medical and Surgical Diseases in Pregnancy

GENERAL MEDICAL DISEASES

◆ Endocrine

✧ *Pituitary*
Enlarges during pregnancy
Numerous physiologic changes
- gonadotropins decreased
- growth hormone release decreased
- ACTH increased but shows diminished response to metyrapone
- TSH unchanged
- prolactin increased dramatically

✳ *Pituitary tumors*
Microadenomas are common
- monitor during pregnancy with visual fields in every trimester
- MRI or CT if symptoms develop or if changes are noted in visual field
- treatment with bromocriptine is safe during pregnancy
- prolactin levels are not helpful

✳ *Sheehan syndrome*
Postpartum pituitary necrosis resulting from obstetric hemorrhage
Incomplete or irregular functional impairments possible
Symptoms
- failure to lactate
- chronic fatigue
- oligomenorrhea
- cold intolerance
- coarse skin and hair
- inability to concentrate
- hypoglycemia
- weight loss

Treatment requires replacement of thyroid and adrenocorticosteroid hormones

✧ *Thyroid*
* *Maternal thyroid function*
  Normal changes in thyroid function tests noted (Table 25-1)
  * mostly result of increased thyroid-binding globulin
  No changes in thyroxine turnover
  T_3 uptake still an important aspect of the evaluation
  * elevated total T_4 and decreased RT_3U is normal

* *Maternal thyrotoxicosis*
  Complicates 1/500 pregnancies
  Clinical diagnosis in pregnancy may be difficult
  * lab criteria better
    * total T_4 >15 μg/dL
    * elevated free T_4 or free thyroxine index (FT_4I)
  Treatment
  * radioactive iodine contraindicated
  * usual therapy is PTU or methimazole
    * PTU usually preferred (methimazole may have adverse neo-natal dermatologic effects)
    * blocks thyroxine synthesis and $T_4 \rightarrow T_3$ conversion
    * 100 to 150 mg every 8 hours until symptoms are controlled
  Thyroid storm
  * occasionally seen
  * maternal mortality 10% to 20%

* *Thyroid nodules or cancer*
  Evaluation by ultrasound, needle biopsy or aspiration
  Surgery is safe in pregnancy; radioactive iodine is not

* *Fetal thyroid function*
  Neonatal hyperthyroidism is a serious condition
  Treatment in utero is possible with intraamniotic injection of thyroxine
  Neonatal thyrotoxicosis is less common
  * neonatal mortality of 10% to 16%
  * mild cases require no treatment

TABLE 25-1. Thyroid Function Tests in Late Pregnancy

Test	Nonpregnant	Late Pregnancy	Cord
Serum thyroxine (μg/dL)	4.5-12.0	8-16	6-13
Free thyroxine (ng/dL)	0.6-2.1	0.8-2.4	1.5-3.0
Serum triiodothyronine (ng/mL)	120-230	150-250	40-60
Resin T_3 uptake (%)	25-35	20-25	25-35
Thyroid-binding globulin (mg/L)	5-30	30-50	12-30
Thyroid-stimulating hormone (μU/mL)	0-10	0-10	0-20

⬦ *Adrenal*

Total cortisol concentration increases during pregnancy

Elevation of free cortisol usually seen but competes with progesterone for nuclear receptors

Adrenal function tests usually unaltered
- cortrosyn stimulation test
- metyrapone stimulation test
- dexmethasone stimulation test

✳ *Adrenocortical insufficiency (Addison Disease)*

Chronic or acute

Diagnosis may be difficult
- generally made by cortrosyn stimulation test (Table 25-2)

Etiology
- autoimmune disorder

Therapy
- prednisone
  - usually 5 mg q a.m., 2.5 q p.m.
- 9 α-fluorohydrocortisone
- stress doses needed in labor
  - cortisol hemisuccinate, 25 mg IM every 6 hours prior to delivery
  - cortisol 100 mg IV at time of delivery

✳ *Addisonian crisis*

Glucose containing isotonic saline

Cortisol hemisuccinate, 200 mg IV

Additional 100 mg of cortisol per liter of IV fluid

✳ *Cushing syndrome (hypercortisolism)*

Elevated glucocorticoids from bilateral adrenal hyperplasia, adrenal adenomas, or exogenous corticosteroid therapy

Classical symptoms and features
- round faces, full cheeks (chipmunk cheeks)
- glucose intolerance
- acne
- gynecologic manifestations
- androgenization
- amenorrhea
- irregular vaginal bleeding

Diagnosis (Table 25-3)

✳ *Congenital adrenal hyperplasia*

Enzyme defect in cortisol biosynthesis
- 21-hydroxylase
- 11ß-hydroxylase
- 18-hydroxysteroid dehydrogenase

90% of patients with congenital adrenal hyperplasia in pregnancy have 21-hydroxylase deficiency
- increased risk of masculinization of female fetus
- DNA probes are available

TABLE 25-2. Laboratory Diagnosis of Adrenocortical Insufficiency (Addison Disease) During Pregnancy

Test	Normal	Normal Response	Addison Disease
Corticotropin stimulation		> Doubling of Cortisol at 1 h	< Doubling of cortisol at 1 h
Plasma adrenocorticotropic hormone	23 ± 5 pg/mL in first trimester 59 ± 16 pg/mL in last trimester	Increase during pregnancy	Increased with primary disease; decreased with secondary disease
A.M. Plasma cortisol	9 ± 3 µg/dL in first trimester 27 ± 11 µg/dL in last trimester	Increase during pregnancy	Decreased

TABLE 25-3. Laboratory Diagnosis of Hypercortisolism (Cushing Syndrome) During Pregnancy

Test	Normal	Normal Response	Cushing Syndrome
A.M. Plasma cortisol	9 ± 3 µg/dL in first trimester 27 ± 11 µg/dL in last trimester	Increase during pregnancy	Further increase with loss of diurnal variability
P.M. Plasma	4 ± 2 µg/dL in first trimester 15 ± 6 µg/dL in last trimester		
24-Hour urinary free cortisol	30 – 100 µg/d in first trimester 90 – 140 µg/d in last trimester	Increase during pregnancy	Further increase
Plasma adrenocorticotropic hormone	23 ± 5 pg/mL in first trimester 59 ± 16 pg/mL in last trimester	Increase during pregnancy	Very low or undetectable

Treatment
- prednisone or cortisone at 10 weeks gestation
- add 9α-fluorohydrocortisone if there is any evidence of mineralocorticoid deficiency

✳ *Pheochromocytoma*
  Rare but serious pregnancy complication
  5% to 55% maternal mortality rate
  Diagnosis made by measurement of 24-hour urinary catecholamines
  Localize with CT and selective venous sampling
  Treatment
- surgical removal

◆ Gastrointestinal Diseases

◇ *Nausea and vomiting*
Occurs in 60% to 80% of pregnant women
- 1 to 200/1 to 300 require parenteral hydration

✳ *Hyperemesis gravidarum*
  Etiology unclear
- numerous hormonal (hCG, pituitary excess etc.) and psychologic theories
  Treatment
- small frequent meals
- reassurance
- medication
  - pyridoxine 10 to 30 mg/day
  - meclizine 12.5 mg BID
  - prochlorperazine 5 to 25 mg every 4 to 6 hours
  - chlorpromazine 10 to 25 mg every 4 to 6 hours
- hydration for ketones, electrolyte abnormalities
- hyperalimentation has been used in severe cases

◇ *Reflux esophagitis*
Affects over half of pregnant women
Etiology
- enlarging uterus
- decreased gastroesophageal sphincter tone
- decreased propulsive activity in distal esophagus
Treatment
- liquid antacids
- elevation of head in bed
- other medications
  - cimetidine and metoclopramide
    - fetal effects unknown

◇ *Gastric and duodenal ulcer disease*
Associated with high acid production, helicobacter pylori infection
Pregnancy usually ameliorates ulcer
Treatment

- antacids
- possibly cimetidine

◇ *Cholelithiasis and biliary disease*
Frequency not increased by pregnancy
Symptoms are the same as nonpregnant state
- postprandial right upper quadrant pain
- nausea and vomiting
Diagnosis
- ultrasound 95% to 99% accurate in diagnosing cholelithiasis
- only 50% of patients are asymptomatic
Management
- same as nonpregnant state
- cholecystectomy indications
  - obstructive jaundice
  - recurrent/persistent pancreatitis, acute abdomen

◇ *Pancreatitis*
Most common cause during pregnancy is cholelithiasis
Most common symptom is epigastric pain with radiation to the back
Serum amylase is usually greater than 1000 IU/L
Diagnosis confirmed by ultrasound
Management
- enteric rest
- NG suction
- IV hydration
- analgesics (meperidine 75 to 100 mg every 4 hours)
- preterm labor surveillance
- can represent a grave illness

◇ *Inflammatory bowel disease*

✳ *Ulcerative colitis*
Confined to colorectal mucosa
Continuous pattern (no skip lesions)
Bloody diarrhea common

✳ *Crohn disease*
Entire thickness of bowel wall involved
Most common site is distal ileum
Pregnancy complications more common in face of active disease

✳ *Treatment*
High-calorie diet, low-roughage diet
Medical therapy
- sulfasalazine
- prednisone
- diphenoxylate (Lomotil)

◆ Liver Disease

◇ *Nonpregnancy-specific liver diseases*

✱ *Viral Hepatitis*
See Chapter 26

◇ *Pregnancy-specific liver diseases*

✱ *Intrahepatic cholestasis of pregnancy*
Presents with pruritis, 50- to 100-fold increase in bile acids
  • moderate increase in transaminases
  • only 20% have increased bilirubin
Increased risk of poor fetal outcome
  • antepartum surveillance should be initiated
Treatment
  • symptomatic relief suboptimal
  • cholestryamine 4 g every 4 to 6 hours
  • administer vitamin K as well
  • phenobarbital

◆ Neurologic Diseases

◇ *Headache*

✱ *Muscle tension*
Most common type of headache in pregnancy
Tends to worsen as pregnancy progresses
Funduscopic neurologic examination normal
Treat with local care and acetaminophen

✱ *Migraine*
80% of women with known migraines experience relief in pregnancy
Propranolol 10 to 40 mg every 6 hours or 80 mg of long-acting every day may be helpful
Other medications
  • acetaminophen
  • midrin
  • narcotic analgesics
  • phenothiazine, antiemetics
  • avoid NSAIDs

◇ *Seizure disorders*
22% experience improvement
24% experience exacerbation
54% unchanged
Drug therapy
  • requirements usually increase by 30% to 50% during pregnancy
  • increased requirement for folic acid
Pregnancy may decrease seizure threshold in poorly controlled patients
Onset of seizure is a special concern in pregnancy

- structural abnormalities are common

Status epilepticus is a true emergency

✳ *Teratology of drugs*

Several factors to consider

- increased incidence of anomalies in infants of mothers with seizure disorders
- nonexposed mothers also exhibit fetal-hydantoin type abnormalities themselves
- risk may be related to specific enzyme defects

Specific contraindications

- trimethadione and valproic acid
- 1% to 2% syndrome of malformations
  - offer amniocentesis if the drug is truly required

✳ *Vitamin K deficiency*

Administer 10 mg to women in labor and probably during last weeks of pregnancy

Administer 1 mg to all infants of mothers with seizure disorders

◆ Muscle Disease

✧ *Leg cramps*

Affects 25% of all pregnant women

More common at night

Etiology unclear

Treatment

- calcium supplementation

✧ *Myasthenia gravis*

Autoimmune disease characterized by IgG antibody against striated muscle acetylcholine receptors

Mild disease may require no specific therapy

More severe disease

- treat with pyridostigmine or neostigmine
  - safe in pregnancy

Normal response to oxytocin

Drugs to avoid

- curare
- succinylcholine
- magnesium sulfate
- aminoglycoside antibiotics
- antiarrhythmics (quinine, quinidine, procaine)
- procaine anesthetics
- large doses of narcotics

Neonatal symptoms present in 10%

- usually transient (2 weeks)

✧ *Peripheral nerve disease*

✳ *Back pain*

Reported by as many as 50% of pregnant women

Generally a musculoskeletal response to shifting center of gravity
- treat with restricted activity, local heat, gestational support undergarment, and a firm mattress

Occasionally lumbar sacral nerve root disease
- radicular pattern
- treat with bedrest, rarely surgery

✴ *Entrapment-compression syndromes*
Carpal tunnel syndrome is most common
- usually bilateral
- median nerve distribution
  - treat with splinting
    - rarely steroid injection
    - 15% will progress and may require surgical release

Bell's palsy
- risk in pregnancy increased threefold
- early prednisone use may be helpful
- major hazard is corneal or conjunctival damage
- no increased risk of obstetric complications

◆ Dermatologic Diseases

◇ *Physiologic changes during pregnancy*
Hyperpigmentation
Prominent vascular changes
Striae gravidarum
Scalp hair growth slowed

◇ *Pregnancy-specific dermatologic diseases*

✴ *Melasma*
Mask of pregnancy
Exacerbated by sun exposure
May also be seen with oral contraceptives, suggesting hormonal etiology

✴ *Herpes gestationis*
Intensely pruritic dermatosis
Not related to herpes virus
- results from a complement fixing IgG antibasement membrane autoantibody

May be associated with placental vilositis and poor outcome
- fetal surveillance indicated

Treatment
- systemic corticosteroids
- antihistamines
- antipruritics (topical)

Generally subsides 3 to 6 months postpartum
Recurrence rate 75%

✴ *Impetigo herpetiformis*
Rare systemic disease
May represent pustular psoriasis during pregnancy

Treatment is supportive
Monitor fluid and electrolyte balance and correct hypocalcemia

Pruitic urticarial papules and plaques of pregnancy (PUPPS)
Pregnancy-specific syndrome
Third trimester onset
Involves abdomen, thigh; rarely involves chest; never involves
    face, palm, soles, and mucous membranes
Responds well to systemic and topical steroids

SURGICAL DISEASES IN PREGNANCY

◆ Acute Abdomen

◇ *Definition*
Nonobstetric emergency abdominal surgery
Complicates 0.2% to 2.2% of pregnancies

◇ *Physical findings*
Intestinal tracts displaced by uterus
Incisional hernias are more common during pregnancy
Always perform pelvic and rectal examination
Consider other etiologies
- pyelonephritis
- pneumonia
- renal calculi
- myocardial infarction
- acute gastroenteritis
- inflammatory bowel disease
- abdominal crisis associated with medical disorders
    - sickle cell anemia
    - porphyria
    - vaculitis
    - drug withdrawal

◇ *Laboratory and radiologic findings*
Baseline laboratory studies
- CBC
- chemistry panel
- UA
- arterial blood gas
Abdominal ultrasonography may be helpful
Plain x-ray
- may be very helpful
    - usual dose of ionizing radiation less than 0.005 Gy (terato-
      genic dose 0.05 to 0.1 Gy)

◆ General Preoperative Considerations

◇ *Anesthesia*
No evidence of teratogenicity

Aspiration always possible

Regional anesthetic not without risk

◇ *Premature labor*

Not a frequent complication except in the presence of peritonitis (increases from 5% to 20% to 35%)

Prophylactic tocolysis is not proven efficacious

◆ Specific Conditions

◇ *Appendicitis*

Most common surgical complication of pregnancy

- 1/1500 to 2000 pregnancies

Equal frequency in all trimesters

Diagnosis remains clinical and surgical

Optimum results occur in series in which the incidence of false-negative laparotomies is about 20%

Choice of incision should allow for adequate exposure

◇ *Cholecystitis*

Acute cholecystitis requiring surgery is not common (1/4000 to 1/5000)

Patients usually can be managed medically

Maternal mortality is rare

Fetal loss rate <5% in absence of pancreatitis

◇ *Pancreatitis*

Treatment is primarily medical

◇ *Intestinal obstruction*

Uncommon in pregnancy

May be associated with previous appendectomy or gynecologic surgery

Diagnosis may be difficult

Medical therapy usually initial approach, but aggressive surgical intervention may minimize morbidity

Premature labor 30% to 50%

Maternal mortality 10% to 20% in some series

◇ *Gynecologic emergencies*

Adnexal torsions or rupture

- corpus luteum may be involved
  - if removed in first 12 weeks of pregnancy, supplement with progesterone vaginal suppository 25 to 50 mg BID

Ovarian tumors can coexist in pregnancy

- surgical intervention for tumors that are solid, increasing in size, bilateral, hormonally active, or symptomatic
- luteoma of pregnancy does not require surgical removal

◇ *Maternal trauma*

Leading cause of maternal mortality

Most common

- motor vehicle accident
- falls
- assaults

Follow ABCs of resuscitation

- aggressively treat blood loss to avoid shock
- increase circulating volume

Check Kleihauer-Betke screen

Administer RhoGAM to Rh-negative women

Appropriately treat head injuries and chest injuries

Evaluate for intraabdominal bleeding

Exploratory surgery for intraabdominal gunshot wounds or stab wounds

After maternal stabilization, electronic fetal monitoring for 12 to 24 hours (based on clinical judgment) for risk of abruption, fetal injury, or fetomaternal hemorrhage

26

◆ Perinatal Infections

BACTERIAL INFECTIONS

◆ Intraamniotic Infection (IAI)

Presents clinically in 1% to 4% of pregnancies

Most often seen during labor with prolonged rupture of membranes

30% of patients in preterm labor (with intact membranes) may have positive amniotic fluid cultures

Clinical Presentation is varied may include:
- maternal temperature >38.5C
- maternal or fetal tachycardia
- uterine tenderness
- foul-smelling amniotic fluid
- leukocytosis
- premature labor
- PROM
- indirect markers may be helpful

◇ *Treatment*

* *Antibiotics and delivery*

Perform cesarean for obstetric indication, not solely for diagnosis of amnionitis

Intrapartum treatment offers substantial reduction in neonatal sepsis
- ampicillin (2 g IV 4 to 6 h) and gentamicin (1.5 mg/kg IV q 8 h)
- add clindamycin (900 mg IV q 8 h) after cesarean delivery

Oxytocin requirements may increase

Endomyometritis may occur after delivery
- 2% after vaginal delivery
- 7.5% after cesarean

◆ Postpartum Endomyometritis

Most common infectious complication in puerperium (5%)
- higher for cesarean vs. vaginal delivery (10 to 50% vs. 2%)

Polymicrobial infection

Risk factors (Table 26-1)

TABLE 26-1. Risk Factors for Postpartum Endomyometritis

Cesarean section
Lengthy duration of ruptured membranes
Prolonged labor
Low socioeconomic status
Multiple vaginal examinations
Internal fetal monitoring (?)
Bacterial vaginosis (?)

⬦ *Symptoms*
Usually presents on second to seventh postpartum day
Fever, malaise, and lower abdominal pain

⬦ *Treatment*
Clindamycin, gentamicin, and usually ampicillin
- ampicillin especially usefully if cephalosporin prophylaxis may have resulted in enterococcus selection
Aztreonam
Extended spectrum cephalosporins (cefoxitin, cefotetan)
Extended spectrum penicillins (piperacillin, mezlocillin)

⬦ *Response*
Usually within 48 hours
Consider further evaluation in treatment failures
- abscess
- hematoma
- pelvic septic thrombophlebitis
Surgery rarely indicated except in cases of *C perfringens* infection (hysterectomy usually required)

⬦ *Prophylactic antibiotics*
Has reduced puerperal morbidity by 50%
Little difference between choices
- first generation cephalosporins as effective as second or third generation

◆ Mastitis

Occurs in 1% to 5% of lactating mothers
Epidemic vs. endemic
- epidemic now rare
- *S aureus* most frequent pathogen
- <10% of cases complicated by breast abscess
Prompt antibiotic therapy usually results in clinical resolution within 48 hours
Treatment choices
- dicloxacillin or cephalosporin
- erythromycin or trimethoprim-sulfamethoxazole if penicillin allergic

Usually all cases can be managed on an ambulatory basis
Continue breast feeding or pumping as long as no breast abscess
present

◆ Group B Streptococcal Infections

Most common cause of neonatal sepsis in the United States
• 15,000 cases, 1600 deaths
Vaginal colonization in 5% to 40% of pregnant women
• most effective culture technique is introital, anorectal swab
Rate of transmission increased in heavily colonized women
• only 1% to 2% of neonates develop sepsis

✧ *Early onset infection*
0.7 to 3.7/1000 live births
Usually first 2 days of life
Presents with pneumonia, bacteremia, sepsis, and meningitis
Normal at delivery with rapid deterioration
Mortality 13% to 37% (66% in preterm infants)

✧ *Late onset infection*
0.9 to 1.9/1000 live births
Primarily term infants
Onset 6 to 90 days after delivery
Most often presents as meningitis
Mortality 5% to 25%
• survivors may have significant neurologic sequelae

✧ *Endomyometritis and other maternal infections*
Group B steptococci is frequent pathogen
Sudden onset with high-spiking fever is usually seen
Asymptomatic bacteriuria has been associated with preterm
delivery and clear risk of pyelonephritis

✧ *Prevention*

✳ *Antepartum treatment*
Not effective in reducing vertical transmission

✳ *Intrapartum*
Use of penicillin in high-risk groups reduces mortality of early
onset disease by 95%
ACOG Recommendations
1. Routine screening of all pregnant patients NOT recommended
   • no colonization site in the genitourinary and lower intestinal tract is exclusively predictive of infection
   • over the course of pregnancy, a positive culture site may become negative and vice versa
   • combination of screening culture with intrapartum chemprophylaxis for women with positive culture fails to prevent 25% to 30% of early neonatal sepsis and 10% of deaths.

2. In absence of screening culture, the following risk factors identify women who should receive intrapartum antibiotic chemoprophylaxis (ampicilin 2 g q 6 h or penicillin G 5 million U q 6 h):
   - preterm labor or PROM <37 weeks
   - fever during labor
   - ruptured membranes >18 hours
   - previous infant affected by symptomatic GBS
3. Selective or routine cultures can be considered in populations with high incidence of GBS infections:
   - women with threatened or arrested premature labor
   - women with PROM remote from term
   - women undergoing surgical procedures of the cervix

American Academy of Pediatrics (AAP) Recommendation

1. Screening of all pregnant women at 26 weeks. Antepartum treatment of colonized women is not indicated except in women with clinical GBS bacteriuria.
2. Maternal GBS carriers either identified antepartum or intrapartum by culture or antigen tests and with one or more risk factors should be given intrapartum ampicillin 2 g IV then 1-2 g IV q 4 to 6 h or penicillin G 5 million units q 6 h until delivery. Patients with penicillin allergy should receive clindamycin or erythromycin. Risk factors include:
   - preterm labor or PROM <37 weeks
   - fever during labor
   - ruptured membranes >18 h
   - multiple birth
   - GBS bacteriuria during pregnancy
3. If maternal GBS status is unknown and risk factors identified, chemoprophylaxis is given.
4. Mothers who have previously given birth to an infant with invasive GBS should receive antibiotics regardless of carrier status or risk factors.
5. The management of infants born to mothers given prophylaxis will vary according to clinical circumstances. Symptomatic neonates need to be evaluated fully and treated. Asymptomatic neonates whose mothers have received a single dose of ampicillin <1 h prior to delivery and preterm infants <34 weeks should probably receive therapy. Antibiotics should be discontinued after 72 h with negative cultures unless clinical course is strongly suggestive of sepsis.

◆ Listeria Infections

Small gram-positive rod
One half of all reported cases are pregnancy related
Clinical presentation
- asymptomatic
- flu-like illness

High risk for preterm delivery, intrauterine infection
Transplacental transmission is primary means of spread
High index of suspicion required
- obtain blood, cervical cultures, and Gram stains

Treatment
- IV ampicillin and gentamicin
- TMP-SMX or erythromycin in penicillin-allergic patients

Prevention
Avoid unpasteurized dairy products

VIRAL INFECTION

◆ HIV

250,000 cases reported in the United States
Fifth leading cause of death of women of reproductive age
6000 pregnancies complicated by HIV yearly
- 1800 cases of perinatal transmission in 1992

Can present with persistent candidiasis
Effects of pregnancy unclear
- risk of severe infection increased with women of low CD4+ counts ($<300/mm^3$)

Perinatal transmission (25% to 35%)
- antepartum transmission
- has been documented in first trimester abortuses
- intrapartum transmission
- first-born twins more likely to be infected
- breast-feeding

Antiviral treatment may reduce transmission rates
Recommended testing (Table 26-3)
- PCP prophylaxis when CD4+ counts $<200/mm^3$
- antiviral therapy when CD4+ counts $<500/mm^3$

Obstetric care
- avoid procedures that increase fetal exposure to maternal blood (PUBS, amniocentesis, fetal scalp electrode)
- cesarean section for obstetric complications

Follow-up
- infants should be tested regularly
- advise against breast-feeding

◆ Hepatitis

◇ *Hepatitis A*

Transmitted by the fecal-oral route
Self-limiting disease
Exposed women should be immunized even if pregnant with immunoglobulin 0.02 mL/kg IM

TABLE 26-2. Vertical Transmission of Hepatitis B from
HB$_s$ Ag-Positive Mothers

Maternal Status	Neonatal Infection Rate
HB$_e$Ag positive	90%
HB$_e$Ag negative	10%–20%
anti-HB$_e$ positive	0–10%
Acute HBV in first trimester	10%–20%
Acute HBV in third trimester or within 1 month of delivery	80%–90%

◇ *Hepatitis B*
   More serious infection
   Sexually or blood-borne transmission
   • vertical transmission possible (Table 26-2)
   • marked elevation of liver function tests
   Confirm by serologic testing
   Fetal risk based on maternal disease
   Supportive therapy
   Neonatal therapy
   • infants require HBIG and HBV within 12 hours of delivery

◇ *Herpes simplex virus*
   DNA virus with two major serotypes
   HSV-1, HSV-2
   Classic lesions involve skin and mucous membranes
   • after primary infection, lesions remain latent in dorsal root ganglia
   • 50% of patients experience recurrent outbreaks
   • 30% to 35% of U.S. population has serologic evidence of HSV-2 infection
   • diagnosis
   • history and viral culture

◇ *Fetal infection*

✳ *Intrapartum attack rate*
   Primary infection 50%
   Symptomatic recurrent infection 5% to 10%
   Asymptomatic <1%
   • 70% of infants with severe HSV infection are born to asymptomatic mothers

✳ *Prevention*
   Careful history and examination
   Cesarean delivery if lesions present
   • regardless of duration or presence of ruptured membranes
   • preterm PROM can probably be managed expectantly (possible with acyclovir treatment)

✳ *Neonates*
  Should be isolated in nursery
  Mothers with lesions should wear mask, gown, and gloves as
    appropriate
  Routine antiviral therapy not currently recommended

◆ Cytomegalovirus

Double-stranded DNA virus
Most common congenitally acquired infection in the United
  States
• incidence 0.5% to 2.5%
Maternal infection typically asymptomatic
• 55% to 85% of pregnant women immune
• usually acquired by infected children

◇ *Diagnosis*
Confirm by viral culture or serology
CMV IgM present in 80% of primary infection, 20% recurrent
  infection
Fourfold rise in CMV titer considered evidence of acute infection

◇ *Perinatal transmission*
Transplacental in utero transmission (1%)
Intrapartum exposure or breast-feeding
Rarely results in serious infection

◇ *Congenital CMV*
30% to 40% risk of vertical transmission from maternal primary
  infection
25% of children have sequelae
Highest risk during first and second trimester
  • third-trimester infection is usually without sequelae

◇ *Presentation*
10% symptomatic (poor prognosis) morbidity 20% to 30%
Diagnosed by viral culture
90% asymptomatic
• 15% develop late complications

◇ *Treatment*
No effective agents

◆ Varicella

Herpes virus responsible for varicella (chickenpox) and herpes
  zoster (shingles)
Most adults previously infected
• 95% pregnant women seropositive
Pneumonia can develop in adults with primary infection
• pregnant women are at higher risk (35% vs. 11%)
  • mortality 10%
  • acyclovir treatment may be helpful

Diagnosis
- clinical examination
- serologic testing (ELISA usually)

✧ *Congenital varicella*
Fetal risk 2% to 5%
Rare in second half of pregnancy

✧ *Neonatal infection*
Maternal infection 5 to 20 days prior to delivery: mild infection
Maternal infection <5 days, 2 days postpartum: 30% risk of disseminated VZV
- administer VZIG

✧ *Maternal exposure*
Check for immunity
Nonimmune patients should be given VZIG
- 125 IU/10 kg (maximum 625 IU/10 kg)
- administration within 30 to 96 hours reduces maternal morbidity
- fetal protective benefit unknown

◆ Rubella (German Measles)

Documentation of acute infection
- rubella-specific IgM
  - positive one week after appearance of rash
  - present for four weeks
  - absence does not exclude infection
- fourfold rise in IgG or seroversion of IgG evidence of infection
All women of child-bearing years should be checked for immunity
- vaccination recommended in nonpregnant susceptible patient
  - avoid pregnancy for 3 months after vaccine
Congenital rubella syndrome
- first month of pregnancy: 50% risk
- second month of pregnancy: 25% risk
- third month of pregnancy: 10% risk
- second trimester: 1% risk
- no documented cases after 20 weeks

◆ Parvovirus

DNA virus
Parvovirus B19 is only known human pathogen from Parvoviridae family of DNA viruses
- causes fifth disease in children
  - childhood exanthum (slapped cheeks)
- 50% of adults immune
- can cause intrauterine infection (rarely)
  - hydrops
  - stillbirth
- exposed pregnant women

- check for IgG, IgM
- both negative: susceptible
- IgM positive: acute infection
- monitor fetus closely
- may require intrauterine transfusion
- IgG positive: immune

◆ Vaginitis in Pregnancy

✧ *Candida*
Symptomatic candida vulvovaginitis occurs in 15%
- treat with topical antifungal agents

✧ *Bacterial vaginosis*
Most common (20% of pregnant women)
- may be associated with increased rate of preterm delivery, intraamniotic infection, and endometritis

Treatment
- ampicillin (60% cure rate)
- clindamycin vaginal cream
- metronidazole
- avoid in first trimester

✧ *Trichomonas vaginalis*
Frothy green discharge
Confirmed by wet-mount
Found in 12% to 30% of pregnant women
- associated with preterm delivery, low birth weight, PROM

Treat with metronidazole, 2 g single dose or 250 mg TID for 1 week

OTHER INFECTIONS

◆ Toxoplasmosis
Intracellular parasite transmitted to human through contact with cat feces or ingestion of raw meat
- 50% of pregnant women in the United States are immune

Primary infection
- 0.1% in pregnancy
- congenital infection can occur but often is asymptomatic
- 90% of symptomatic neonates will be neurologically impaired

✧ *Diagnosis*
Maternal infection
- fourfold rise in IgG from paired serum
- IgM may be present for many years

✧ *Treatment and prevention*
- some success reported with 3 g of spiramycin daily
- 746 cases of maternal toxoplasmosis

All women treated with 3 g of spiramycin daily

- 39 fetuses diagnosed with congenital toxoplasmosis
- 15 mothers continued pregnancy
- treated with pyrimethamine, sulfonamides, folinic acid
- severity of congenital toxoplasmosis apparently reduced
- avoid handling cat litter
- wash hands after touching cat
- cook all meat thoroughly

Nonpregnant infected women should delay pregnancy for 6 months

Routine screening has not been proven to be cost effective

◆ Syphilis

Incidence is on the rise
- 4000 cases of congenital syphilis in the United States 1991

Sexually transmitted spirochete (*Treponema pallidum*)

Congenital infection associated with poor prenatal outcome

Screen all pregnant women with serologic test (VDRL, RPR)

Rescreen high-risk patients in third trimester and after delivery

Positive screening test requires specific treponema test (MHATP)

◇ *Treatment*

Penicillin G benzathine 2.4 million units IM
- use three weekly doses if late syphilis (greater than 1 year duration)
- allergic pregnant patients should undergo penicillin desensitization
- Jarish-Herxheimer reaction occurs in most treated patients
  - pyrexia
  - malaise
  - headache
  - musculoskeletal pain
  - exacerbation of primary lesions
- pregnant women may demonstrate decreased fetal movement, contractions, preterm labor, and recurrent late decelerations

Monitoring
- follow VDRL, RPR
- successful treatment should result in fourfold decrease in level within 3 months
- eightfold decrease within 6 months
- check titers every 3 months for 1 year
- fourfold increase indicates treatment failure, reinfection, and need for retreatment

◆ Chlamydia Infection

Most prevalent sexually transmitted organism
- 4 million infections annually
- urethritis, cervicitis, and PID

Subclinical infection in 70%

Influence on pregnancy is controversial

- many confounding factors

Neonatal risks are clear

- pneumonia
- conjunctivitis

✧ *Diagnosis*

Tissue culture

Imunoassay

- PCR

✧ *Treatment in pregnancy*

Erythromycin, 500 QID for 7 days

Erythromycin ethylsuccinate, 800 mg QID for 7 days

Amoxicillin, 500 TID for 7 days

Treat partner

Test of cure, 4 weeks after treatment

◆ Gonorrhea

2 million infections annually in the United States

Most women asymptomatic

Increased risk for adverse pregnancy outcome

Neonatal infection may occur

- ophthalmia prevention with occular application of erythromycin or tetracycline ointment

✧ *Treatment*

Ceftiaxone, 250 mg IM

- plus 7 days erythromycin

Test of cure, 1 month after treatment

Alternative treatment, spectinomycin for penicillin-and ampicillin-allergic patients

27

◆ Placenta Previa and Placental Abruption

INTRODUCTION

Bleeding during second half of pregnancy occurs in 3% to 4% of
women
Warrants immediate evaluation
Lesions of the vagina and cervix should be considered
Most common causes are placenta previa and placental abruption
- potentially fatal to both mother and fetus

SECOND-TRIMESTER BLEEDING

More common than generally appreciated
Perinatal mortality rate 23% to 32%
- higher than third-trimester bleeding
5 major categories
  1. placenta previa
  2. premature placental separation
  3. molar gestation
  4. cervical/vaginal lesion
  5. undermined
Proper evaluation
- hospitalization
- stabilization
- placental localization by ultrasound
- fetal monitoring
- speculum examination
  - less dangerous than in third trimester-bleeding
Conservative management almost always indicated (except in
molar pregnancy)

PLACENTA PREVIA

Defined as implantation of the placenta in the lower uterine segment, overlying or reaching the cervix
Traditionally categorized into 3 types (Fig. 27-1)

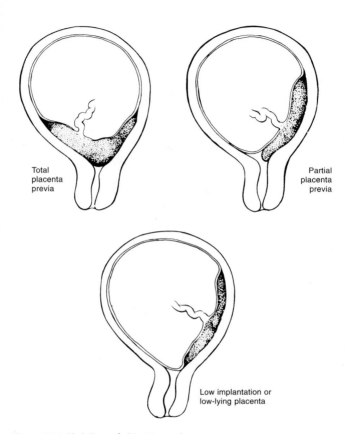

Figure 27-1. Variations of placenta previa.

1. total previa—internal os entirely covered
2. partial previa—os partially covered
3. marginal previa—placenta reaches edge of os

◆ Incidence

1/200 births
More common in parous women (1/20 in grand multiparity)
Incidence decreasing in U.S.

◆ Etiology

Specific cause is unknown
Implantation may be affected by
- abnormality of endometrial vascularity
- delayed ovulation
- prior endometrial trauma
- multiple pregnancy
- previous uterine surgery (cesarean, myomectomy)

◆ Clinical Course

Usually presents as painless vaginal bleeding in third trimester
- can occur as early as 20 weeks
- uterine activity can be evident
Blood loss from first bleeding is rarely fatal
Mean gestational age at diagnosis is 32.5 weeks
- one third of patients present before 30 weeks
- one third after 36 weeks
Associated with increased risk of congenital abnormalities and IUGR

◆ Diagnosis

Painless vaginal bleeding is placenta previa until proven otherwise
- less than 50% of patients actually have previa
Ultrasound is diagnostic technique of choice (93% to 97% accurate)
- some difficulties can arise
  - obese patient
  - posterior previa
  - overdistended bladder
Placental migration can result in inaccurate diagnosis
Transvaginal ultrasound may be preferred to transabdominal for initial resolution
Definitive diagnosis by direct palpation of placenta is not recommended

◆ Management

Hospital admission
High intensity care area (labor and delivery)
Intravenous access
Type and screen
Serial hematocrit
Vital signs
- 20% to 40% increase in blood volume in late pregnancy may result in deceptively minor changes in pulse and blood pressure
Physical examination
- defer vaginal or rectal exam

Ultrasound
Remote from term
- expectant management
  - patient selection
    - maternal hemodynamic stability obviously a requirement
  - preterm contractions/preterm labor
    - tocolytics have been used ($MgSO_4$ tocolytic of choice)
    - no proven efficacy
  - replace blood loss to keep hematocrit greater than 30%
  - steroids have been shown to be beneficial to aid fetal lung maturity
  - serial ultrasound examinations every 2 to 3 weeks
  - bed rest in hospital with bathroom privileges
  - home care only under ideal circumstances
    - highly-motivated patient
    - full understanding of risks
    - ability to maintain bed rest
    - location near hospital
    - 24-hour transportation available

◆ Delivery

The ideal is a well-planned elective cesarean section at 36 to 37 weeks
- amniocentesis useful for timing of delivery

Vaginal approach considered in rare circumstances
- dead fetus
- major fetal malformations
- previability
- active labor with engagement of fetal head
- uncertainty about degree of previa

◆ Double Setup

Inconclusive ultrasound or only low-lying placenta noted
Patient prepped and draped for cesarean section
Wide-bore IV in place
Anesthesia backup present
Sterile speculum examination performed first
If uncertain, gently palpate fornix for fullness
Gently probe cervix with one finger
- gritty texture equals placenta, stop examination
- if no placental tissue felt, then 360 degree rotation inside os

If greater than 3 cm dilated and no placenta covering os, then perform amniotomy

◆ Cesarean Section

Type of incision
- low transverse or low vertical incision

- posterior placenta previa
- polar lie
- classical or extended low vertical incision
  - anterior placenta
  - transverse lie

Try to avoid incising placenta
- find edge of placenta and rupture membranes
- quickly clamp cord
- pediatrician should assess infant's hematocrit level

◆ Complications

Maternal mortality less than 1%
Perinatal mortality less than 5%
Placenta accreta, percreta, or increta in 15% of cases
- cesarean hysterectomy may be needed to control hemorrhage

RUPTURED VASA PREVIA

Rare cause of bleeding
Often associated with placenta previa or multiple gestation
- umbilical vessels course through membranes

Fetal exsanguination can occur rapidly
- 50% fetal mortality rate

Signs
- significant vaginal bleeding and fetal distress with rupture of membranes
  - fetal tachycardia
  - sinusoidal pattern
  - variable decelerations

Prompt cesarean needed to save the infant

PLACENTAL ABRUPTION

Premature separation of the normally implanted placenta
Most often occurs in third trimester
- can happen anytime after 20 weeks

Complicates approximately 1% of pregnancies
- most common cause of intrapartum fetal death
  - 15% of perinatal mortality
  - permanent neurologic impairment in 14% of surviving infants

Separation can be complete, partial, or marginal (Fig. 27-2)
Grading
- 48% mild (grade I)
- 27% moderate (grade II)
- 24% severe (grade III)

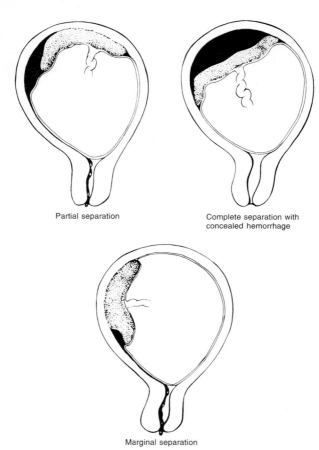

Partial separation

Complete separation with
concealed hemorrhage

Marginal separation

Figure 27-2. Various degrees of separation of a normally implanted placenta.

◆ Pathophysiology

Separation is initiated by bleeding into decidua basalis
- decidua splits and placenta sheared off
- blood may extravasate into and through myometrium (couvelaire uterus)

Fetal effects depend on degree of separation

◇ *Etiology/risk factors*
  • maternal hypertension
  • PIH
  • cocaine-induced
  • chronic hypertension
  Maternal smoking
  Short umbilical cord
  Uterine anomalies
  Advanced maternal age
  Physical work
  Poor nutrition
  Trauma
  Sudden decompression of overdistended uterus
  • amniotomy in patient with polyhydramnios
  • delivery of first twin

◇ *Recurrence risk*
  Tenfold increase in second pregnancy over population risk
  • perinatal mortality 15%
  With two previous abruptions, 25% chance of third abruption

◆ **Signs and Symptoms**

  Clinical diagnosis
  Classical findings (Fig. 27-3)

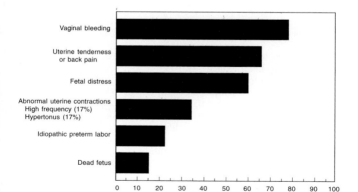

Figure 27-3. Prevalence of signs and symptoms of placental abruption. (Hurd WW, Miodovnik M, Hertzberg V, Lavin JP. Selective management of abruptio placentae: a prospective study. Obstet Gynecol 1983;61:467.)

- vaginal bleeding (80% of patients)
  - may cause port wine stained amniotic fluid
  - blood remains concealed (20% of patients)
- abdominal pain
- uterine contractions
- uterine tenderness

Differential diagnosis
- previa
- bloody show
- uterine rupture

Ultrasonography
- retroplacental mass in 20% to 25% of cases

Do not waste time if fetal distress present or mother unstable

◆ Consumptive Coagulopathy

Most common cause is abruption
- seen in 30% of severe abruption

Hypofibrinogenemia (less than 150 mg/dL)
Increased level of fibrin degradation products
Decrease in other coagulation factors

◆ Renal Failure

Seen in severe form of abruption
Etiology is unclear
- probably from reduced renal perfusion

◆ Management

Close observation
- at least 4 to 6 hours or until signs/symptoms have subsided
  - abruption rare in trauma patients who have no contractions
  - 20% incidence in those with contractions

Fetomaternal hemorrhage
- incidence is low in abruption
  - greatly increased in cases with trauma
  - usually less than 15 mL
    - 300 mg of Rh immune globulin sufficient to prevent sentization in Rh(-) mother

Goals of therapy
- maternal urine greater than 30 mL/hr
- hematocrit greater than 30%

Induction of labor
- evidence or concern regarding maternal or fetal compromise
- greater than 37 weeks gestation
- no placenta previa
- perform vaginal examination and amniotomy
- oxytocin may be useful if labor does not progress

- 48% of patients will deliver vaginally

Cesarean section
- continued bleeding
- fetal distress
- may be dangerous in setting of coagulation defect

Hemorrhagic shock
- blood products
  - 3 units of packed red blood cells available
- wide-bore IV in place
- repeat coagulation test
  - clot formation in red-topped tube
    - should clot within six minutes
- fetal monitoring
  - distress will develop in 60% of patients with moderate abruption

◆ Complications

Excessive bleeding
- clotting defect
  - hypofibrinogenemia, thrombocytopenia
- poor contractile efficiency
  - often seen with couvelaire uterus
  - may require hypogastric artery ligation or hysterectomy
- renal failure
  - avoid hypotension
- pituitary necrosis (Sheehan syndrome)
  - lactation and return of menses indicates pituitary has escaped serious damage
  - consider a follow-up endocrine testing of thyroid and adrenal at 4 to 6 months after severe abruption

CIRCUMVALLATE PLACENTA

Can cause second- or third-trimester bleeding
- bright red, painless, moderate bleeding

Can result in preterm labor
- some increase seen in perinatal mortality (prematurity)

Diagnosis made after delivery of placenta

UTERINE RUPTURE

Very poor outcome for the fetus
- usually dies if extruded into peritoneal cavity

Major causes
- weakness of myometrium secondary to previous surgery
  - cesarean section
  - myomectomy
  - metroplasty

- difficult operative delivery
  - breech extraction
  - difficult forceps
- trauma
  - gunshot wound
  - motor vehicle accident
- inappropriate use of oxytocin

Signs and symptoms
- pain usually precedes tear
  - pain may decrease following rupture
- bleeding may be scant or heavy

Treatment
- repair uterus if possible
- supracervical hysterectomy if defect too extensive

SUMMARY

Bleeding in pregnancy is not normal and should be carefully evaluated

Wide range of etiologies exist and each have specific aspects which distinguish them (Table 27-1)

Good outcomes are possible with prompt, careful treatment

TABLE 27-1. Differential Diagnosis of Bleeding Late in Pregnancy

	Placenta Previa	Marginal Separation	Moderate Abruption	Severe Abruption	Antepartum Rupture of Scarred Uterus
External Bleeding	Mild to severe	Mild	None to moderate	None to severe	None to mild
Pain	None to mild	None to mild	None to moderate	None to severe	None to severe
Myometrial Tone	Normal	Normal	Increased	Hypertonic	Normal to increased
Uterine Tenderness	None	Usually none	Marked, usually diffuse	Marked and diffuse	None to moderate
Fetal Status at First Examination	Alive	Alive	Frequently alive; in jeopardy	Dead or in jeopardy	Dead or in jeopardy
Presentation	High incidence of breech, oblique, transverse	Normal distribution	Normal distribution	Normal distribution	Normal distribution if not extruded
Station of Presenting Part	High	Variable	Variable	Variable	High
Shock	Uncommon	None	Frequent	Usual	Frequent
Coagulopathy	None	None	Occasional	Frequent	Rare
Association With Hypertention	Normal distribution	Normal distribution	Increased	Increased	Normal distribution

28

◆ Malpresentations and Umbilical Cord Complications

BREECH PRESENTATION

Most common obstetric malpresentation (4% of deliveries)
Fetal buttocks present at maternal pelvic inlet

◆ Frank Breech

Fetal hips flexed, knees extended (Fig. 28-1)
Buttocks most dependent
- good dilating wedge
- 60% to 65% of breech presentations: more common at term

◆ Incomplete Breech

One or both hips incompletely flexed
- lower extremity most dependent
  - single footling
  - double footling
Poor dilating wedge
25% to 35% of breech presentations: more common in premature infant

◆ Complete Breech

Fetal hips and knees flexed
Buttocks most dependent
- can convert to incomplete breech in labor
Least common breech presentation (5%)

◆ Terminology

Fetal position described in reference to sacrum
Spontaneous breech delivery: no manual assistance
Assisted breech delivery (partial breech extraction)
- spontaneous delivery to level of umbilicus; then manual assistance
Complete breech extraction

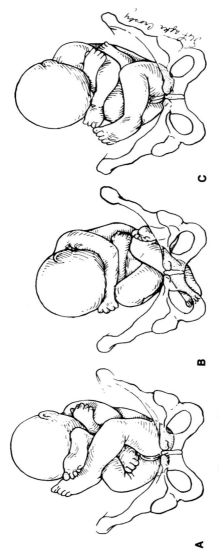

Figure 28-1. Fetal attitude in (A) frank, (B) incomplete, and (C) complete breech presentations.

   • manual assistance by traction on lower extremity before complete delivery of buttocks

◆ Incidence

Clearly associated with birth weight
• 4% overall
• 15% in <2500 g infants
• 30% in 1000 to 1500 g infants
• 40% <1000 g infants
Only 70% of infants with breech presentation are >2500 g

◆ Cause

Many recognized factors (Table 28-1)
Fetal anomalies should be emphasized (Table 28-2)
• 17% in premature infants
• 9% in term
Association with cerebral palsy recognized
• cause and effect may be reversed with cerebral palsy resulting in breech presentation as opposed to traumatic breech delivery resulting in cerebral palsy
No causative factor recognized in 50%

◆ Diagnosis

Leopold's maneuvers
Vaginal examination
Ultrasound

TABLE 28-1. Factors Predisposing to Breech Presentation

Fetal anomalies
　Head anomalies
　　Anencephaly
　　Hydrocephalus
　Chromosomal anomalies
　　Autosomal trisomies
　Multiple anomaly syndromes
Uterine anomalies
　Septate
　Bicornuate
　Unicornuate
Uterine overdistension
　Polyhydramnios
　Multiple gestation
High parity with lax abdominal
　　and uterine musculature
Pelvic obstruction
　Placenta previa
　Myomata
　Other pelvic tumors

TABLE 28-2. Congenital Malformations Among Term Infants in Breech Presentation

Type of Malformation	Incidence (%)
Central nervous system	1.7
Hydrocephalus	0.6
Anencephaly	0.4
Trisomy 21	0.5
Cardiovascular	0.6
Gastrointestinal	0.5
Genitourinary	0.1
Overall	9.0
Overall among term infants who die	50.0

Kaupilla O: Acta Obstet Gynecol Scand 1975;39(Suppl):1

TABLE 28-3. Incidence of Cord Prolapse

Presentation	Incidence (%)
Vertex	0.14
Breech	2.5-3.0
Frank	0.4
Complete	5.0
Incomplete	10.0
Shoulder (transverse lie)	5.0-10.0
Compound	10.0-20.0
Face-brow	Rare

◆ Perinatal Mortality

Much higher in breech presentation (fourfold greater in term; twofold to threefold greater in preterm)
- much of this is unpreventable
  - only one third of perinatal deaths possibly preventable

Head trauma

Musculoskeletal trauma

Cord prolapse with asphyxiation (Table 28-3)
- 0.4% in frank breech
- 5% to 6% in complete breech
- 10% in incomplete breech

◆ Antepartum Management

<32 weeks gestation → expectant management
>32 weeks gestation → schedule close follow-up

External cephalic version
36 weeks nulliparae
38 weeks multiparae

Performed in labor and delivery suite
Consider preprocedure tocolysis
Absolute contraindications
- active labor
- ruptured membranes

Relative contraindications
- engaged presenting part
- estimated fetal weight >4000 g

External cephalic version in cases of previous cesarean section
probably safe

◆ Management of Labor and Delivery

Cesarean delivery does not guarantee atraumatic birth
Universal cesarean delivery may not reduce rate of adverse outcomes

✧ *Term breech presentation*

Under strict selection criteria, this is a safe alternative to cesarean delivery
- more than 60% of term breech infants can be delivered satisfactorily vaginally

✧ *Premature breech*

No randomized prospective data
Retrospective data suggests that cesarean delivery may benefit fetuses <1500 g
Strict adherence to protocol needed

✧ *Incomplete breech*

Incidence of cord prolapse is 10%
Trial of labor still should be considered if other criteria met (Fig. 28-2)

✧ *The primigravida*

No data to suggest that primagravida with breech infants are at higher risk for fetal injury
Multipara also need to be evaluated critically for planned breech delivery

✧ *Extension of the fetal neck*

Hyperextension of the fetal neck (>90 degrees) associated with poor outcomes with vaginal deliveries
Radiographic or ultrasound evaluation of the attitude of the fetal neck is mandatory prior to trial of labor
Arm extended over the normally flexed head should also be delivered by cesarean

◆ Management of Labor

Membranes intact
- defer amniotomy as long as fetal monitoring adequate

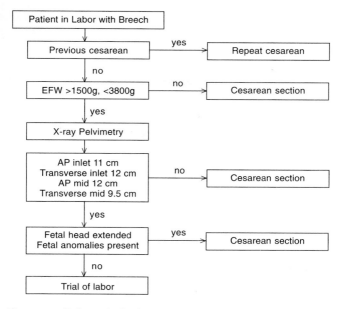

Figure 28-2. Patient selection for trial of labor.

Membranes ruptured
- apply internal monitoring

Progression of labor
- nulliparae 1 cm/hr
- multiparae 1.5 cm/hr

Descent
- should occur with dilation
- failure to descend to below spine at onset of second stage is indication for cesarean delivery

Arrest disorders
- oxytocin should be considered contraindicated

Second stage
- 30 minutes in multiparae
- 1 hour in nulliparae

Anesthesia
- epidural is an excellent choice
- very useful to prevent maternal loss of control

◆ Management of Vaginal Delivery

Obstetrician, anesthesiologist, and pediatrician all should be
present

◇ *Technique*
Fetus delivered spontaneously up to umbilicus
Loop of cord (4 inches) brought down to avoid compression
Legs delivered by flexing knees and sweeping lower extremities
Towel placed around fetal pelvis and gentle downward traction
applied
Fetus delivered up to fetal scapulae
Fetal body rotated so that shoulders are in anteroposterior position
Anterior arm flexed and swept out under symphysis
Fetus rotated 180 degrees to keep breech towards symphysis
Delivery of the head best accomplished with Piper's forceps (Fig.
28-3)
Generous episiotomy should be routine

◆ Presentation with Imminent Breech Delivery

Rapid assessment required
Three points to determine
1. abdominal examination for estimated fetal weight
2. pelvic examination to check for complete dilation
3. ultrasound to determine that fetal neck is not extended

◇ *Indications for emergency cesarean*
Estimated fetal weight >3800 g
Neck extended

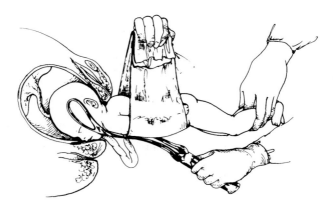

Figure 28-3. Breech delivery is accomplished with Piper forceps applied to
the aftercoming head. Note that the infant's body is being supported
parallel to the floor.

◆ Management of Cesarean Delivery

Abdominal delivery does not guarantee atraumatic birth
Head entrapment by the uterus can occur
- consider low vertical incision for preterm fetus and poorly developed lower segment

Obtain cord pH
- useful index of fetal condition prior to delivery

◆ Practical Considerations

Management of vaginal breech delivery requires skill and patience
Inexperienced obstetricians can best serve their patients by performing cesarean deliveries

FACE PRESENTATION

Fetal neck hyperextended (occiput touches the back)
Presenting part is fetal face between orbital ridges and chin
Incidence 1/550 births

◆ Cause

No identifiable causative factor in approximately 38%
Associated with anencephaly
Nuchal cord is not a cause of face presentation
LGA, SGA infants occur in similar proportion to general population
Possibly an associated with high parity, but 34% occur in primagravida

◆ Diagnosis

Usually made in labor by vaginal examination with confirming ultrasound
- 3% diagnosed antepartum
- 35% diagnosed during first stage labor
- 27% during second stage labor
- 35% at delivery

Position
- 60% mentum anterior
- 15% mentum transverse
- 25% mentum posterior

◆ Mechanism and Course of Labor

Presenting diameter is tracheloparietal (trachelobregmatic), which is 0.7 cm longer
Initial rotation occurs at lower station
- engagement does not occur until face at +2 station

Safe vaginal delivery of mentum posterior impossible
- 35% will rotate to mentum anterior (range up to 50% to 65%)

◇ *Management*

No contraindication to oxytocin

Forceps acceptable

Old adage "if a face is progressing, leave it alone" applies

Heart rate abnormalities increased

- only 14% have normal tracings in labor

BROW PRESENTATION

Fetal head mid-way between flexion and hyperextension

Presenting part is head between orbital ridges and anterior fontanelle

Less common than face presentation (1/1400 deliveries)

◆ **Cause**

Difficult to determine specific causative factors

Cephalopelvic disproportion more commonly associated with brow presentation rather than face presentation

◆ **Diagnosis**

Nearly always made by vaginal examination or ultrasound

◆ **Mechanism and Course of Labor**

Spontaneous conversion to face or vertex (50% or more)

- 30% convert to face
- 20% convert to vertex

Persistent brow presentation

- vaginal delivery impossible

Course of labor similar to face/vertex after conversion

- prolonged in case of persistent brow

◇ *Management*

Same as for face presentation: expectant management

Fetal heart rate abnormalities common

SHOULDER PRESENTATIONS (TRANSVERSE LIE)

Fetal long axis perpendicular to maternal long axis

1/300 births

◆ **Definitions**

Fetal head lies in one maternal iliac fossa; breech lies in the other

One fetal pole in iliac fossa and the other in upper quadrant represents an oblique or unstable lie

◆ **Cause**

High parity with lax abdominal wall and uterine musculature

Prematurity, polyhydramnios
Obstructed pelvis
- previa
- myoma
- ovarian tumor

◆ Diagnosis

Physical examination of maternal abdomen
Very high or unreachable presenting part on vaginal examination
Confirmation by ultrasound

◆ Mechanism of Labor

No known normal mechanism of labor possible

◇ *Management*

Incidence of cord prolapse 10% to 15%
Consider hospital bedrest for patient not at term with cervix
    dilated >3 cm
External version may be considered prior to labor or in early
    labor without ruptured membranes and no fetal part in the
    pelvis
Cesarean delivery required in active labor or in patient with rup-
    tured membranes
Neglected transverse lie is an obstetric emergency

COMPOUND PRESENTATIONS

Fetal extremity prolapsed along presenting part
- most commonly vertex/hand, vertex/arm
Incidence 1/400 to 1/1200

◆ Cause

Most common cause in prematurity
- greatly decreased with increasing fetal weight

◆ Diagnosis

Vaginal examination
At least 50% diagnosed in second stage

◆ Management

Expectant; do not attempt replacement (risk of cord prolapse)
Three outcomes possible
1. prolapsed part withdraws
2. delivery occurs with arm or hand along side of head
3. progression in labor will cease requiring cesarean delivery

Special cases
- vertex/foot should probably be delivered by cesarean
- no role for version and extraction

UMBILICAL CORD COMPLICATIONS

Mean cord length 55 to 60 cm
- related to fetal activity in the first two trimesters

◆ Cord Prolapse

Incidence 0.2% to 0.6%
- 4% to 6% with cords >80 cm

Other causes
- malpresentation 50%
- low birth weight (<2500 g) 30% to 50%
- grand multiparity 10% to 20%
- multiple gestation 10%
- obstetric manipulation (amniotomy) 10% to 15%

Nearly 50% occur during second stage

✧ Diagnosis

Fetal heart rate abnormalities should lead to vaginal examination

✧ Management

Avoid palpation of cord

Prevent compression, Trendelenburg position, or knee-chest position

Prompt delivery within 10 minutes usually leads to perinatal mortality <5%

◆ True Knots

Incidence 0.3% to 2.1%

Associated with antepartum stillbirth

No association with neurologic abnormalities

◆ Nuchal Cord

Incidence 24.6% (21% >one loop; 3.5% >two loops)

Maximal number recorded is nine

No increase in fetal death, neurologic abnormalities, abnormal cord pH

◆ Body Coils of Cord

Incidence 0.5% to 2%

More common with long cords

No increase in low Apgar scores, perinatal mortality, or neonatal morbidity

◆ Cord Entanglement with Monoamniotic Twins

Perinatal mortality approaches 50%

Previously, cesarean delivery was advocated; more recent data suggest vaginal delivery may be attempted after 30 weeks gestation

Induction appropriate at 37 weeks

Antenatal monitoring initiated at 28 weeks

29

◆ Practical Diagnosis and Management of Abnormal Labor

INTRODUCTION

Cesarean birth rate increased from 5.5% in 1970 to 25% in 1987

Dystocia (abnormal labor progress) accounts for one third of all cesarean births, one half of all primary cesarean deliveries

Threat of liability has produced changes in physician behavior without commensurate improvements in quality of intrapartum outcomes

• higher cesarean rate occurs in private patient populations

Increased use of conduction anesthesia may also contribute to operative delivery rates

RISKS FOR DYSTOCIA

Three categories
1. passage (pelvic architecture)
2. passenger (fetal size, presentation, position)
3. powers (of uterine action, cervical resistance)

PELVIC FACTORS

Pelvic cavity can be considered as an open cylinder with a curve to it

Four diameters used to describe the inlet
1. obstetrical conjugate [(AP) diameter]
2. diagonal conjugate
3. transverse diameter
4. oblique diameter

Midpelvis
• AP diameter greater than or equal to 11.5 cm
• intraspinous diameter >10 cm
  • <9 cm, definitely contracted

Outlet
• rare to find outlet contraction without midpelvis contraction

Caldwell-Malloy classification system (Table 29-1)
- 50% or more are gynecoid
- android: one third of Caucasian population, one sixth of non-Caucasian population
  - can present with deep transverse arrest
- anthropoid: 25% Caucasian population, 50% non-Caucasian population
  - sacrum contains six segments as opposed to five
- platypelloid found in 5%
  - head often engages as occiput transverse (OT)

◆ Clinical Pelvimetry

Best performed close to 34 to 36 weeks (See Figs. 29-1 through 29-4)

◆ X-ray Pelvimetry

Current indications
- anticipated vaginal breech delivery
- history of disease or trauma affecting the bony pelvis

FETAL FACTORS

◆ Malposition and Malpresentation

Breech face and brow presentation are discussed in Chapter 28

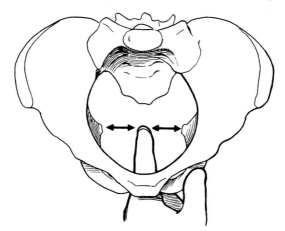

Figure 29-1. Evaluation of the transverse diameter. Lateral motion of the fingers is restricted in a transversely narrowed pelvis. (Steer CM. Moloy's evaluation of the pelvis in obstetrics. 2nd ed. Philadelphia: WB Saunders, 1959.)

TABLE 29-1. Characteristics of the Four Basic Types of Pelves of Average Size

Characteristic	Type of Pelvis			
	Gynecoid	Android	Anthropoid	Platypelloid
Anteroposterior diameter of inlet	11 cm	11 cm	12+ cm	10 cm
Widest transverse diameter of inlet	12 cm	12 cm	<12 cm	12 cm
Forepelvis	Wide	Narrow	Narrow	Wide
Sidewalls	Straight	Convergent	Divergent	Straight
Ischial spines	Not prominent	Prominent	Not prominent	Not prominent
Sacrosciatic notch	Medium	Narrow	Wide	Narrow
Inclination of sacrum	Medium	Forward (lower one third)	Backward	Forward
Subpubic arch	Wide	Narrow	Medium	Wide
Transverse diameter of outlet	10 cm	<10 cm	10 cm	10 cm
Bone structure	Medium	Heavy	Medium	Medium

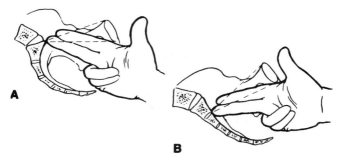

Figure 29-2. Measurement of the diagonal conjugate. (**A**) When the promontory is reached, the index finger marks the undersurface of the symphysis. The distance from this point to the tip of the extended middle finger is the length of the diagonal conjugate; subtracting 1.5 cm is thought to provide the length of the true conjugate. (**B**) The promontory may be difficult to reach in early pregnancy, before the vagina and its supports are relaxed, and in late pregnancy, it may be impossible to reach without disengaging the presenting part. If the head is engaged, this information is not needed. Even if accurately measured, there is great variation in the diagonal conjugate's relation to the true conjugate. Because it is rarely useful and often impossible to determine, this measurement should be discarded from modern obstetric practice. (Steer CM. Moloy's evaluation of the pelvis in obstetrics. 2nd ed. Philadelphia: WB Saunders, 1959.)

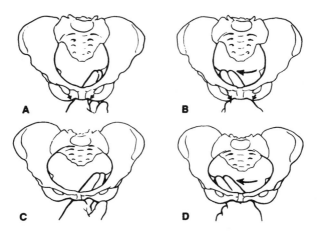

Figure 29-3. Estimation of the width of the subpubic arch and interspinous diameter by the act of pronation. (**A,B**) Transversely narrowed diameters in the mid- and lower pelvis. (**C,D**) Wide transverse diameters in the mid- and lower pelvis. (Steer CM. Moloy's evaluation of the pelvis in obstetrics. 2nd ed. Philadelphia: WB Saunders, 1959.)

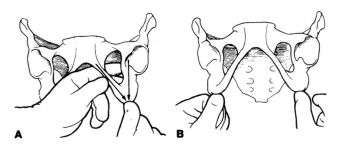

Figure 29-4. Estimation of the intertuberous diameter. (**A**) Identification of the ischial tuberosity at the point of convergence of the pubic rami and pelvic sidewalls. (**B**) Measurement of the intertuberous diameter. (Steer CM. Moloy's evaluation of the pelvis in obstetrics. 2nd ed. Philadelphia: WB Saunders, 1959.)

✧ *Occiput posterior (OP)*
25% prevalence in early labor
10% to 15% prevalence in active labor
Anthropoid pelvis predisposes to OP
Signs in labor
- slow active phase
- increased maternal backache
- ineffective uterine contractions
- persistent anterior cervical lip
- prolonged second stage with gaping anus
- distinctive maternal abdominal contour

Failure to rotate
- regional anesthesia
- poor voluntary effort
- convergent side walls, prominent spine

Delivery options
- spontaneous delivery as OP
- manual or forceps rotation

✧ *Occiput transverse*
Deep transverse arrest caused by constricted pelvis requires cesarean delivery
- attempt forceps rotation if pelvis is adequate

◆ Fetal Anomalies
Hydrocephalus
- cesarean delivery may be planned

Other anomalies may lead to choice of cesarean section in attempt to improve fetal outcome

◆ Fetal Macrosomia

Increased risk for poor outcome
Usually defined as birth weight >4000 or 4500 g
Labor abnormalities
- protracted active phase
- prolonged deceleration phase
- protracted descent

Risk factors
- multiparity
- diabetes
- maternal obesity
- excessive pregnancy weight gain

◆ Shoulder Dystocia

One half of all cases occur in infants <4000 g
Only 16% of cases are easily predicted
Prophylactic cesarean delivery
- consider in diabetic mother >4000 g estimated fetal weight
- infant of nondiabetic >4500 g

Fetal injuries
- Erb's palsy recovery usually 72% to 92% by end of first year
- other injuries
  - diaphragmatic paralysis
  - broken bones

Maternal complications
- postpartum hemorrhage
- lacerations
- hematoma
- uterine rupture

◇ *Management*

McRoberts maneuver
- flexion of maternal thighs against abdominal wall with light superpubic pressure

Woods screw
- posterior shoulder pushed toward infant's chest
- continue until posterior shoulder becomes anterior shoulder

Delivery of posterior arm
- may result in clavicular/hemoral fracture
- usually heals very well

Zavenelli maneuver
- cephalic replacement

◆ Fetal Weight

Use of ultrasound has greatly improved estimation of fetal weight
Still difficult to evaluate at extremes of weight
- prediction of macrosomia
  - 10% to 15% error inherent
    - false positives still represent a problem

◆ Effects of Anesthesia

Epidural anesthesia associated with prolongation of second stage
Initiation of oxytocin significantly shortens second stage of
labor and reduces operative delivery rate

UTERINE FACTORS

◆ Physiology of Labor

Oxytocin released in pulsative intervals during labor
Oxytocin receptors in myometrium and decidua
• receptor concentration probably controls uterine response
• decidual receptors probably stimulate $PGF_2\alpha$ production
Cervical changes occur prior to labor
Uterine fibers arranged circumferentially
• lower segment thin
• upper segment thickens

◆ Uterine Dysfunction

✧ *Uterine activity*

Internal pressure can be measured directly
Average intensity above resting pressure multiplied by number
of contractions in 10 minute interval
Quantification has limited ability to aid in the management of labor

✧ *Functional dystocia*

Associated with two different types of contraction patterns
• hypertonic pattern—oxytocin may help
• hypotonic pattern—frequently responds to oxytocin
Clinically significant factors
• increased second stage duration in women of advanced maternal age
• morbidly obese patients have discordant pattern
Fetal size inversely proportionate to length of labor
Pelvic contraction, fetal malpresentation
Multiple gestation often results in prolonged active phase
Anxiety and fear decrease uterine activity through action of epinephrine

✧ *Drugs and contractility*

Inhibitory factors
• ß-mimetics
• calcium channel blockers
• magnesium sulfate
• antiprostaglandins

PHARMACOLOGIC STIMULATION OF LABOR

Oxytocin is safe and effective when used appropriately
Timing and dosage schedule varies

Typical uses
- arrest of labor
- failure of descent
- prolonged latent phase
- protracted active phase

◆ Cervical Ripening with PGE$_2$

Most successful and widely used agent is cervical PGE$_2$ gel
- associated with dissociating with collagen and increasing glycosaminioglycans, increased fibroblast activity, reduction of stretch modulus

Recent approval of commercial available product (Prepidil)
- improved Bishop's score of unripened cervix
- decreased duration of labor, induction to delivery interval, oxytocin dose, failure of induction rate

Continuous monitoring for 30 minutes prior to and at least 4 hours after gel application
- hold oxytocin dose until 4 hours after last gel

Side effects
- hyperstimulation in 1% of patients
  - treat with magnesium sulfate, terbutaline or ritodrine
- small incidence of nausea, vomiting, fever, shivering

◆ Oxytocin

Steady state reached in 40 to 60 minutes
- in vivo half-life 10 to 15 minutes

Increases in dose of less than 40 minute intervals can result in hyperstimulation
- minimally effective dose is preferable
- 0.5 to 2 mU/minute increase by 1 to 2 mU/minute every 30 minutes

Preterm uterus less sensitive to oxytocin

Pulsed oxytocin delivery offers similar efficacy but less hyperstimulation

◇ *Active management of labor*
Effective at reducing cesarean delivery rates

◇ *Key points*
Nulliparous women
Accurate diagnosis of labor required
Early amniotomy performed
Oxytocin administration
- 6 mU/m
- increase every 15 minutes if dilation less than 1 cm/hour

◇ *Fetal tolerance*
Wide variation of fetal reserve
Change maternal position (left lateral decubitus) in cases of hyperstimulation and fetal distress

- once resolved restart oxytocin at one half of previous rate
- lengthen interval between increases
- pursue close observation

FUNCTIONAL APPROACHES TO LABOR ABNORMALITIES

◆ Labor Graph

Friedman introduced the graphicostatistical method of labor analysis
- chart dilation and station

Vaginal examination is usually recommended every two hours in early labor with examination every hour in active labor

◆ Quantitative Guideline

Definition of abnormal labor (Table 29-2)

◆ Latent Phase

Onset of labor to onset of active phase
Sensitive to analgesia and anesthesia
- may prolong latent phase

May consider treatment with low dose of oxytocin after 12 hours
- 1 to 2 mU/m

◆ Active Phase

✧ *Protracted active phase dilation*

Graphing of labor progress
Complicates 10% to 15% of labors
Cause is uncertain
Increased risk of later dysfunctional patterns
Best treatment option unclear
- consider active management

TABLE 29-2. Dysfunctional Labor Patterns With Diagnostic Criteria for Nulliparous and Multiparous Labor

| | Limits for Abnormality | |
Pattern	Nulliparous Labor	Multiparous Labor
Prolonged latent phase	≥21 h	≥14 h
Protracted active phase of dilatation	<1 cm/h	<1.5 cm/h
Secondary arrest (no change for)	≥2 h	≥2 h
Prolonged deceleration phase	≥3 h	≥1 h
Protracted descent	<1 cmh	<2 cm/h
Arrest of descent (no change for)	≥1 h	≥1/2 h

- careful use of oxytocin
- usually only 8 mU/minute needed
- electronic fetal monitoring should be instituted

✧ *Secondary arrest of dilation*
No change for two hours in active labor
Occurs in 5% to 10% of labors
- more frequent in term labors
Well-recognized association with fetal pelvic disproportion
- however, majority will progress to vaginal delivery
Management
- oxytocin augmentation proven efficacious
- progress should be seen within 2 to 3 hours within initiation of oxytocin

✧ *Deceleration phase*
Third phase of active labor
Engagement should occur at 9 cm for nullipara and at 10 cm for multipara
- failure of engagement may herald a secondary stage abnormality
Incidence of 1% to 3%
- may respond to oxytocin augmentation

◆ Second Stage of Labor
Begins with complete dilation
Median duration
- 1 hour in nullipara
- 1.25 hour in multipara
Clinical limits (not required time to delivery)
- 2 hours in nullipara
- 45 minutes in multipara

✧ *Protracted descent*
May be caused by malposition or mild fetal pelvic disproportion
- also possible relation to conduction anesthesia
Requires adroit management
- oxytocin stimulation in appropriate cases
- abdominal delivery if previous labor had been abnormal
Current management
- fetal monitoring
- low dose oxytocin if otherwise normal labor
- presence of edematous cervical lip significantly reduces chance for vaginal delivery
- rotation from OP to OA
  - manually or with forceps delivery (Scanzoni maneuver)

✧ *Arrest of descent*
In absence of other labor abnormalities it responds well to oxytocin
Cesarean delivery may be indicated if associated with previous abnormal labor

Midpelvic forceps delivery associated with a high incidence of shoulder dystocia

FORCEPS DELIVERY

◆ Preoperative Conditions

✧ *Eight conditions mandatory*
1. cervix fully dilated
2. vertex presentation
3. vertex engaged (station above 0 = high forceps)
4. ruptured membranes
5. position known with certainty
6. no disproportion, consider modified Miller-Hillis maneuver to check for some descent
7. adequate analgesia
8. empty bladder

◆ Choice and Application of Forceps

Classic forceps (Fig. 29-5)
• cephalic and pelvic curves both present

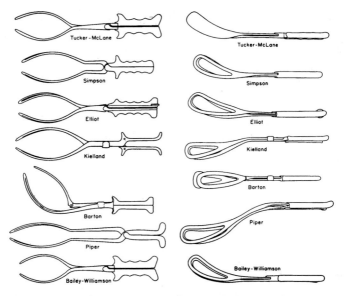

Figure 29-5. Commonly used forceps. (Douglas RG, Stromme WB. Operative obstetrics. New York: Appleton-Century-Crofts, 1957.)

Special forceps
• designed to deal with special problems
Application
• should be applied precisely to occipital middle of the head
Choice of forceps
• OA or OP position
  • Simpson (nulliparous), Elliot (multiparous)
  • Tucker-McLane with Bill's axis traction bar a common choice
• Rotation
  • Kielland (not suited for traction after rotation)
  • Simpson or other classic forceps may also be used

◆ Criteria for Forceps Delivery

Fetal station (defined as −3 to +3 or −5 to +5)
Position of the fetal vertex
Honesty of the clinician and correct documentation
• tendency to misclassify to lower level given medical-legal environment
• redefined by ACOG in 1965 (Table 29-3)
• compared with old classification (Table 29-4)

TABLE 29-3. 1988 American College of Obstetrics and Gynecology Classification of Forcep Deliveries According to Station and Rotation

Outlet	Scalp is or has been visible at the introitus without separating labia; skull has reached pelvic floor; sagittal suture is in the anteroposterior diameter; fetal head is at or on the perineum; rotation ≤45 degrees
Low	Station ≥+2 cm
	With rotation ≤45 degrees
	With rotation >45 degrees
Mid	Station <+2 cm, head engaged
High	Not defined

TABLE 29-4. 1965 American College of Obstetrics and Gynecology Classification of Forcep Deliveries According to Station and Rotation

Outlet	Scalp is or has been visible at the introitus without separating labia; skull has reached pelvic floor; sagittal suture in anteroposterior diameter
Mid	Head engaged, conditions for outlet not met; any rotation; term "low midforceps" disapproved
High	Unengaged

◆ Morbidity Risks of Forceps Deliveries

Risk of midforceps has been described
Outcome should be compared with cesarean outcome as opposed
   to spontaneous delivery or low forceps

✧ *Minimizing the risks*

The key is to know when to quit
Adequate preparation for cesarean should be performed to minimize delay in cases of failed forceps
Other options
* manual rotation
* nonintervention
* vacuum extraction

◆ Vacuum Extraction

Not without complications
* increased rate of retinal hemorrhage compared with forceps
Decreased facial injuries
Low vacuum delivery associated with low maternal morbidity
   and minimal neonatal morbidity

MANAGEMENT RECOMMENDATIONS

Intensive observation with conservative attitude toward intervention is the best choice
Managing labor is an art
* must integrate patient expectations with fetal, maternal, and
   physician distress

30

◆ Cesarean Delivery

INTRODUCTION

Refers to the delivery of a viable fetus through an abdominal incision (laparotomy) and a uterine incision (hysterotomy)

One of the most important operations performed in obstetrics and gynecology
- life saving value to the mother and fetus

Cesarean delivery rate has increased from 5% to 20% in the last 20 years

INDICATIONS

See Table 30-1

TABLE 30-1. Common Indications for Cesarean Delivery

Accepted
Failed induction
Cephalopelvic disproportion
Failure to progress in labor
Proven fetal distress
Placental abruption
Placenta previa
Umbilical cord prolapse
Obstructive benign and malignant tumors
Active genital herpes infection
Abdominal cerclage
Conjoined twins

Controversial (or Selective)
Breech presentation
Repeat cesarean
Immune thrombocytopenia
Severe Rh immunization
Congenital fetal anomalies, major
Cervical carcinoma
Prior vaginal colporrhaphy
Large vulvar condylomata

COMPLICATIONS

25% to 50% complication rate
Maternal mortality 1 to 2/1000
- as many as 25% of maternal deaths related to anesthetic complications

Late complications can occur as well

TYPES OF CESAREAN OPERATIONS

Two major types
1. upper segment (Fig. 30-1)
2. lower segment (Fig. 30-2)

Poor choice of uterine incision type may lead to extension of a low transverse incision

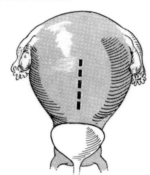

Figure 30-1. Classic incision in the upper segment of the uterus.

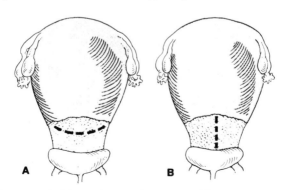

Figure 30-2. Incisions in lower uterine segment. (**A**) Low transverse incision. (**B**) Low vertical incision.

TABLE 30-2. Risk of Uterine Rupture Depending on Scar Location

Previous Uterine Incision	Incidence of Uterine Rupture (%)
Low segment transverse	0.2-2.3
Classic	4.3-8.8
T-shaped incision*	4.3-8.8
Low vertical†	0.5-6.5

*Estimate based on clinical impression.
†Estimate. If scar is truly lower segment, rate is closer to that of the low segment transverse. If scar extends into the upper segment, rate probably approaches that for prior classic incision.

ANESTHESIA

Choice of anesthetic is dictated by several factors (Chapter 7)
Hypotension can result form anesthetic or patient positioning
Induction to delivery time optimally 5 to 15 minutes

◆ Abdominal Incision

Abdominal incision: vertical or Pfannenstiel
Pfannenstiel usually chosen for cosmetic reasons
• transverse uterine incision preferred

◆ Surgical Technique

Abdomen opened in layers
Degree of uterine rotation ascertained
Bladder flap created
Uterine incision made
• extended with scissors or bluntly
Head delivered followed by body
Placenta removed after cord is clamped and cut
Uterus inspected then cleared of debris
Inspection of other organs (tubes, ovaries, appendix)
Closure of fascia

VAGINAL BIRTH AFTER CESAREAN SECTION (VBAC)

◆ Safety

Risks of labor related to risk of scar separation (Table 30-2)
• strongest predictor of safety is location of previous scar
• classical incision has higher rate of rupture
Judicious approach to trial of labor is warranted in all cases

◆ Success of Labor

Varied based on indications for first delivery (Table 30-3)

TABLE 30-3. Incidence of Vaginal Birth After Previous Cesarean Delivery

Indication for Prior Cesarean	Successful Vaginal Delivery (%)
Fetal distress	71-75
Twins	72
Breech	84-88
Failure to progress or dystocia	
Overall	65-68
Latent-phase diagnosis	79
Active-phase diagnosis	61

*Pridjian G. Labor after prior cesarean section. Clin Obstet Gynecol 1992;35:445.

TABLE 30-4. Fetal Meturity Assessment Prior to Elective Repeat Cesarean Delivery*

Fetal heart tones documented for 20 wk by nonelectronic fetoscope or for 30 wk by Doppler

36 wk since a positive serum or urine human chorionic gonadotropin pregnancy test was performed by a reliable laboratory

An ultrasound measurement of the crown-rump length, obtained at 5-11 wk, that supports a gestational age of >39 wk

An ultrasound, obtained at 12-20 wk, that confirms the gestational age of >39 wk determined by clinical history and physical examination

*ACOG Committee Opinion No. 98, September 1991.

Prediction of recurrent dystocia may be aided by use of fetopelvic index
- combines radiographic pelvimetry and fetal ultrasound

◆ Preparation

Evaluation for potential trial of labor should occur early in pregnancy
- global mandates for trial of labor are inappropriate

If elective cesarean section is chosen, fetal maturity should be documented (Table 30-4)

◆ Intrapartum Management

IV access

Blood count and type and screen

NPO

Continuous fetal monitoring

External tocodynamometry, internal monitoring when feasible

Alert anesthesia, obstetric, neonatal personnel

◇ *Oxytocin use*
Optimize uterine contractions, avoid hyperstimulation
Timely diagnosis and management of dystocia is necessary

◇ *Uterine rupture*
Abnormal fetal heart rate in 50% to 70%
Uterine pain, vaginal bleeding in many
Gross hematuria, loss of contraction, recession of presenting part has been described

◇ *Scar palpation*
Routine palpation after vaginal delivery is controversial
Mandatory assessment in cases of excessive bleeding or hypovolemia
Recurrence
- lower section rupture 6.4% recurrence
  - upper section rupture 32% recurrence
  - sterilization may be appropriate

31

◆ Care of the Critically Ill Obstetric Patient

HYPOVOLEMIC SHOCK

Hemorrhage remains a major cause of maternal mortality
Average blood loss
- 500 mL at vaginal delivery
- 1000 mL at cesarean section

Fetus serves as a "miner's canary"
- can see fetal distress in absence of maternal hypoperfusion
- significant shock never seen in presence of reassuring fetal heart rate

◆ Two Goals of Management

1. restore circulating blood volume
2. eliminate source of hemorrhage

Blood products
- improve tissue oxygenation/perfusion
- can result in depletion of labile clotting factors
- give fresh frozen plasma if fibrinogen <100 mg/dL or increased PT/PTT

Platelets
- one unit raises count by 8000 to 10,000/mm^3
- consider in bleeding patient with count less than 50,000/mm^3

SEPTIC SHOCK

Accompanies up to 15% of bacteremias with gram-negative organisms
- 5% of those with gram-positive organisms
- Mortality rate 25% to 50%

Pregnancy may predispose to septic shock
- septic abortion
- chorioamnionitis
- pyelonephritis
- endometritis

◆ Etiology

Endotoxin-releasing gram-negative coliform bacteria
- complex cell wall associated lipopolysaccharide
- activates lymphocytic T cells, mast cells

◆ Early Septic Shock

Classic example of distributive shock
- hypotension, fever, chills
- increased SVR, high normal or elevated cardiac output
- eventually increased arteriovenous shunting

Treatment
- optimize preload
  - crystalloid infusion
- treat infection
  - broad-spectrum antibiotics
  - drain abscess

◆ Progressive Septic Shock

Primary importance
- myocardial dysfunction, ventricular failure
- direct effect of myocardial depressant in sera
- prognosis grave in cases of severely depressed cardiac output

Treatment
- if still hypotensive after preload manipulation, begin dopamine
  - 5 μg/kg/min improves renal blood flow
  - 5 to 30 μg/kg/min causes positive inotropic effect
  - greater than 30 μg/kg/min α-adrenergic vasoconstriction
- capillary injury may lead to lung injury and ARDS
  - major cause of death in patients with septic shock
- acute tubular necrosis (ATN) and disseminated intravascular coagulation (DIC) can also be seen

FETAL RESPONSE TO MATERNAL HEMODYNAMIC INSTABILITY

Fetal well-being depends on maintenance of maternal oxygenation
- no fall in fetal PO_2 as long as maternal $PO_2 > 60$
- fetus operates on steep portion of 0_2 dissociation curve
- further decreases may have significant fetal effects
- maternal oxygen administration may increase fetal oxygen saturation

◆ Uterine Perfusion

500 mL/min near term
- 10% of cardiac output

Little capacity for autoregulation
- maternal blood pressure maintained at expense of uterine flow

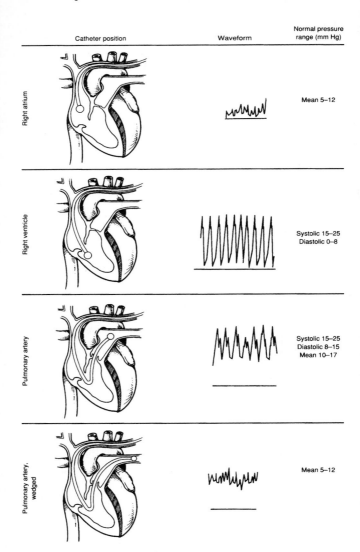

	Catheter position	Waveform	Normal pressure range (mm Hg)
Right atrium			Mean 5–12
Right ventricle			Systolic 15–25 Diastolic 0–8
Pulmonary artery			Systolic 15–25 Diastolic 8–15 Mean 10–17
Pulmonary artery, wedged			Mean 5–12

Figure 31-1. Pulmonary artery catheter placement. Catheter position, corresponding waveforms, and pressures are shown. (Clark SL, Phelan JP. Critical care obstetrics. 2nd ed. Boston: Blackwell Scientific, 1990:67.)

TABLE 31-1. Derived Hemodynamic Parameters

Parameter	Derivation	Normal Nonpregnant Range
Stroke volume index	$\dfrac{CO}{(HR)(BSA)}$	34-45 ml/beat/m^2
Mean arterial pressure	$\dfrac{(Systolic) + 2 \, (diastolic)}{3}$	85-95mm Hg
Systemic vascular resistance	$\dfrac{(MAP - CVP)}{CO} \times 79.9$	900–1200 dynes-sec-cm^{-5}
Pulmonary vascular resistance	$\dfrac{MPAP - PCWP}{CO} \times 79.9$	150–250 dynes-sec-cm^{-5}
Left ventricular stroke work index	$SVI \times (MAP - PCWP) \times 0.0136$	51-61 g-m-M^{-2}

CO, cardiac output; BSA, body surface area; CVP, central venous pressure; HR, heart rate; MAP, mean arterial pressure; MPAP, mean pulmonary artery pressure; PCWP, pulmonary capillary wedge pressure; SVI, stroke volume index.

INVASIVE HEMODYNAMIC MONITORING

Pulmonary artery catheter
- introduced in early 1970s
- important role in managing critically ill patients
- multilumen catheter
- placement confirmed by characteristic pressures and wave forms (Fig. 31-1)
  - lumens should terminate in
    - pulmonary artery
    - superior vena cava or right atrium

Measurement of parameters allows calculation of hemodynamic indices (Table 31-1)

◆ Determinants of Cardiac Output

◇ *Preload*

Volume or pressure generated with ventricles at end diastole

Starling's Law
- ventricular output is directly proportional to ventricular preload

Right ventricular preload = CVP

Left ventricular preload = PCWP
- more clinically useful
- use of CVP pressures presumes equal preload on right and left sides of heart

◇ *Afterload*

Resistance to blood flow during ventricular systole

Calculated as systemic vascular resistance (SVR)

Markedly influenced by preeclampsia and septic shock

◇ *Ventricular stroke work index*

Also a calculated parameter

Assessed on modified Starling Curve

Allows assessment of myocardial function and guides therapy

◆ Indications

Similar indications in pregnancy to all of critical care medicine
- severe cardiac disease
- septic shock
- hemodynamically unstable patients with uncertain volume status
- severe preeclampsia
  - unresponsive to conventional antihypertensive therapy
  - pulmonary edema
  - persistent oliguria
- rarely indicated in obstetric hemorrhage

Normal values well defined (Table 31-2)

DIC ASSOCIATED WITH PREGNANCY

Not a distinct clinical entity
End point of many disease processes (Fig. 31-2)

◆ Pathophysiology

Release of tissue thromboplastin or endothelial disruption
Clotting via intrinsic or extrinsic pathways
Consumption of clotting factors
Destruction of platelets

◆ Diagnosis

Clinically suspected by excessive bleeding from surgical incision or postpartum uterus
• in severe cases, bleeding from IV sites and mucus membranes
Laboratory values variable
• PT/PTT insensitive
  • not prolonged until 40% to 50% of factors consumed
• fibrinolytic split products
  • normal in 10% to 15% with acute DIC

◆ Causes

Most common are placental abruption and dead fetus syndrome

TABLE 31-2. Central Hemodynamic Changes

Parameter	Nonpregnant	Pregnant
Cardiac output (L/min)	4.3 ± 0.9	6.2 ± 1.0
Heart rate (beats/min)	71 ± 10.0	83 ± 10.0
Systemic vascular resistance (dyne-cm-sec-5)	1530 ± 520	1210 ± 266
Pulmonary vascular resistance (syne-cm-sec-5)	119 ± 47.0	78 ± 22
Colloid oncotic pressure (mm Hg)	20.8 ± 1.0	18.0 ± 1.5
Colloid oncotic pressure-pulmonary capillary wedge pressure (mm Hg)	14.5 ± 2.5	10.5 ± 2.7
Mean arterial pressure (mm Hg)	86.4 ± 7.5	90.3 ± 5.8
Pulmonary capillary wedge pressure (mm Hg)	6.3 ± 2.1	7.5 ± 1.8
Central venous pressure (mm Hg)	3.7 ± 2.6	3.6 ± 2.5
Left ventricular stroke work index (g-m-m^{-2})	41 ± 8	48 ± 6

Clark SL, Cotton DB, Lee W, et al. Central hemodynamic assessment of normal term pregnancy. Am J Obstet Gynecol 1989;161:1431.

Amniotic fluid embolism (AFE)
• associated with DIC in 40% of cases
Rarely severe preeclampsia
Septic shock, transfusion disorders

◆ Management

Correction of underlying pathophysiologic process
• usually self-limiting in abruption, dead fetus syndrome, or AFE
• resolution begins with delivery of fetus and placenta
Prevent clinical hemorrhage in short term while delivery is accomplished
• replacement of clotting factors
• fresh frozen plasma
• platelet transfusion
• heparin (5000 units sq BID) may be useful in dead fetus syndrome

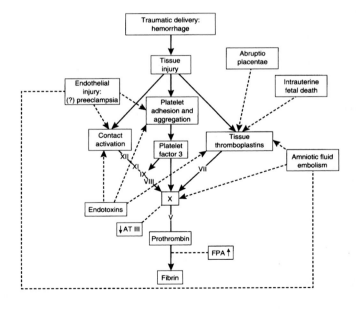

Figure 31-2. Obstetric disorders that initiate disseminated intravascular coagulation. (Clark SL, Phelan JP. Critical care obstetrics. 2nd ed. Boston: Blackwell Scientific, 1990:182.)

BLOOD TRANSFUSION

Indications
- restoration of circulating volume
- improvement of oxygen transport
- correction of coagulation disorders

Incidence
- less than 1% of vaginal deliveries
- 2% to 12% of cesarean deliveries

Type and screen
- ABO and Rh(D) type determined
- 99.99% effective in preventing incompatible transfusions
- less costly than type and cross

◆ Whole Blood

Unit of whole blood contains 450 mL of blood
One unit raises hematocrit by 3% to 4%
Clotting factors maintained during storage
- factor V and VII may be reduced
Red blood cells plus component therapy preferred

◆ Red Blood Cells

Separated from plasma by centrifugation or sedimentation
Hematocrit of 70% to 75%
Same number of erythrocytes as unit of whole blood

◆ Platelets

Prepared from whole blood by centrifugation
Donor plasma must be ABO compatible with recipient
One unit raises count 8000 to 10,000/mm^3
- available in packs of 8 to 10 units
Transfusion indications controversial
- <10,000/mm^3 in nonbleeding patients
- <50,000/mm^3 in bleeding or surgical patients

◆ Fresh Frozen Plasma (FFP)

Contains all soluble clotting factors (similar to whole blood)
Significant amounts of factor V and VIII
One unit = 250 mL
Indications
- consumption or dilution coagulopathy
- bleeding patient with fibrinogen less than 10 mg/dL and prolonged PT/PTT

◆ Cryoprecipitate

Prepared by thawing one unit FFP, removing supernatant plasma, and refreezing precipitate

Contains factors VIII, VIIIc, von Willebrand factor, fibrinogen, fibronectin

Sole advantage over FFP
- large amount of factors in small volume

◆ Transfusion Reactions

Acute reaction delayed in 7%

Signs and symptoms
- lumbar pain
- facial flushing
- chest pain
- fever, tachycardia
- hypotension
- shock
- DIC (acute tubular necrosis, ARDS)

Laboratory values
- decrease in plasma haptoglobin
- increase in free serum hemoglobin
- hemoglobinuria if plasma level is greater than 25 mg/dL

✧ *Management of hemolytic transfusion reactions*

Goals of therapy
- maintain blood pressure
- avoid respiratory failure or acute tubular necrosis

Stop transfusion

Maintain IV with normal saline

Pressors as needed

Oxygen and assisted ventilation as necessary

Maintain urine output
- mannitol 20 to 25 mg IV over 5 minutes
  - repeat up to four times in 24 hours

Send transfused blood to blood bank for analysis

Check recipient plasma for hemolysis

ARDS

Primary lung epithelial injury
- airways or capillary injury

Physiologic criteria (Table 31-3)
- increased capillary permeability
- loss of lung volume
- arterial hypoxemia

Final common pathway of alveolar, epithelial, or endothelial injury

---

**TABLE 31-3. Physiologic Criteria for Adult Respiratory
Distress Syndrome**

Po_2 <50 with $F10_2$ >0.6
Pulmonary capillary wedge ≤12 mm Hg
Total respiratory compliance <50 mL/cm (usually 20-30 mL/cm)
Functional residual capacity reduced
Shunt (Q_s/Q_t) >30%
Dead space (V_D/V_t) > 60%
Alveolar-arterial gradient on 100% oxygen ≥ 350 mm Hg

$F10_2$, fraction of inspired oxygen; Po_2, partial pressure of oxygen: Q_s, blood flow
to nonventilated areas; Q_t total blood flow to both ventilated and nonventilated
areas; VD, dead space volume; V_T, tidal volume.

Clark SL, Cotton DB, Hankins GDV, Phelan JB, eds. Critical care obstetrics. 2nd
ed. Boston; Blackwell Scientific, 1991:342.

◆ Clinical Management

Four considerations essential
1. oxygen delivery and tissue extraction
2. pulmonary compliance
3. intrapulmonary shunt fraction
4. eradication of underlying cause

✧ *Oxygen delivery/tissue extraction*
Maintain CO_2, correct anemia
Maintain CO_2, 60 to 79 mm Hg
Avoid drop in body temperature
Correct respiratory alkalosis

✧ *Pulmonary compliance*
Calculate by ventilatory parameters
PEEP may have positive effect

✧ *Intrapulmonary shunting*
Normal shunt 2% to 5%
Greater than 25% suggests ARDS
Arterial oxygen pressure should be greater than 500 mm Hg in
   intubated patient on 100% oxygen
• less than 300 mm Hg suggests severe shunting
Underlying Cause
• while searching for underlying cause and correction early
   intubation essential (Table 31-4)

◆ Mortality

Adults still have greater than 50% mortality rates despite optimal
   management

TABLE 31-4. Guidelines for Instituting Ventilator Therapy

	Normal	Intubate
Respiratory rate	12-20	>35
Vital capacity (mL/kg)	65-75	<15
FEV_1 (mL/kg)	50-60	<10
Inspiratory force (cm H_2O)	75-100	<25
Pao_2 (mm Hg)	100-75 air	<70 mask 0.4
		<300 $F1O_2$
$Paco_2$ (mm Hg)	35-45	>55
V_D/V_T	0.25-0.40	>0.6

FEV_1, forced expiratory volume in 1 second; $F1O_2$, forced inspiratory oxygen concentration; $Paco_2$, arterial carbon dioxide pressure: P_aO_2, arterial oxygen pressure: VD/VT, ratio of dead space volume to tial volume.

Clark SL, Cotton DB, Hankins GDV, Phelan JB, eds. Critical care obstetrics. 2nd ed. Boston; Blackwell Scientific, 1991:357.

AMNIOTIC FLUID EMBOLISM

Uncommon
Mortality as high as 80%
Sudden release of amniotic fluid or fetal debris into maternal venous circulation
Most common presentation
- sudden dyspnea
- hypotension
- cardiorespiratory arrest
- 10% to 20% seizure activity
- 70% chest x-rays reveal some degree of pulmonary edema
- 50% die within 1 hour
- 40% to 50% with hemorrhagic phase
Most cases occur during labor
- abruption present in up to 50% of cases
Etiology unclear
- possible biphasic model of hemodynamic injury (Fig. 31-3)
- may be result of altered release of endogenous substances in susceptible women
- recurrence in survivors has not been documented

◆ Differential Diagnosis

Septic shock
Aspiration pneumonitis
Acute MI
Pulmonary embolism
Placental abruption (coagulopathy)

Treatment

Maintain oxygenation
Support cardiac output
- rapid infusion of crystalloid
- dopamine as needed
Pulmonary artery catheterization
Resolution of coagulopathy
Blood component therapy

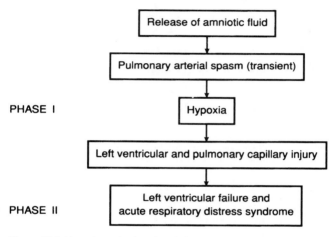

Figure 31-3. Hemodynamic alterations in human amniotic fluid embolism. Phase I is resolved within 30 minutes of the acute event, whereas phase II has been documented 1 or more hours after presumed embolization. (Clark SL, Phelan JP Critical care obstetrics. 2nd ed. Boston: Blackwell Scientific, 1990:400.)

32

◆ Gynecologic History, Examination, and Diagnostic Procedures

PHYSICIAN-PATIENT RELATIONSHIP

◆ Patient Motivation and Comfort

Physician needs to determine the unstated fears and concerns of a patient

An understanding attitude and a matter-of-fact approach are reassuring

Physician demeanor is crucial
- mood should not necessarily be somber
- adjusts to the patients attitude and personality

Avoid vague and superficial responses

✧ *Five ways to reduce patient anxiety*
1. attain history with the patient fully dressed and in a comfortable and private setting
2. initial points of the interview should cover neutral and nonmedical subjects
3. physician should not make assumptions about the patient's background (e.g., sexual preference)
4. schedule an appropriate length of time
5. the patient should feel like an equal partner in the decision-making process

◆ Psychosocial Reactions to Disease

✧ *Disease*
Refers to a pathophysiologic condition often associated with objective anatomic deformities

✧ *Illness*
Refers to subjective distress a person experiences as a result of a real or perceived disease

✧ *Different patients perceive diseases in different ways*
Loss
Punishment
Gain

Relief

Challenge

✳ *Disease as a loss*

Can be real or symbolic

Depression often occurs from sense of loss of self-worth

Patients often cope with grief and depression poorly

- withdrawal
- hostile confrontation
- helpless attention seeking
- noncompliance
- suicide

✳ *Disease as a punishment*

Patients may regard disease as a just or unjust punishment for real or imaginary transgressions

If judged as a just punishment

- acceptance and surrender are usual responses

If judged as unjust punishment

- anger and bitterness
- paranoia, hostility, litigious behavior

✳ *Disease as a threat*

Likely to view disease with anxiety, fear, or anger

May become angry, hostile, or paranoid

✳ *Disease as gain or relief*

Often unconscious rationalization

May be noncompliant with treatment

A physician may feel helpless and ineffectual

✳ *Disease as a challenge*

Patient approaches disease in a rational and flexible way

Aggressively seeks medical care

Educates herself and complies with treatment

This view should be encouraged

◆ Factors That Influence Reactions to Disease

◇ *Four major factors influence psychologic reaction to disease*

1. intrapersonal
2. interpersonal
3. disease related
4. socioeconomic

◇ *Coping with disease*

Two major cognitive coping styles

1. minimization
2. vigilant focusing

Three behavior coping styles

1. actively dealing
2. denial
3. submission

◆ Principles of Effective Communication

Establish a good relationship
- empathy
- respect
- warmth
- genuineness, caring

✧ *Effective communicating style*
Maintain eye contact
Have a relaxed and open posture
Face and lean towards the patient
Show facial expression consistent with the patient's emotion
Have a modulated nonmechanical speaking tone

PATIENT HISTORY

◆ Overview

History is perhaps the most important part of the gynecologic examination
Office chart is a legal document

✧ *Major parts of the history*
Presenting complaint
Gynecologic and menstrual history
Obstetric history
Medical history
Surgical history
Review of systems
Social history
Family history

✧ *Presenting complaint*
Open-ended questions are usually best
Patient should describe the problem in her own words

✧ *Menstrual history*
Cycle length, symptoms, changes
PMS symptoms
Sexual history
- screening history unless this is the chief problem
- begin with nonthreatening questions such as, "Are you having any sexual problems?"
Sexually transmitted diseases

✧ *General medical history*
Genetic disorders
Endocrine and metabolic diseases
Cardiovascular disorders
Hematologic disorders
Renal disease
Neurologic disorders

Genitourinary disorders
Gastrointestinal disorders
Social factors/habits

PHYSICAL EXAMINATION

Should be part of initial evaluation of all patients
Presence of a female nurse or aid should be routine
Psychologic support for the patient
Medical/legal implications
General aspects
- general appearance
- nutritional state
- skin and hair
- head and neck
- eye examination
- otoscopy
- posterior cervical and supraclavicular nodes
- thyroid

Cardiopulmonary System
- cardiac disease is important in reproductive health
- presence of clicks, rubs, or murmurs
- pulmonary disease
- wheezes, rubs, etc.

Breast Examination
- detailed examination very important to the gynecologist (see Chapter 38)

Abdominal Examination
- knees elevated and flexed
- check for masses, ascites, inguinal nodes

Extremities
- edema or varicosities
- peripheral pulses

◆ Pelvic Examination

◇ *Patient preparation*
Dorsal lithotomy position
Head elevated to allow eye contact
Empty bladder

◇ *External genitalia*
Inspect vulva
Spread labia and examine hymen and clitoris
Palpitation of Bartholin gland, urethra, and labia
Patient should strain and relax to determine presence and degree of prolapse

◇ *Vaginal examination*
Inspection with the aid of speculum
Insert warm speculum lubricated with water

Oblique orientation

Assess discharge, erosion, and possible tumors

✧ *Bimanual examination*

Systematic sequence of examination steps (Fig. 32-1, a to e)

Key to examination is careful directed evaluation of the uterus and adnexal

Rectovaginal examination is important

　Confirmation of bimanual examination

　Checking for gastrointestinal tract lesions

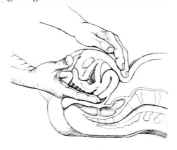

Figure 32-1-a. Bimanual examination, first step. The vaginal fingers feel the consistency and symmetry of the cervix and its axis in relation to the axis of the vagina. They then elevate the uterus toward the abdominal wall, so the total length of the uterus can be determined. (Duncan AS. In: Bourne A, ed. British gynaecological practice. Philadelphia: FA Davis, 1955. Figure drawn by G. McHugh.)

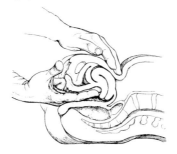

Figure 32-1-b. Bimanual examination, second step. The vaginal fingers are moved into the anterior fornix to permit palpation of the uterine corpus. If the abdominal wall is thin and well relaxed, it is possible to define even minor irregularities in the contour or consistency of the uterus. Third step: with the vaginal fingers still in the anterior fornix and with the aid of the abdominal hand, the uterus is moved gently toward a retroverted position and then from side to side to determine its mobility and the presence or absence of pain on movement of the uterus. (Duncan AS. In: Bourne A, ed. British gynaecological practice. Philadelphia: FA Davis, 1955. Figure drawn by G. McHugh.)

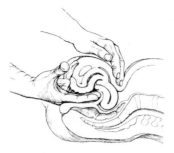

Figure 32-1-c. If the fingertips of the abdominal and vaginal hands come together when carrying out the second step of the bimanual examination, it can be concluded that the uterus is retroverted; the vaginal fingers are then moved to the posterior fornix to outline symmetry, consistency, and mobility of the retroverted corpus. (Duncan AS. In: Bourne A, ed. British gynaecological practice. Philadelphia: FA Davis, 1955. Figure drawn by G. McHugh.)

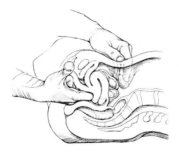

Figure 32-1-d. Bimanual examination, fourth step. To outline the adnexia, the vaginal fingers are moved to the right fornix, fingers together at a point presumed to be superior to the fallopian tube and ovary. (Duncan AS. In: Bourne A, ed. British gynaecological practice. Philadelphia: FA Davis, 1955. Figure drawn by G. McHugh.)

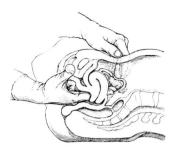

Figure 32-1-e. Bimanual examination, fifth step. When the fingers of the abdominal and vaginal hands are quite close together (it is desirable but not always possible to approximate these fingers), they are then moved gently toward the examiner so the adnexa slip between the fingers as they can be outlined. (Duncan AS. In: Bourne A, ed. British gynaecological practice. Philadelphia: FA Davis, 1955. Figure drawn by G. McHugh.)

✧ *Recording the findings*

I. Perineum
    A. old lacerations
    B. lacerations

II. External genitalia
    A. stage of development
    B. color
    C. evidence of lesions
    D. Bartholin glands

III. Vestibule
    A. Skene glands
    B. urethral orifice
    C. hymenal ring

IV. Vagina
    A. presence of leukorrhea
    B. color
    C. lesions
    D. tone
    E. rugae

V. Cervix
    A. shape
    B. consistency
    C. mobility
    D. state of parity
    E. lesions

VI. Uterus
    A. position
    B. mobility
    C. size
    D. shape
    E. consistency

VII. Adnexa
- A. position and mobility of ovaries and tubes
- B. presence of masses or tenderness

VII. Rectovaginal examination
- A. degree of confirmation of previous findings
- B. statement about additional pathology

IX. Rectal examination
- A. occult blood

DIAGNOSTIC PROCEDURES

◆ Pap Smear

Described in detail in Chapter 48
Should be performed annually
- young women
- women with previous hysterectomy for cervical carcinoma

Other intervals to be determined by physician discretion after three normal examinations

◆ Colposcopy

Described in detail in Chapter 48

◆ Endometrial Sampling

Obtain informed consent first
Rule out pregnancy
Determine size and position of uterus
Clean cervix and upper vagina with Betadine
- tenaculum may be needed to straighten uterus

Local anesthetic should be applied before tenaculum application
Insert biopsy instrument to the fundus
- sounding first is unnecessary

Vasovagal syncope can occur
- treat with atropine

Bleeding complications are rare

◆ Vulvar Biopsy

Colposcopy is a useful adjunct
Always infiltrate with local anesthetic
Use 3 to 4 mm Keyes punch biopsy
Control bleeding with Monsel solution or silver nitrate sticks

◆ Ovulation Detection

Basal body temperature charting
Serial ultrasound examinations have now become more popular
Home urinary LH kits predict ovulation 1 day in advance

◆ Office Hysteroscopy

Quick and simple procedure

Perform early in cycle to avoid disrupting pregnancy or encountering menstrual flow

Paracervical block usually very effective

Flexible CO_2 hysteroscope may not require placement of tenaculum

◆ Transvaginal Ultrasonography

May enhance and extend the pelvic examination

Provides objective information

Can help in the following situations:

- pelvic mass
- monitoring follicular growth in ovulation induction
- diagnosis and sizing of leiomyomata
- differentiating ectopic from intrauterine pregnancy
- evaluating pelvic inflammatory disease (abscess)
- evaluating endometrium in patient with abnormal bleeding

33

◆ Puberty and Pediatric and Adolescent Gynecology

INTRODUCTION

Puberty is the period between childhood and the adult state
Characterized by profound somatic changes
- development of secondary sexual characteristics
- acceleration of linear growth
- bone maturation
- changes in body composition

◆ Somatic Development

Secondary sexual characteristics
- described by Tanner (see Fig. 3-4 and Fig. 3-5 in Chapter 3)
- influenced by genetic and nutritional state
- breast development (thelarche)
  - usually the first external manifestation of puberty
  - pubic hair development can reach stage 3 or 4 before breast development
  - estrogen: duct growth
  - progesterone: lobuloalveolar development
  - prolactin: lactation
- pubic and axillary hair (adrenarche)
  - under influence of adrenal androgens
  - normal development requires passage through each stage
  - axillary hair development usually begins at breast development stage 3 or 4
- genital changes
  - prepubertal labia and vulvar membrane is bright red
  - epithelial layer is thin
  - early signs of estrogen stimulation
    - thickening of labia minora epithelium
    - presence of mucoid vaginal secretion
    - change in coloration from red to pink
- puberty usually occurs between 8.5 and 13 years-of-age
  - <7.5 years-of-age: precocious
  - >14 years-of-age: delayed

- interval from first manifestation to completion is 1.5 years to 6 years
- timing of events
  - menarche usually occurs during breast development stage 3 or 4
  - breast development reaches mature stage between 11.8 and 18.9 years-of-age
  - interval from first sign of puberty (usually breast development stage 2) to menarche is 2.3 years (range, 6 months to 5.75 years)
  - mean age of menarche is 12.3 years to 12.8 years
- acceleration of linear growth
  - occurs early in puberty in girls
    - usually breast development stage 2 or 3
  - peak growth spurt before menarche
  - 25 cm of growth during spurt
  - sex steroids and growth hormone play important roles
- body composition
  - lean body mass, skeletal mass, and body fat mass are equal in prepubertal children
  - men have 1.5 times the lean body mass, muscle mass, and skeletal mass of women
  - women have 2 times the body fat of men

GYNECOLOGIC EXAMINATION OF INFANTS, CHILDREN, AND YOUNG ADOLESCENTS

Ability to establish trust is crucial for successful examination
Examine child in comfortable position
- on mother's lap
- frog-legged on table
- mother and child together on table
- knee-chest
  - requires significant cooperation
Anatomic parameters different than sexually mature woman
- vaginal mucosa thin, bright red
- hymeneal opening changes little until puberty
- cul-de-sac shallow
- posterior fornix short
- uterus parallel to long axis of body
  - total length 2 to 3 cm
  - two thirds is cervix
- rectal examination may be more useful
- vaginal examination is best performed with vaginascope

CONGENITAL ANOMALIES

Often unrecognized until adolescence

◆ Hymenal Anomalies

Typically isolated occurrences
Imperforate hymen
- recurrent pelvic pain
- bulging hymen
- hematocolpos
- correct surgically with cruciate incision

Cribriform hymen
- often presents with difficulty on tampon insertion
- correct by opening still intact hymen

VAGINAL ANOMALIES

Congenital absence usually presents with primary amenorrhea
Uterus usually also absent
Evaluate by rectal examination and sonography

✧ *Uterus absent*

- check chromosomes
- check testosterone level

Mayer-Rokitansky-Küster-Hauser Syndrome
- normal testosterone, normal karyotype
- congenital absence of Müllerian system
- perform IVP to screen for renal anomalies
- lengthen vagina (surgical or nonsurgical methods)

Androgen insensitivity syndrome (testicular feminization)
- male karyotype
- male levels of testosterone
- remove intraabdominal testes after puberty
- defect is at receptor levels

✧ *Uterus present*

Transverse vaginal septum
- can occur at any level
- primary amenorrhea or cyclic pelvic pain
- frequently found at junction of upper two thirds of vagina
- surgical correction with simple excision and reanastomosis
- more extensive septum may require split-thickness skin graft

Longitudinal vaginal septum
- often occurs in association with coital difficulties
- can present with menstrual bleeding around tampon placed on one side of septum
- usually simple surgical excision
- evaluate for obstructive lesion
  - may predispose to endometriosis
- evaluate with pelvic examination, ultrasound, IVP, and possibly HSG

GYNECOLOGIC DISORDERS IN PREMENARCHAL CHILDREN

◆ Vaginal Discharge

Vulvovaginitis is most common gynecologic complaint of children
* hypoestrogenic state makes them more susceptible

Perform Gram stain, wet prep, and appropriate cultures

Many causes
* physiologic discharge prior to menses (no inflammation present)
* poor hygiene
  * coliform bacteria
  * more common in obese children
  * therapy
  * vulvar hygiene
  * remove chemical irritants (soap)
  * local or systemic antibiotics as indicated
  * topical steroids
  * topical estrogen (short course)
* foreign body
  * commonly toilet paper or toy
  * treatment is vaginoscopy with copious lavage
* sexual abuse
  * perform cultures
  * gonorrhea produces severe local inflammation
  * chlamydia, HSV, trichomonas, and syphilis raise issue of sexual abuse
* pin worm (enterobius vermicularis)
  * vaginitis associated with perianal pruritis
  * diagnosis by cellophane tape test
* lichen sclerosus
  * uncommon in children
  * avoid use of topical testosterone
* labial adhesions
  * may be associated with vulvovaginitis
  * apply estrogen cream for 1 to 2 weeks

◆ Bleeding

Can be associated with vulvovaginitis or foreign bodies

Trauma

Dystrophic vulvar lesions

Vaginal or cervical adenocarcinoma or sarcoma botyoides

Urethral prolapse
* treat with local estrogen or excision (rarely)

Multiple endocrine causes
* exogenous hormones
* precocious puberty
* gonadotropins
* thyroid function

- estradiol levels
  - steroid secreting ovarian neoplasm

◆ Genital Injuries

Straddle injuries common
Small hematomas
- ice pack
Larger hematomas
- incise and drain under anesthetic
- may require packing
- careful inspection needed to rule out penetration injury

◆ Genital Neoplasm

Rare in children
DES daughters are an increasingly rare exception
- 80% incidence of vaginal or cervical adenosis
- clear cell adenocarcinoma rare
- DES no longer used in pregnancy so incidence is now very low
Benign vaginal and vulvar tumors
- retention cysts
- Gartner duct cysts
- no treatment unless very large
Botyoid sarcoma
- mesenchymal tumor
- most common in children <3 years-of-age
- chemotherapy and radical excision (50% cure rate)
Ovarian tumors
- abdominal mass or pain
- dermoid most common

DISORDERS OF SEXUAL MATURATION

◆ Accelerated Maturation

Less than 7.5 years-of-age, premature
Premature pseudopuberty
- exogenous estrogens
- estrogen-secreting neoplasm
- not dependent on gonadotropin secretion
- exogenous GnRH agonist ineffective
Precocious puberty
- can be either pituitary-dependent or pituitary-independent
- GnRH agonist useful in cases of pituitary dependent
- most common is pituitary-dependent idiopathic (constitutional) puberty
- need to consider CNS lesions as etiology
- McCune-Albright syndrome
  - polyostotic fibrous dysplasia

- gonadotropin-independent
- café au lait spots
- bone lesions

◆ Delayed Maturation

Lack of evidence of puberty by 14 years-of-age or of menarche by 16-years-of-age
Determine presence or absence of uterus
- absent
  - Müllerian agenesis, androgen insensitivity syndrome
- present
  - check gonadotropins
    - hypergonadotropic hypogonadism
      - perform karyotype
    - hypogonadotropic hypogonadism
      - complete androgen evaluation
        - adrenal hyperfunction
        - hypothyroidism
        - hyperprolactinemia
      - CNS lesions
        - image sella turcica
      - Kallman syndrome
        - associated with anosmia
      - functional causes diagnosed by exclusion
        - constitutional delay
        - weight loss
        - excessive exercise
        - stress

ADOLESCENT PREGNANCY

Increasing problem in United States
Teens may lack access to contraception
Significant social issues at play
Adolescent pregnancies fall into high-risk category
- premature labor
- low birth weight
- substance abuse
- increased incidence of CPD

Prevention
- emotional support
- school curriculum
- contraceptive instruction and advice

34

◆ Control of Human Reproduction: Contraception, Sterilization, and Pregnancy Termination

CONTRACEPTIVE USE IN THE UNITED STATES

Greater than 50% of the 6 million pregnancies per year are unintended

According to 1987 data, 6% to 8% of women use no method
- 24% use sterilization
- 23% use oral contraceptives (OCPs)
- 12% use condoms
- 2% use intrauterine devices (IUDs)

CONTRACEPTIVE EFFICACY

Method effectiveness refers to failure rate with correct use (method failure)

Effectiveness refers to failure with both correct and incorrect use (patient failure)

Coitally related methods less effective (Table 34-1)
- greater discrepancy between effectiveness and method effectiveness

Failure rates inversely related to the user's level of motivation

PERIODIC ABSTINENCE

Based on three assumptions
1. human ovum is capable of fertilization for only 24 hours postovulation
2. spermatozoa retain fertilizing ability for only 48 hours
3. ovulation occurs 12 to 16 days prior to onset of next menses

Calculating fertile period by the calendar method
- subtract 18 days from length of shortest cycle (e.g., 25 days → 7)
- subtract 11 days from length of longest cycle (e.g., 30 days → 19)
- abstain from cycle days 7 to 19

Women with irregular menses cannot utilize this method

**TABLE 34-1. Estimated Percentage of Women That
Experience an Unintended Pregnancy in First
Year of Use**

Method	Effectiveness	
	Method	Use
No method (chance)	85.0	85.0
Periodic abstinence		
Calendar method	9.0	19.0
Postovulation	3.0	
Symptothermal	3.0	
Ovulation detection	3.0	
Withdrawal	4.0	24.0
Condom	2.0	16.0
Diaphragm	6.0	18.0
Cervical cap	6.0	18.0
Sponge, parous	9.0	28.0
Sponge, nulliparous	6.0	18.0
Spermicides	3.0	30.0
IUD, copper	0.8	4.0
IUD, progestin alone	0.5	6.0
Oral contracepties		
Combination	0.1	6.0
Progestin alone	0.5	6.0
Norplant (six rods)	0.04	0.05
Depot medroxyprogesterone acetate	0.3	0.4
Tubal sterilization	0.2	0.5
Vasectomy	0.1	0.2

IUD, intrauterine device

Harlap S, Kost K, Forrest JD. Preventing pregnancy, protecting health: a new
look at birth control choices in the United States. New York: Alan Guttmacher
Institute, 1991:35.

Other methods of natural family planning
- temperature method
  - abstain until third consecutive day of postovulatory basal
    body temperature (BBT) rise
- cervical mucus method
  - abstain during menses
  - abstain every other day until first day of increased mucus
  - abstain every day thereafter until 4 days after peak mucus
    day
  - method failure rates are 20% to 24%, discontinuation rates
    are 72% to 74%
  - 3.5% failure rate with motivated couples in random
    clinical trials
- symptothermal method
  - uses multiple indices: calendar, cervical mucus, and BBT
    rise
  - more effective with higher motivation rates

MECHANICAL BARRIER METHODS

◆ Condoms

Reduces transmission of STDs
- gonorrhea, chlamydia, HSV, HIV

Reduces cervical dysplasia

Use with OCP in <25 years-of-age (high-risk group for PID and pregnancy)

Correct method of use
- applied prior to vaginal penetration
- covers entire length of penis
- reservoir tip at end to collect semen
- adequate lubrication to prevent breakage
  - do not use petroleum jelly
- condom and penis withdrawn together after ejaculation

Failure rates 1% to 4% (>30 years-of-age), 10% to 33% (<30 years-of-age)

◆ Diaphragm

Cervix completely covered
- correct sizing critical

User and her partner should be unaware of diaphragm once it is in place
- user needs to be comfortable with insertion and removal

Correct use
- use contraceptive jelly or cream
- left in place minimum of 8 hours after last coitus

Failure rates are age related, 4% (25 to 29 years-of-age), 1% (35 to 39 years-of-age)

Increased rate of UTIs reported by users and also with foamed condoms

◆ Cevical Cap

Can be left in place longer than diaphragm (not >48 hours)
- always use with spermicides

Available cap: Prentif cavity rim cervical cap
- manufactured in four sizes
- correct-sizing critical
- requires training in fitting procedure

Failure rates 6% to 17%

Use only with normal pap smear

◆ Spermicides

Foams, creams, jellies, and suppositories

Contain a spermicidal agent—usually nonoxynol 9

Contraceptive sponge
- 1 mg of nonoxynal 9

- effective for 24 hours
- failure rates 15% (may be higher in parous women)
- increase incidence of Toxic Shock Syndrome
  - do not use during menses or puerperium
- antibacterial and antimicrobial activity
  - no evidence of teratogenesis in failures

ORAL CONTRACEPTIVE PILLS

More than 30 combination pills and 2 progestin-only pills available
Combination pills include mono- and multi-phasic preparations—5 progestins, 2 estrogens (Table 34-2)
- all have 21 days of steroid-containing pills. The 28-day packets also have 7 days of steroid-free pills to allow withdrawal bleeding
Progestin-only pills have daily low-dose progestin with no steroid-free interval
All steroids used in pills are 17 ethinyl derivatives (both estrogens and progestins)
- ethinyl group reduces hepatic metabolism
- most frequent dose is 30 to 35 µg of ethinyl estradiol
  - fewer side effects
  - same efficacy as 50 µg preparations
Effect on reproductive system
- inhibits midcycle gonadotropin surge → no ovulation
- cervical mucus thick, scanty, viscid → retards sperm access to uterus
- alteration of uterine and tubal motility → decreases gamete transport
- decreased glycogen production in endometrial glands → impairs blastocyst survivial
- does not produce hypoestrogenic state
  - levels of estrogen similar to early follicular phase
- progestin-only preparations do not consistently inhibit ovulation
  - less effective
  - ingest at same time daily to aid in maintaining steady state

◆ Adverse Effects

Nausea, breast tenderness, fluid retention, depression
- probably estrogen-related
Increased body weight, acne, amenorrhea, nervousness
- probably progestin-related
Breakthough bleeding, cholasma
- probably related to both
Cholelithiasis
- users of OCPs for less than 4 years have increased risk
- after 4 years, risk decreases to normal
- pills with <50 µg of ethinyl estradiol do not increase gallbladder disease

TABLE 34-2. Representative Examples of Available Oral Contraceptives

Monophasics	Progestin		Estrogen	
Demulen 1/35	ED	1.0 mg	EE	0.035 mg
Demulen 1/50	ED	1.0 mg	EE	0.050 mg
Desogen	DS	0.15 MG	EE	0.030 mg
Levlen	L-NG	0.15 mg	EE	0.030 mg
LoEstrin 1/20	NEA	1.0 mg	EE	0.020 mg
LoEstrin 1.5/30	NEA	1.5 mg	EE	0.030 mg
LoOvral	DL-NG	0.3 mg	EE	0.030 mg
Modicon	NE	0.5 mg	EE	0.035 mg
Nordette	L-NG	0.15 mg	EE	0.030 mg
Nornyl 1+35	NE	1.0 mg	EE	0.035 mg
Ortho-cept	DS	0.15 mg	EE	0.030 mg
Ortho-cyclen	NO	0.25 mg	EE	0.035 mg
Orthonovum 1/35	NE	1.0 mg	EE	0.035 mg
Orthonovum 1/50	NE	1.0 mg	EE	0.050 mg
Ovcon 35	NE	0.4 mg	EE	0.035 mg
Ovcon 50	NE	1.0 mg	EE	0.050 mg
Ovral	DL-NG	0.5 mg	EE	0.050 mg
Jenest 28				
Day 1-7	NE	0.5 mg	EE	0.035 mg
Day 8-21	NE	1.0	EE	0.035 mg
Triphasics				
Ortho Tri-Cyclen				
Day 1-7	NO	0.180 mg	EE	0.035 mg
Day 8-14	NO	0.215 mg	EE	0.035 mg
Day 15-21	NE	0.250 mg	EE	0.035 mg
Orthonovum 7/7/7				
Day 1-7	NE	0.5 mg	EE	0.035 mg
Day 8-14	NE	0.75 mg	EE	0.035 mg
Day 15-21	NE	1.0 mg	EE	0.035 mg
Triphasil (Trilevlen)				
Day 1-6	L-NG	0.050 mg	EE	0.030 mg
Day 7-11	L-NG	0.075 mg	EE	0.040 mg
Day 12-21	L-NG	0.125 mg	EE	0.030 mg
Trinorinyl				
Day 1-6	NE	0.5 mg	EE	0.035 mg
Day 7-15	NE	1.0 mg	EE	0.035 mg
Day 16-21	NE	0.5 mg	EE	0.035 mg
Progestin Only				
Micronor (NorQD)	NE	0.35 mg	None	
Ovrette	DL-NG	0.075 mg	None	

ethinyl estradiol (EE)
norethindrone (NE)
levonorgestrel (L-NG)
dl-norgestrel (DL-NG)
ethynodiol diacetate (ED)
desogestrel (DS)
norgestimate (NO)

◆ Cardiovascular Disease

Arterial cardiovascular disease directly related to progestin
- dose of progestin has greatly diminished in last 30 years

Subhuman primate studies suggest protective effect of estrogens against atherosclerotic disease

Incidence of cardiovascular disease does not correlate with duration of use
- suggests a thrombotic process

More recent epidemiologic studies are reasuring
- newer lower-dose preparations are safer
- exclusion of high-risk groups adds to safety
  - a smoker >35 years → discontinue OCPs
  - a healthy non-smoker >40 years may benefit from OCP use

◆ Neoplasia

✧ *Breast cancer*

At least 27 epidemiologic studies, 5 large cohort studies, 17 case-control studies

Premenopausal breast cancer
- may increase risk if OCPs used for >4 years before 25 years of age or before first full-term pregnancy
- largest U.S. study revealed NO increased risk in women with high-risk factors
  - family history of first-degree relative
  - benign breast disease
  - use of OCPs prior to first pregnancy

Preliminary data from perimenopausal women suggests possible decreased incidence of breast cancer in former users
- reduction greater with younger onset and greater duration of use.

✧ *Cervical cancer*

May be associated with increased dysplasia and cancer

Modulated by confounding factors
- includes number of sexual partners, more frequent pap smears

Current recommendations are for annual pap smear

✧ *Endometrial cancer*

50% reduction in risk after 1 year of use

Protective effects last for at least one decade after ceasing use

Nulliparous women experience greatest benefit

✧ *Ovarian cancer*

Risk is reduced by OCP use

Magnitude related to duration of use
- 6 months confers protection for 1 decade

Reduction occurs only in women of low parity (<4)

✧ *Liver adenoma and cancer*

Hepatocellular adenoma rare (1/30,000 to 1/250,000)

Increased incidence for >5 years of pill use

Regresses once OCP is withdrawn

✧ *Pituitary adenoma*
   No effect

✧ *Malignant melanoma*
   Many confounding factors
   Any effect is a small one

◆ **Pregnancy After Discontinuation of OCPs**

One fifth of users have 2- to 3-month delay in return of fertility
   compared with barrier users
• after 2 to 3 years, there is no difference between method users
No adverse pregnancy effects
Early pregnancy exposure
• no significant increase in congenital anomalies
Breast-feeding
• estrogen inhibits action of prolactin at receptor level in breast
   tissue
• progestin-only pill better choice in puerperium

◆ **Noncontraceptive Benefits**

Lower incidence of functional ovarian cysts
Decreased risk of ovarian and endometrial cancer
Decreased dysmenorrhea and PMS
Decreased menstrual flow
Decrease in benign breast disease
Decreased incidence of PID (50% reduction in acute salpingitis)

◆ **Contraindications to OCP Use**

✧ *Absolute*
   History of deep vein thrombosis (DVT) or pulmonary embolus (PE)
   Presence of cerebrovascular or coronary artery disease
   Untreated hypertension (HTN)
   Diabetes with vascular complications
   History of congestive heart failure (CHF)
   Over 35 years-of-age and smoker
   Estrogen-dependent neoplasm
   Undiagnosed/abnormal genital bleeding
   Pituitary prolactinoma
   Known/suspected pregnancy
   Active liver disease
   Intestinal malabsorption
   Rifampin use

✧ *Relative*
   Migraines
   Oligoamenorrhea
   Depression

◆ Conditions Which are NOT Contraindications to Use of OCPs

History of pregnancy-induced hypertension (PIH)
Varicose veins
Previous liver disease with normal hepatic function
Sickle cell trait
Asymptomatic mitral valve prolapse

◆ New Progestins

Three new progestins (desogestrel, gestodene, norgestimate)
- 19-nortestosterone derivatives, as are all of progestins
- chemically related to levonorgestrel
- comparable efficacy, less androgenic
- minimal effects on protein, carbohydrate, lipid metabolism

NORPLANT

Approved by FDA in 1990
Six rods (34 mm × 2.4 mm) with 36 mg of levonorgestrel in each rod
Inserted subcutaneously under local anesthetic, usually upper, inner arm
Mechanism of action
- ovulation suppression, cervical mucus changes, and endometrial growth suppression

Effectively equivalent to sterilization for 5 years
- noncoitally related
- useful in lactating women

Irregular bleeding in two thirds of women

DEPOT MEDROXYPROGESTERONE ACETATE (DEPOPROVERA)

Used by >11 million women in 90 countries
Injection of aqueous suspension (150 mg)
- 3-month interval between injections

Inhibits ovulation, forms atrophic endometrium
Amenorrhea in 50% of women by end of first year
Return of fertility delayed (long-term fertility unaffected)
No increase in breast, ovarian, and hepatic cancer
Decrease in endometrial cancer

INTRAUTERINE DEVICE

Two different IUDs currently available
Progesterone-releasing
- 65 µg/day
- must be replaced annually

- less blood loss than with copper IUD
- higher incidence of ectopic pregnancy if conception occurs, overall incidence decreased

Copper T380A

- 308 mg of copper
- highly effective for at least 8 years, 1.9 cumulative pregnancy rate
- prevents fertilization
  - impedes sperm transport
  - may increase sperm cytolysis in uterus, and ova cytolisis in fallopian tubes

◆ Timing of Insertion

Usually done at time of menses
Can be done on any cycle day, if pregnancy excluded
Postpartum insertion at 4 to 8 weeks

◆ Bleeding/Pain

Nearly 50% of removals are for excessive bleeding
Copper IUD mean monthly blood loss equals 50 to 60 mL
Progesterone IUD mean monthly blood loss equals 25 mL
OCP mean monthly blood loss equals 20 mL

◆ Perforation

Associated with insertion procedure
Properly inserted IUDs do not migrate through endometrium into/ through myometrium
Rate of perforation is 1/1000 to 1/2000 insertions
"Lost" IUD usually detected by missing strings on follow-up visit
- possible explanations
  - undetected expulsion
  - strings have retracted inside uterine cavity
  - extrauterine location of IUD
Management
- exclude pregnancy
- gently probe uterus
  - if unsuccessful, perform imaging study (x-ray, ultrasound)
  - may require hysteroscopic retrieval

◆ Infection

Earlier studies flawed
Risk of salpingitis inversely related to time elapsed since placement (Fig. 34-1)
Highest risk is during initial 20 days after IUD placement
Emphasis on aseptic insertion
Major risk factor is exposure to sexually-transmitted diseases
Some doctors advocate prophylactic antibiotics at time of insertion
- IUD appropriate for parous women in mutually monogamous relationships

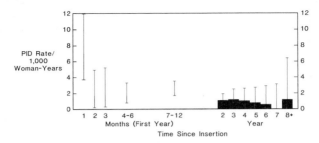

Figure 34-1. Incidence of pelvic inflammatory disease (PID) by duration of intrauterine device use. The 95% confidence intervals are shown. Farley TMW, Rosenberg MJ, Rowe PJ, et al. Intrauterine devices and pelvic inflammatory disease: an international perspective. Lancet 1992; 339:785.)

- nulligravid women should not be excluded if they meet other criteria

◆ Pregnancy-Related Complications

If user is pregnant and string is visible, remove IUD
- reduces threefold incidence of spontaneous abortion

If string is not visible, perform ultrasound
- IUD in uterus → remove at time of delivery
- IUD extrauterine → remove at time of delivery (if cesarean), or postpartum
- IUD does increase risk of preterm labor and premature rupture of membrane (PROM), if maintained during pregnancy
- IUD does NOT increase risk of ectopic compared with nonusers of contraception
- IUD does increase ratio of ectopic:intrauterine pregnancy in users (but most never conceive)

STERILIZATION

According to 1988 data, 36% of all married couples use it as method of choice

Should be considered permanent
- 1% of women request reversal
- 10% of young women with low parity regret decision

◆ Male Sterilization

Transection of vas deferens

Can be done under local anesthetic

Hematomas occur in 5% of men

Not considered sterile until after two sperm-free ejaculates 1 month apart

6% to 7% of men request reversal (45% to 60% success rate)

◆ Female Sterilization

Usually performed using general or regional anesthestic
Can be performed immediately postpartum
Failure rate for laparoscopic sterilization, 1/1000
- not decreased by transection of tube
- usually fulguration or application of occlusive devices (clips, rings)
Overall ectopic pregnancy rate if conception occurs, 16%
- rises to 50% if method used was laparoscopic fulguration

EMERGENCY CONTRACEPTION

90% effective if started within 72 hours of exposure
Most common regimen
2 tablets of 0.5 mg dl-norgestrel and 50 μg ethinyl estradiol
   (Ovral), repeat once in 12 hours
Most common side effect is nausea

PREGNANCY TERMINATION

First-trimester procedure, usually suction or sharp curettage
>12 weeks gestation, use laminaria preoperatively to gently
   dilate cervix
Second trimester
Overall complication rate (any method) three to four times higher
   than first trimester
- surgical procedure (D&E)
  - quicker, equally safe in experienced hands
  - incidence of bowel injury, perforation of the uterus higher
    than induction of labor
- vaginal prostaglandin E_2 or IM prostaglandin F_{2a}
  - complications
    - hyperthermia
    - bronchoconstriction
    - tachycardia
    - gastrointestinal distress
- intraamniotic saline
  - late second trimester
  - may result in DIC type consumptive coagulopathy

◆ Mifepristone (RU-486)

19-norsteroid with affinity for progesterone receptor
Efficacy 96% when used with prostaglandin E_2
- can be used up to 49 days of amenorrhea (9 weeks gestation)
- not yet available in United States

35

◆ Pelvic Infections and Sexually Transmitted Diseases

INTRODUCTION

Many pelvic infections are sexually transmitted (Table 35-1)

TABLE 35-1. Sexually Transmitted Infections

Organisms	Diseases
Bacteria	
Neisseria gonorrhoeae	Gonorrhea
Chlamydia trachomatis	Chlamydial infection
Treponema pallidum	Syphilis
Haemophilus ducreyi	Chancroid
Calymmatobacterium granulomatis	Granuloma inguinale
Gardnerella vaginalis, anaerobes	Vaginitis
Group B β-hemolytic streptococcus	Group B infection
Mycoplasmas	
Mycoplasma hominis	Mycoplasmal infection
Ureaplasma urealyticum	Mycoplasmal infection
Viruses	
Herpes virus hominis	Genital herpes
Cytomegalovirus (CMV)	CMV infection
Hepatitis B virus	Hepatitis
Human papillomavirus	Condyloma acuminatum
Molluscum contagiosum virus	Molluscum contagiosum
Human immunodeficiency virus	Acquired immunodeficiency syndrome
Protozoa	
Trichomonas vaginalis	Vaginitis
Entamoeba histolytica	Proctitis
Fungi	
Candida albicans	Vaginitis
Parasites	
Sarcoptes scabiei	Scabies
Phthirus pubis	Pediculosis pubis

VULVA

◆ Herpes

One third of women 25 to 40 years-of-age have serologic documentation of HSV-2 infection
- 60% to 85% of these women report no clinically recognized symptoms

Primary infection
- 3 to 7 days following exposure
- multiple vesicles coalescing into ulcers
- constitutional symptoms of fever, malaise, headache

Recurrent shedding
- virus present on 1% of days without symptoms

Recurring lesions
- usually less painful and more localized

75% to 85% of genital infections are HSV-2

✧ *Diagnosis*
Viral isolation
Serologic testing

✧ *Treatment*
Pregnancy concerns (see Chapter 26)
Oral acyclovir shortens ulcerative phase and can reduce number of recurrences in patients suffering less than six episodes per year

◆ Human Papillomavirus

Infection is common and typically subclinical
PCR testing of college-age women revealed >45% positive on the vulva and >30% on the cervix
- only 1% had a wart and only 9% had a prior wart

Incubation period for gross warts is approximately 3 months
>50 serotypes identified
Must distinguish between condyloma accuminata and syphilitic condyloma latum

✧ *Treatment*
Podophyllin (not in pregnancy)
TCA
Cryotherapy
Laser ablation

◆ Furunculosis

Infection of hair follicles on vulva
Local therapy or antistaphylococcal antibiotics if large area involved

◆ Bartholinitis

Acute infection

- often *Neisseria gonorrhoeae* or *Chlamydia trachomatis*
Duct obstruction can lead to abscess formation

✧ *Treatment*
Incision and drainage for 3 to 6 weeks with Word catheter

◆ Chancroid

Painful ulcer with ragged edge, raised border
"Kissing ulcers" across the vulva can occur
Unilateral, tender adenopathy in 50%
Incubation period 2 to 5 days
Etiologic agent: *Haemophilus ducreyi*

◆ Granuloma Inguinale

Sexual or gastrointestinal transmission
Soft, red, painless granuloma
Nodes enlarged, painless, not suppurative
Etiologic agent: *Calymmatobacterium granulomatis*
- intracellular parasite
- difficult to isolate
Diagnosis
- biopsy specimen with Donovan bodies present (bipolar staining bacteria within mononuclear cells)

◆ Lymphogranuloma Venereum

Incubation period is 2 to 5 days
Primary, painless, genital or anorectal ulcer
2 to 3 weeks later multiple confluent suppurative nodes
Etiologic agent: L_{1-3} chlamydia immunotypes
Diagnosis
- microimmunofluorescent antibody test
- complement fixation (CF) test lacks specificity

VAGINITIS

Most common gynecologic complaint
At least four types of vaginitis infections
- candidal, trichomonal, bacterial vaginosis, and gonococcal (in
children)

◆ Examination

External genitalia may be normal or inflamed
Vaginal pH should be obtained
KOH odor test and microscopic examination performed
- check for amine odor (BV)
- observe for presence of hyphae (Fig. 35-1)

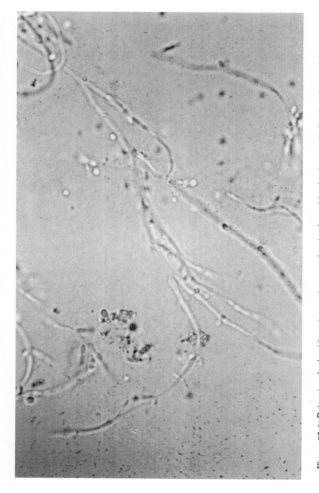

Figure 35-1. Potassium hydroxide wet-mount smear showing branching hyphae, an indication of yeast infection. (Original magnification × 400.)

◆ Candidal Vaginitis

Vulvar and vaginal pruritus
Curd-like vaginal discharge
Candida albicans causes more than 90% vaginal yeast infection

✧ *Etiology*

Changes in host resistance or local bacterial floor
Pregnancy
Diabetes
Antibiotic therapy
• immunosuppressive drugs
PH is normal
Diagnosis is made by wet mount examination

✧ *Therapy*

Local antifungal agents
• imidazole agents
Oral therapy
• 150 mg fluconazole one time dose
Frequent recurrent infection
• assess HIV status and screen for diabetes
• extended 2- to 3-week vaginal therapy
• treatment of male partner
• gentian violet (1%)
• suppressive therapy
  • 100 mg ketoconazole daily
  • vaginal treatment with imidazole or boric acid either twice weekly or daily for 5 days once per month

◆ Trichomonas Vaginitis

Profuse yellow, malodorous discharge
Vulvar pruritis
>50% asymptomatic
• often carried in male partners
pH greater than 4.5, amine odor present with KOH
Wet mount reveals trichomonads (Fig. 35-2)

✧ *Treatment*

Metronidazole, 2 g single dose
• 95% cure rate
Some increased resistance to metronidazole observed
Avoid this drug during first 20 weeks of pregnancy

◆ Bacterial Vaginosis

Overgrowth of aerobic and anaerobic bacteria (*Gardnerella vaginalis*)
Vaginal epithelium appears normal
Fishy amine odor present
Sexual transmission unproven

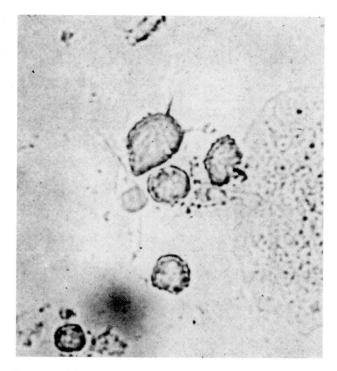

Figure 35-2. Saline wet-mount smear showing the characteristic appearance of a trichomonad, a slightly pear-shaped microorganism that is larger than the surrounding white blood cells. (Micrograph electronically enhanced, original magnification x 400.)

✧ *Diagnosis (three of the following should be present)*
pH greater than 4.5
Homogeneous thin discharge
Amine odor with KOH
Clue cells

◆ Treatment

Symptomatic women
Pregnancy
Preoperative
Metronidazole
• 2 g single dose or 0.75 metronidazole gel
Clindamycin 2% cream

◆ Toxic Shock Syndrome

Acute illness caused by toxin-producing *Staphylococcus aureus*
Associated with tampon use

◇ *Clinical features*

High fever (greater than 38.9°C)
Diffuse rash
Hypotension
Skin desquamation (1 to 2 weeks later)
GI, renal, skin, and neurologic effects

◇ *Treatment*

Hospitalize
IV fluids
Possible ICU treatment

SYPHILIS

Spirochete *Treponema pallidum* enters the lymphatic system after
   exposure
Primary chancre develops in 3 weeks
• painless, firm ulcer
• serologic test is positive 1 to 4 weeks later
Secondary syphilis
• 6 weeks later
• symmetric, macular, papular rash
• highly infectious
• serologic test positive
Latent phase
• no clinical or physical manifestations
VDRL and RPR tests are nonspecific
• confirmatory FTA test is required
• follow titers after treatment

GONORRHEA

Sexually transmitted
Symptoms usually develop 2 to 5 days after exposure
• urinary frequency
• dysuria
• vaginal discharge
Disseminated infection occurs in 2%
• fever
• septicemia
• dermatitis, arthritis, endocarditis
May ascend to upper genital tract
• especially during menstruation

◆ Diagnosis

Culture of *N gonorrhea*
Gram-negative diplococci intracellular on cervical and urethral
  Gram stain

◆ Treatment

Identification of male counterpart
Several treatment options available (see Table 35-2)

CHLAMYDIA INFECTION

Assuming an increasing importance
3 to 5 times more common than gonorhea
Often asymptomatic

◆ Diagnosis

Culture
Direct monoclonal antibody slide test
ELISA

GENITAL MYCOPLASMS

Organisms in search of a disease
Role in fertility unclear
Possible role in puerperal endometritis

SALPINGITIS

Occurs exclusively in sexually active menstruating nonpregnant
  women
Chlamydia and gonorrhea are evident in 50% to 60%
15% occur after instrumentation of genital tract
Unfortunately a common event (1% of women 15 to 39 years-of-
  age)

◆ Risk Factors

Multiple sexual partners
Previous salpingitis
Age
Previous cervical gonorrhea or chlamydia
Barrier contraceptives and oral contraceptives are protective
IUD use (highest rate at time of insertion)

◆ Pathogenesis

Menstrual flow facilitates gonorrheal infection of upper genital
  tract

TABLE 35-2. Treatment Regimens for Sexually Transmitted Diseases

Uncomplicated Gonoccocal Infections
A single dose of:
Ceftriaxone 125 mg IM, or
Cefixime 400 mg orally, or
Ciprofloxacin 500 mg orally, or
Ofloxacin 400 mg orally
PLUS
A regimen effective against coinfection with *C trachomatis*, such as doxycycline 100 mg orally 2 times/day for 7 days or azithromycin 1 g orally in a single dose.

Chancroid
Recommended:
Azithromycin 1 g orally in a single dose, or
Ceftriaxone 250 mg IM in a single dose, or
Erythromycin base 500 mg orally 4 times/day for 7 days
Alternative:
Amoxicillin 500 mg plus clavulanic acid 125 mg orally 3 times/day for 7 days, or
Ciprofloxacin 500 mg orally 2 times/day for 3 days

Chlamydia
Recommended:
Coxycycline 100 mg orally 2 times/day for 7 days, or
Azithromycin 1 g orally in a single dose
Alternative:
Ofloxacin 300 mg orally 2 times/day for 7 days, or
Erythromycin base 500 mg orally 4 times/day for 7 days, or
Erythromycin ethylsuccinate 800 mg orally 4 times/day for 7 days, or
Solfisoxazole 500 mg orally 4 times/day for 10 days

Genital herpes
First clinical episode:
Acyclovir 200 mg orally 5 times/day for 7-10 days
Daily suppressive therapy for frequent recurrences (≥6 per year)
Recommended regimen: Acyclovir 400 mg orally 2 times/day
Alternative: Acyclovir 200 mg orally 3-5 times/day

Syphillis
Patients with primary, secondary, or latent syphilis of <1 year's duration:
Benzathine penicillin G, 2.4 million units IM in a single dose
Patients with latent syphilis of >1 year's duration or of unknown duration:
Benzathine penicillin G 7.2 million units IM given as 3 weekly doses of 2.4 million units

- chlamydia not as dependent on menses

Fitz-Hugh-Curtis syndrome
- perihepatic inflammation
- pleuritic pain
- may result from either chlamydia or gonorrhea

◆ Diagnosis

Findings are often variable
- only 45% with laparoscopic confirmed salpingitis have temperature >38°C
- 50% have normal WBC
- 25% have normal sedimentation rate

Ultrasound can be helpful

Laparoscopy most accurate and particularly useful if diagnosis is unclear or if patient fails to improve on antibiotic therapy

20% will have normal laparoscopic finding with clinical diagnosis of PID

◆ Treatment

Hospitalization
- severe peritonitis
- nausea and vomiting
- temperature >38°C
- suspected abscess
- outpatient failure
- uncertain diagnosis

Outpatient therapy
- reexamine within 2 to 3 days; then at 7 and 21 days

Presence of IUD
- remove 24 to 48 hours after treatment has begun

Surgery
- ruptured pyosalpinx or ovarian abscess
- unilateral salpingo-oophorectomy in young patient with localized disease
- percutaneous drainage may also be successful

36

◆ Menstruation and Disorders of Menstrual Function

NORMAL MENSTRUATION

◆ Follicular Phase

Rapid endometrial growth induced by ovarian estradiol production

Regeneration begins in region of glandular stumps

Fibrinolytic activity aids in dissolution of fibrin clot

Sloughing of endometrium → total reepithelialization in 4 to 6 days

Endometrium increases in thickness

Maximum thickness in late follicular phase

◆ Luteal Phase

Further thickness inhibited by progesterone

Angiogenesis continues in functional layer

Well-differentiated microvasculature

◆ Menstrual Phase

Initiated by precipitous fall in progesterone

Prolonged vasoconstriction

• followed by vasodilation and hemorrhage

Vasoactive substances released

• prostaglandin $F_{2\alpha}$

• specific roles remain to be elucidated

Hemostasis attained through several mechanisms

• platelet plugs in spiral arterioles

• progressive vasoconstriction in basal layer

• prompt regeneration of functional layer

◆ Normal and Abnormal Menses

Normal duration = 5.2 days

Normal blood loss = 35 to 43 mL

Definition of abnormalities as below

AMENORRHEA

Primary: no menarche by 16 years-of-age or within 4 years of thelarche
Secondary: cessation of menses for at least 6 months
Four major subgroups
1. hypothalamic dysfunction
2. pituitary dysfunction
3. ovarian failure
4. anatomic (outflow) abnormality

◆ Hypothalamic Dysfunction

Abnormally low FSH and LH
Failure of withdrawal bleeding in response to progesterone challenge
10 mg medroxyprogesterone daily for 7 days

◇ *Specific disorders*
Kallman syndrome
- congenital failure of development of CNS structures
  - arcuate nucleus and olfactory bulbs
- deficient GnRH secretion and anosmia
- administration of pulsatile GnRH restores normal gonadal function
  - impractical from clinical standpoint
- therapy
  - estrogen to stimulate breast development
  - cyclic hormone replacement to prevent hypoestrogenism
  - ovulation induction to achieve fertility
Other syndromes (Prader-Willi, Lawrence-Moon-Biedl)
Systemic stress
- weight loss
- excessive exercise
- severe emotional stress
CNS tumors
- hamartomas
- craniopharyngiomas
- may be associated with hyperprolactinemia secondary to withdrawal of negative hypothalamic feedback
Other illness (sarcoidosis, encephalitis)

◆ Pituitary Dysfunction

Destructive or neoplastic process
Gonadotropins low; other anterior pituitary hormones variable

◇ *Specific disorders*
Hyperpituitarism (AM fasting)
- benign adenoma of lactotrophes
  - Forbes-Albright syndrome (amenorrhea, adenoma with hyperprolactinemia)

- drugs
  - usually mild increase (<50 ng/mL)
- hypothyroidism
- follow yearly after treatment

Hypoprolactinemia
- Sheehan syndrome
- head trauma
- neoplasm
- hypopituitarism
- provocative testing
  - TRH stimulation test
- initiate replacement therapy promptly
  - corticosteroids
  - thyroid replacement

◆ Ovarian Failure

Serum FSH >40 mIU/mL on two occasions
Increased FSH resulting from lack of sex steroid negative feedback
15% primary amenorrhea, 85% secondary amenorrhea
Evaluation
- karyotype (<30 years old) → gonadal dysgenesis, mosaicism
- TSH, T_4 → thyroid dysfunction
- morning cortisol → adrenal dysfunction
- Ca+2, PO_4 → parathyroid dysfuntion

✧ *Specific etiologies*
Gonadal dysgenesis
- accelerated loss of ovarian follicles in early life and embryogenesis
- streak gonads
- most common: monosomy X (XO)
- others
  - excessive X chromosomes (47XXX)
  - Swyer syndrome
    - phenotypical female
    - 46XY karyotype
Other causes
- chemotherapy/XRT
- 17 α-hydroxylase deficiency

✧ *Treatment*
Absent secondary sex characteristics
- conjugated estrogens 3.75 to 5 mg daily until breast development progresses or spotting begins
1.25 mg daily is maintained with monthly progesterone withdrawal (10 mg for 10 days)

◆ Anatomic Abnormalities

◇ *Outflow tract obstruction* (often associated with causation of endometriosis)

Imperforate hymen

Transverse vaginal septum

Cervical atresia

Müllerian agenesis (Mayer-Rokitansky-Küster-Hauser)

- associated with renal and skeletal anomalies

If normal secondary sexual characteristics, there is no need for karyotype or other tests

◇ *Asherman syndrome*

Obliteration of endometrial cavity by scar tissue

- usually associated with postpartum D&C

HSG or hysteroscopy

Hysteroscopic treatment usually successful

ABNORMAL UTERINE BLEEDING

Frequently prompts medical attention

Excessive menstrual blood loss is single most common indication for hysterectomy

Evaluation can usually yield accurate diagnosis

◆ Evaluation

Determination of anovulatory versus ovulatory bleeding

Anovulatory bleeding demands endocrine evaluation

- TSH, FSH, LH, prolactin, DHEAS
- 17-OHP and T in cases of hirsutism
- may also require ACTH stimulation test to rule out nonclassic CAH
- bleeding usually occurs with chronic oligoanovulation or Polycystic Ovary Syndrome
- perform endometrial biopsy to rule out hyperplasia or neoplasm

Ovulatory bleeding

- consider endometritis (chronic)
  - diagnosis by endometrial biopsy (plasma cell infiltrate)
- anatomic abnormalities common
  - hysteroscopy very effective
    - increased yield over "blind" D&C
  - HSG associated with high false-positive rate
  - transvaginal sonography also useful
- coagulation disorders can present with excessive menstrual flow
- adenomyosis usually a diagnosis of exclusion confirmed at hysterectomy

◆ Treatment

Successful therapy depends on accurate diagnosis

✧ *Chronic anovulation*

Endometrial biopsy precedes therapy
Cyclic progestins in absence of hyperplasia
- medroxyprogesterone 10 mg/day for 10 days/month
- norethindrone 2.5 to 5 mg/day for 10 days/month

Simple or complex hyperplasia without atypia
- progesterone withdrawal 10 mg for 10 days
- continuous progesterone 10 to 20 mg/day for 2 to 3 months
- repeat endometrial biopsy

Hyperplasia with atypia
- hysterectomy often recommended

Cancer
- staging laparotomy with TAH/BSO

Extremes of reproductive age may represent hypoestrogenic state
- treat with conjugated estrogens 12.5 mg IV; repeat in 12 hours
- other choice: high-dose oral ethinyl estradiol or OCP
- use combination OCPs once initial bleeding is controlled

✧ *Anatomic anomalies*

Submucous fibroids or polyps → resect with hysteroscope
Intramural fibroids → myomectomy or hysterectomy
Pretreatment with GnRH agonist allows patient to recover from
    anemia (no long term benefit)

✧ *Chronic menometrorrhagia*

Frequent indication for hysterectomy
Endometrial ablation is a newer option
- initial biopsy without hyperplasia or neoplasia
- several different techniques
  - Nd : YAG laser
  - resectoscope
  - roller ball electrode
- pretreatment with GnRH agonist or danocrine for 4 to 6 weeks
- treatment must cover entire endometrium
- operating time should be 35 to 45 minutes
- volume of distention media must be carefully monitored
  - fluid deficit of 2000 mL can result in pulmonary edema
- results excellent
  - 50% amenorrhea
  - 40% hypomenorrhea
  - 10% persistent menorrhagia (consider repeat procedure)

PREMENSTRUAL SYNDROME (PMS)

No specific definition universally accepted
Most require three findings (Table 36-1)

1. symptom complex consistent with PMS (see below)
2. symptoms must occur exclusively in luteal phase
3. symptoms must be severe enough to cause disruption of lifestyle
- review 2 months of symptom charts

Neuroendocrine mechanisms may play important role
- abnormalities of serotonin secretion

Treatment
- exercise, dietary alterations (no salt, caffeine, or alcohol)
- stress reduction
- trial of anxiolytics (buspirone, alprazolam)
- antidepressants as indicated (clomipramine, nortriptylene, fluoxetine)
- suppression of ovarian function
  - OCPs
  - progestins
  - GnRH agonist (with add-back therapy)

DYSMENORRHEA

Primary dysmenorrhea
- usually nulliparous young women with normal pelvic examination
- etiology is increased $PGF_{2\alpha}$
- treat with NSAIDs

Secondary dysmenorrhea
- may be symptom of endometriosis
- can be associated with increased menometrorrhagia
- can also be associated with cervical stenosis
- often following treatment of cervical dysplasia
- surgical evaluation and treatment should be considered
  - laparoscopy with fulgaration or excision of endometriosis
  - presacral neurectomy (mid-line pain)
  - hysterectomy (last resort)

TABLE 36-1. Symptoms of Premenstrual Syndrome

Psychologic	Somatic
Irritability	Mastalgia
Emotional lability	Bloating
Anxiety	Headache
Depression	Fatigue
Hostility	Insomnia

Cognitive	Social Behavior
Inability to concentrate	Craving carbohydrates
Confusion	Withdrawal
	Arguing

37

◆ Androgen Excess

INTRODUCTION

◆ Hirsutism

Most common finding associated with androgen excess
Excessive hair growth in androgen-dependent areas of skin
Frequently accompanied by acne vulgaris

◆ Virilization

Regression of female body characteristics and acquisition of male
  body characteristics
Severe hirsutism
Male pattern temporal balding
Acne
Increased muscle mass
Clitoromegaly
Deepening voice
Always associated with pathologic state of androgen excess

ANDROGENS

Unique group of steroids
Principle androgens
- dihydrotestosterone (DHT)
- testosterone (T)
- androstenedione (A'D)
- dehydroepiandrosterone (DHEA)
- dehydroepiandrosterone sulfate (DHEAS)

Stimulate primary and seconday male sexual characteristics and
  secondary female sexual characteristics
Initiate pubarche and adrenarche

STEROIDOGENESIS

Occurs in specialized tissues

Cholesterol (C-27) is basic structural molecule of all steroid classes

Rate-limiting step is cholesterol → pregnenolone (C-21)

Pregnenolone metabolized by two alternative pathways
- Δ^5 (DHEA, DHT)
- Δ^4 (androstenedione, testosterone)

Sites on C-19 androgen determine potency

less potent → more potent

C-17 ketogroup (A'D) → 17β-hydroxyl (T)

C-3 (DHEA) → C-3 ketogroup (A'D)

C-5 (T) → C-5 hydrogen (DHT)

Binding proteins
- sex hormone-binding globulin (SHBG) (100,000 times greater affinity of T binding compared with albumin)
- albumin

Tissue responsiveness
- fetus at 12 to 22 weeks equally able to convert T → DHT regardless of sex
- male fetus: testicular production of T
- female fetus: absence of T, or inadequate receptor for T

HAIR PATTERN

Vellus hair: light, finely textured, short

Terminal hair: dark, coarse, may grow quite long
- androgens stimulate conversion of vellus to terminal
- excess androgen may have reverse effect on scalp (temporal balding)

Cyclic growth
- anagen: growth phase
  - prolonged by androgens
- telogen: resting phase
  - shedding of hair
- catagen: transition phase

SOURCES OF ANDROGENS AND METABOLISM

◆ DHT

Most potent (twice the potency of T)

Rapidly cleared from serum (bound by SHBG)

Primarily derived from peripheral conversion of A'D

Androstenediol glucuronide (3α-diol G) may reflect androgen activity in hirsute women

Androsterone glucuronide (andros-G) may also be useful marker

◆ T

Second most potent

1% circulates as free hormone

Ovarian production 5% to 20%
>50% from conversion of A'D

◆ A'D

Obligate intermediate of estrone
Can be converted to T
20% androgenic activity of T
Equal contributions from ovary and adrenal
10% from peripheral conversion DHEA→ A'D
Diurnal variation

◆ DHEA, DHEAS

Weak androgens (3% activity of T)
Almost entirely adrenal secretion (85%, 95% respectively)
DHEA varies with circadian rhythm
DHEAS less cyclic

ANDROGEN EXCESS SYNDROME

Development of hirsutism and acne are earliest signs
90% of hirsute women have an increase in one or more androgens

◆ Ovarian-Related Causes

✧ *Polycystic ovarian syndrome (PCO)*
Most common cause with ovarian etiology
70% prevalence of hirsutism in patients with PCO
Classic ovarian finding
- multiple small follicular cysts
  - poor granulosa cell development
  - thickened luteinized theca
Biochemical parameters
- increased DHEAS, T, prolactin
- reversal of estradiol/estrone ratio
- LH-FSH ratio is ≥3 to 1
Etiology
- may reflect abnormal LH response to GnRH
- infers abnormal GnRH pulse amplitude and frequency
- infers abnormal opiod/dopaminergic interactions
Physiology
- elevation of LH, preferential inhibition of FSH (may be inhibin-related)
- LH induced excess of T and A'D
- Normal granulosa cell aromatization of A'D and T to estradiol is reduced without requisite FSH levels

✧ *Hyperthecosis*
Similar clinical features to PCO
Associated with severe hirsutism, often virilization

Numerous islands of luteinized cells in proximity to hilum of ovary

Therapy: wedge resection, possibly bilateral salpingo-oophorectomy (BSO)

✧ *Obesity, insulin resistance, acanthosis nigricans*

Androgen levels increased by obesity
- decreased SHBG
- increased production

Often coupled with PCO

Acanthosis nigricans
- hyperpigmentation of skin over neck, axilla, below breasts
- marker of insulin resistance

✧ *Neoplasms*

Rare cause of hyperandrogenism

Commonly present with amenorrhea, rapidly progressive virilization

Sertoli-Leydig (arrhenoblastoma)
- most common
- unilateral
- frequently palpable
- produces large amount of T (200 ng/dL)

Hilar cell, mixed gonadal stromal (gyneandroblastoma)
- rarer
- nonpalpable
- usually postmenopausal

Other tumors (nonspecific stromal activity)
- dysgerminomas, teratomas, Brenner, serous cystadenoma, Krukenberg
- typically associated with increased A'D

Luteoma of pregnancy
- rare
- benign, solid, frequently bilateral
- spontaneously regresses following pregnancy

◆ Adrenal Causes

✧ *Classic congenital hyperplasia (CAH)*

21-hydroxylase deficiency (Fig. 37-1)
- most common congenital enzyme defect in hyperandrogenism
- usually manifests at birth
  - genital ambiguity
  - severe salt loss (rarely)
- inability of adrenal gland to produce sufficient glucocorticoids or mineralocorticoids
- increased ACTH and adrenal precursor steroids
- linkage association with HLA Bw47, DR7

11 β-hydroxylase deficiency
- second most common
- 11-deoxycorticosterone produced in excess

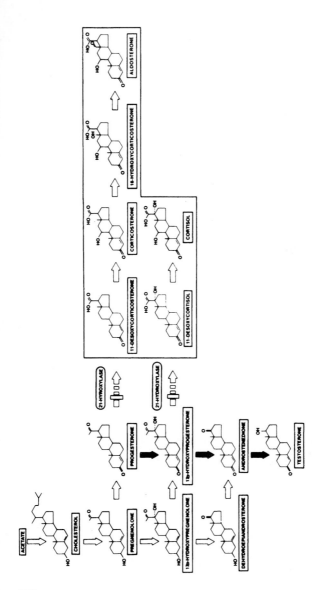

Figure 37-1. Adrenal steroidogenesis: consequences of 21-hydroxylase deficiency. (Adashi EY, Levin PA. Seminars in reproductive endocrinology, vol. 4, New York: Thieme, 1986.)

- potent mineralocorticoid
- salt retention, hypertension
- increased 11-deoxycortisol is diagnostic of CAH 11

3β-hydroxysteroid dehydrogenase, 4-5 isomerase deficiency
- decreased production of all three steroid classes
- salt-wasting
- inadequate virilization of male fetus
- female without secondary sex characteristics (deficient estrogen)
  - may present with hirsutism because of DHEA overproduction

◇ *Nonclassic CAH*
Also called late-onset, attenuated, acquired CAH
Manifests before or after puberty, not at birth
Great phenotypic variability
Nonclassic 21-hydroxylase deficiency
- 17-OHP levels >300 µg/dL basal level with increase to over 800 µg/dL with ACTH
- confirmed by ACTH stimulation test

Nonclassic 3β-hydroxysteriod dehydrogenase (3 hsd) deficiency
- excessive production of Δ^5 steroids
- 17-OH pregnenolone, DHEA, DHEAS elevated basal levels and with ACTH
- compare with elevation of Δ^4 steroids (17-OHP, A'D, T)

Nonclassic 11β-hydroxylase deficiency
- uncommon
- increased 11-deoxycortisol

◆ Neoplastic Disorders

◇ *Cushing disease*
- Cause of 70% of adrenal hyperandrogenism
- Usually result of ACTH-producing pituitary tumor
- Mild hirsutism
- Rarely virilizing

◇ *Cushing syndrome*
- 20% occurance
- Cortisol-secreting adrenal adenoma or carcinoma
- 20% incidence of virilization

◇ *Androgen-secreting adenoma or carcinoma*
- Combination of Δ^4 Δ^5 androgens
- DHEAS >800 µg/dL
- No suppression with dexamethasone
- Rarely a pure T-producing adrenal tumor
- Often responsive to hCG

◆ Mixed Ovarian-Adrenal Hyperandrogenism

30% of hirsute patients have both sources
Adrenal gland influences ovarian steroid production

Indirectly via estradiol conversion with increasing LH secretion
Directly by inhibition of 3 hsd and aromatase

✧ *Clinical evaluation*
History
- onset/velocity of hair growth
- menstrual history
- iatrogenic causes excluded

Physical examination
- scoring methods: Farriman-Galloway (FG) scale (Fig. 37-2)
- normal score=4
- hirsute >8

Other features
- clitoromegaly
- hypercortisolism
- abdominal or pelvic mass

Laboratory studies
- DHEAS, T, prolactin

✧ *PCOS*
T 60 to 150 ng/dL (>200 ng/dL not always tumor)
DHEAS >450 µg/dL
Prolactin >30 ng/mL (10% to 30% of patients)
Ultrasound with multiple ovarian cysts

✧ *Ovarian tumor*
T >200 ng/dL
Unilateral mass
Rapid signs of androgen excess
Consider retrograde ovarian vein catheterization

✧ *CAH*
Basal/stimulated 17-OHP levels
A'D and Δ^5 androstenediol (CAH 3 hsd)
11 deoxycortisol (CAH 11)
CT scan for adrenal tumors

✧ *Cushing disease or syndrome*
Overnight dexamethasone suppression test
- 1 mg PO at 11 PM

Cortisol level obtained at 8 AM
    <6 µg/dL normal
    >10 µg/dL suggests Cushing
- if elevated or indeterminant
    - 24-hour urinary levels of free cortisol (72 µg/24 hours normal)
    - 24-hour urinary 17-hydroxycorticosteroids (8 mg/24 hours)

Low-dose suppression test (0.5 mg q 6 hr for 2 days)
- rules out Cushing syndrome

High-dose suppression test (2 mg q 6 hr for 2 days)
- may suppress cortisol in Cushing disease
- adrenal neoplasms and ectopic ACTH-secreting tumors

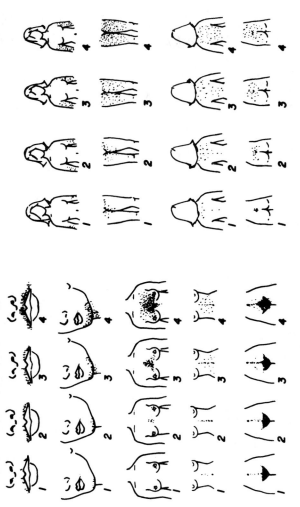

Figure 37-2. Hirsutism scoring from 1 (i.e., mild hirsutism) to 4 (i.e., severe hirsutism) in nine areas. A total score exceeding 8 indicates hirsutism. (Hatch R, Rosenfeld RL, Kim MH, Tredway D. Hirsutism: implications, etiology, and management. Am J Obstet Gynecol 1981; 140:815.)

(Cushing syndrome) do not suppress cortisol

Adrenal CT/MRI more accurate for identification of abnormalities that cause excess cortisol secretion

◇ *Peripheral metabolism*

Normal T, DHEAS, prolactin in menstruating woman with mild or moderate hirsutism

Treatment without further evaluation usually indicated

Elevation of 3α-diol G

* difficult assay
* commercial availability increasing

Elevated prolactin

* 20% to 30% of hyperprolactimemic women have increased DHEAS levels, but not A'D or T
  * prolactin-induced increased DHEAS not a cause of hirsutism
* multiple androgen-related effects
  * inhibits SHBG
  * decreases 5α-reductase activity

TREATMENT

Based on cause/source of androgen

Tumor requires surgery

◆ OCP

Oral contraceptive pill (OCP)

* suppresses LH drive of ovarian androgens
* estrogen component stimulates SHBG
* also lowers adrenal androgen secretion (through pituitary suppression)

Medroxyprogesterone

* suppresses LH secretion
* competes with T for 5α-reductase
* topical treatment being explored

◆ CAH

Steroids

* dexamethasone 0.5 mg q hs
* monitor for adrenal suppression
  * AM cortisol >3 μg/dL assures lack of suppression

Antiandrogens

* cyproterone acetate
  * works at cellular level
  * not available in United States
  * used in oral contraceptives (OCPs) in Europe
  * ACTH inhibition
* spironolactone (100 to 200 mg/day)
  * ideal for cases with increased peripheral conversion

- occupies DHT binding site
- inhibits cytochrome P-450 required for C-19 synthesis
- needs contraception

Flutamide (250 mg BID)
- selective antiandrogen in clinical trials

38

◆ The Breast

EPIDEMIOLOGY

Breast cancer is leading cause of death among American women 40 to 55 years-of-age

Most patients seeking medical attention for breast symptoms have benign conditions

PREGNANCY

After puberty, breasts are quiescent until pregnancy

During pregnancy, several changes occur
- insulin responsiveness
- lobular alveolar growth
- formation of functional secretory cells

Human placental lactogen necessary for lactation
- 6000 ng/mL at term

Prolactin increases to greater than 200 ng/mL

Lactation inhibited by estrogen and progesterone
- milk production results from rapid disappearance of sex steroids after delivery
- suckling decreases prolactin inhibitory factor
- oxytocin is released from the posterior pituitary

FIBROCYSTIC CHANGES

Exaggerated response to changing hormonal environment

Epidemiology is poorly understood
- peak incidence occurs between 30 and 50 years-of-age
- probably related to continued estrogen stimulation
- most women experience fibrocystic change

Treatment regiments
- salt restriction, analgesics, well-fitted bra
- restriction of methylxanthines
- use of danazol (100 to 400 mg daily)

Nipple discharge may be spontaneous or provoked (5% of women)

- usually white or green
- serosanguinous must be investigated
  - most commonly intraductal papilloma
  - breast cancer in 5% to 15%
- provocative stimuli
  - jogging
  - aerobic with weight lifting

Nomenclature should be restricted to those cases with documentation of cyst aspiration or open biopsy

BENIGN NEOPLASMS AND MISCELLANEOUS CONDITIONS

◆ Fibroadenoma

Most common benign lesion
Young women
Firm, painless, mobile
Multiple, bilateral in 10% to 20%
No changes in the menstrual cycle
Removal usually recommended

◆ Lipomas

Superficial and easily documented by mammography
Seen both in young and elderly patients
Removal possible under local anesthesia

◆ Adenoma of Nipple

Located directly beneath the nipple
May be uncomfortable
Remove under local anesthetic

◆ Fat Necrosis

Irregular, tender, dominant mass
May be related to trauma
Mammogram, ultrasound nonspecific
If clear cut history of trauma, observe
Otherwise, open biopsy

◆ Mondor Disease (Superficial Angiitis)

Distinct cord or dimpling with erythematous margins
Self-limited condition
Confirm diagnosis by mammography and reevaluation
- biopsy should be performed if any uncertainty exists

◆ Inflammation

May be from rupture of macrocyst

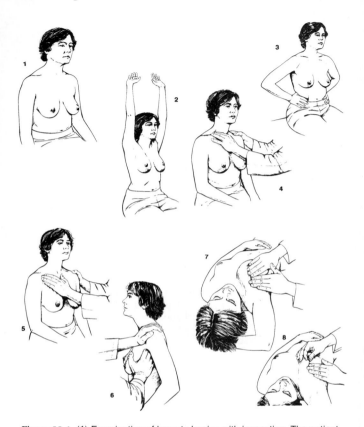

Figure 38-1. (**1**) Examination of breasts begins with inspection. The patient is disrobed to the waist and comfortably seated facing the examiner. Asymmetry, prominent veins, and skin changes may be signs of disease. (**2**) The patient raises her arms above her head, thereby altering the position of the breasts. Immobility or abnormal cutaneous attachments may become evident. (**3**) Inward pressure on the hips tenses the pectoralis major muscle. Abnormal attachments to its overlying fascia and skin can produce retraction or dimpling of the skin. (**4**) Palpatory examination of the supraclavicular lymph nodes. (**5**) The deltopectoral triangle is palpated for evidence of infraclavicular nodal enlargement. (**6**) Each axilla is examined for nodal enlargement. Proper placement of the examiners hands and of the patient's arm is important. (**7**) Thorough palpatory examination of entire breast for masses is performed with patient in supine position. A fine rotational movement of the hands is useful to appreciate the consistency of the underlying tissues. (**8**) The nipple is compressed to elicit discharge.

Marked breast tenderness
Erythema but no dominant mass
Mammography is negative
Lesions resolve within a few days to 2 weeks
Exclude inflammatory carcinoma

BREAST EXAMINATION

Figure 38-1 illustrates breast examination by physician

CYST ASPIRATION

Aspirate with 23- or 24-gauge needle (Fig. 38-2)
If fluid is clear or cloudy, the mass resolves
• follow up examination in 1 month
Bloody fluid or residual mass
• open biopsy recommended
Solid mass
• open biopsy or excisional biopsy in teenager

◆ Fine-Needle Aspiration (Fig. 38-3)

Becoming more popular
Local anesthetic is helpful
Most useful in obvious dominant mass with signs and symptoms suggestive of carcinoma
Negative finding may be unreliable
Mammography may be performed first to avoid distorting anatomy

OTHER DIAGNOSTIC STUDIES

Ultrasonography is useful to confirm macrocyst
• unsuitable for screening
Mammography
• screening examination or confirmation of findings on examination
• access additional lesions in patient with cancer
• false-negative usually 10% (may reach 25% to 30%)
Mass screening
• controversial in regard to cost effectiveness, indications, and frequency
• consensus guidelines
   1. clinical examination of the breast and mammography are best detection methods.
   2. screening process should begin by 40 years-of-age and consist of clinical examination with mammography at 1 to 2 year intervals.
   3. beginning at age 50, both clinical examination and mammography should be performed yearly.

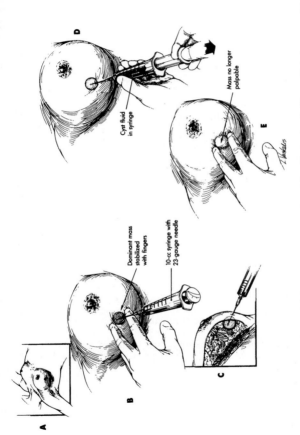

Figure 38-2. Aspiration of cyst. (**A**) The mass is palpated, and the skin is wiped with an alcohol sponge. (**B,C**) The needle penetrates the cyst without passing through the opposite wall. No local anesthesia is necessary. (**D,E**) Fluid is withdrawn until the mass disappears. (Nichols DH. Gynecologic and obstetric surgery. Chicago: Mosby Year Book, 1993.)

Cyst fluid in syringe

Mass no longer palpable

Dominant mass stabilized with fingers

10-cc syringe with 23-gauge needle

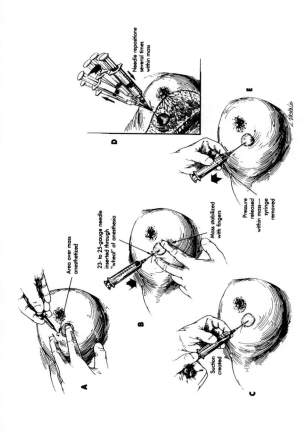

Figure 38-3. Fine-needle aspiration. (**A**) After the mass is located, local anesthetic (1% lidocaine without adrenalin) is applied. (**B**) The mass is stabilized, and the needle is inserted. (**C**) Suction is created as the needle is withdrawn. (**D**) The needle is repositioned several times. (**E**) Suction is released as the needle is withdrawn. (Nichols DH. Gynecologic and obstetric surgery. Chicago: Mosby Year Book, 1993.)

4. These recommendations apply to women without symptoms of breast cancer.

The above are guidelines only

- patients with risk factors may begin screening process earlier

Occult lesions

- 15% to 20% represent early cancer
- some difficulties
  - radiologist fails to define the lesion
  - surgeon fails to remove it
  - removal complicated by inadequate margins or postoperative induration, infection, or hematoma

BREAST CANCER

182,000 new cases in 1993

Decline since 1987 especially in women over 50-years-of-age

Lifetime risk increased to 1 in 8 from 1 in 9 in 1992

- increase in risk associated with increase in life expectancy
  - by 40-years-of-age, 1/217
  - by 50-years-of-age, 1/50
  - by 60-years-of-age, 1/24
  - by 95-years-of-age, 1/8
- risk factors explain only 21% (30 to 54 years-of-age), 29% (55 years-of-age and older)
  - bilateral salpingo-oophorectomy prior to menopause reduces risk
    - 70% reduction if ovaries removed before age 35

◆ Staging

Pretreatment chest x-ray, blood studies (including liver functions)

Bone scan for invasive disease

Clinical staging using TNM system (see Appendix)

- does not adequately segregate patients and select appropriate surgical treatments
- clinical nodal status incorrect in many patients

◆ Treatment Options

Untreated breast cancer has predictable survival

- 20% at 5 years
- 5% at 10 years

Halsted radical mastectomy is now replaced by lesser surgical procedures

- modified radical mastectomy
- segmental resection with axillary dissection and radiotherapy

Multicentricity in 74% of cases

- efforts at local control radiotherapy or radical treatment
  - influence on natural history of the disease and survival is debatable

Multidisciplinary approach needed
Mammography in even most obvious cases
- 4% to 5% synchronous cancers

◆ Surgical Options for Local Treatment

Support for conservative treatment with radiotherapy is increasing
Four criteria
    1. patient selection
    2. surgery of the primary tumor
    3. radiotherapy of the primary tumor
    4. surgery of the axilla
Major benefit is cosmetic
Adequate resection implies grossly clear margins
- re-resect if microscopically positive
Radiotherapy
- begin as soon as wounds are healed
- 1.8 to 2.0 Gy/day for a total of 45 to 50 Gy
Modified radical mastectomy
- postoperative care similar
Simple mastectomy
- ductal, lobular in situ cancer
- recurrence after partial mastectomy and axillary dissection or irradiation
- bulky and ulcerated lesions with distant metastases
- elderly patients with no evidence of axillary adenopathy or distant disease
- prophylactic removal of opposite breast
Subcutaneous mastectomy
- no longer recommended
- removal of at least 80% of breast tissue necessary
Saline implants recommended for reconstruction
Silicone breast implants
- moratorium on January 6, 1992
- no higher incidence of cancer
- less than 100 of 2 million women with implants suffer immune system disorders
- available on research protocol only

◆ Adjuvant Treatment

Use in node-negative now recognized

Low Risk	High Risk
duct cancer in situ	aneuploid tumor
tumor less than 1cm	high S-phase fractions
diploid tumors	high cathepsin D levels
low S-phase fraction	absent estrogen receptors
nuclear grade 1	tumors greater than 3 cm
tumor 1 to 2 cm without high risk features	

50%, decision is straightforward
- 25% have small tumors, histologically favorable
- 25% have large tumors with poor prognosis

50% intermediate
- use above risk factors
- chemotherapeutic agents (CMF or tamoxifen)
  - Cyclophosphamide 100 mg/m^2 orally on days 1 through 14
  - methotrexate 40 mg/m^2 IV on days 1 through 8
  - 5FU 600 mg/m^2 IV on days 1 through 8
  - tamoxifen 10 mg PO BID

◆ Breast Cancers With Unique Features

Lobular neoplasia
- 30% develop susequent carcinoma after long-term follow-up
- surgery or watchful waiting
  - bilateral mastectomy (bilaterality in 50%)

In situ ductal carcinoma
- carcinoma will develop in 50%
- incidence has increased to 25% of mammographically detected lesions

Intraductal carcinoma with microinvasion
- standard treatment is total mastectomy with or without axillary dissection
- cure in nearly 100%
- wide local excision and radiation may be appropriate

◆ Breast Cancer in Pregnancy

2.2/10,000 pregnancies
1.72% of all breast carcinoma
- 7% in premenopausal breast cancer patients

Major problem is delayed diagnosis
Many of these cancers are estrogen receptor negative
- therapeutic abortion does not improve chances cure

Treatment
- first trimester
  - mastectomy and axillary node dissection
- second trimester
  - treatment without delay
- third trimester
  - consider observation until delivery

Adjuvant therapy
- no adverse fetal effects known

Recurrence is usually within 2 years
- at least 2 years of clinical disease-free survival is recommended before pregnancy is attempted

Hormonal replacement therapy
- not routinely recommended

39

◆ Infertility

INTRODUCTION

Infertility is a much abused term

Definition should be clearly stated (Table 39-1)

A couple with relatively normal fertility should conceive in 1 year with regular coitus

- no conception implies infertility
  - cycle fecundity is most useful single decision-making parameter

2.5 million married couples suffer infertility

- not significantly changed from 1970s
  - number of physician visits have risen significantly

TABLE 39-1. Definitions of Terms Used in Human Fertility

Term	Literal Definition*	Practical Definition
Fertile/fertility	Capable of conceiving and bearing young	Spontaneous conception in less than 1 year†; usually implies progression of pregnancy beyond the first trimester; may imply delivery of living infant
Sterile/sterility	Bearing no progeny	Incapable of conception
Infertile/ infertility	Diminished or absent fertility; does not imply as irreversible a con- dition as sterility	No conception in 1 year or more†
Fecund/ fecundity	Pronounced fertility; capability of repeated fecundation (impregnation)	Probability of achieving pregnancy each menstrual cycle; also called cycle fecundity or fecondability
Prolific/ prolificacy	Bearing many children	Number of fetuses or living infants per conception

*Stedman's Medical Dictionary. 22nd ed. Baltimore: Williams & Wilkins, 1972.
†Assumes that the couple is not practicing contraception.

EVALUATION

Infertility categories can be defined by diagnostic test groups
- male gamete factor
- female gamete factor
- female genital tract factor

DIAGNOSIS AND TREATMENT

◆ Male Gamete Factor

No sperm (azoospermia) means sterility
Compromised spermatogenesis
- decreased numbers (Table 39-2)
- decreased motility
- decreased fertilizing ability
Men with poor counts can have surprising fertility
Fertile men demonstrate great variability in counts

◆ Female Gamete Factor

Periodic shedding of an ovum is necessary for conception
- conception or observation of egg outside of ovary is only direct proof of ovulation
- indirect evidence
  - menstrual rhythm
  - BBT charts
  - cervical mucus changes
  - ultrasound monitoring of follicular growth
  - endometrial biopsy
  - serum progesterone
Fecundity rate profoundly decreased in abnormal cycles

TABLE 39-2. Standard Semen Analysis

Parameter	Average Values
Consistency	Fluid (after liquefaction)
Color	Opaque
Liquefaction time	≤20 min
pH	7.2-7.8
Volume	2-6 mL
Motility (grades 0-4)	≥50%
Count (millions/mL)	20-100
Viability (eosin)	≥50%
Morphology (cytology) cell types	≥60% normal oval
Cells (white blood cells, others)	None to occasional
Agglutination	None
Biochemical studies (e.g. fructose, prostaglandins, zinc) if desired	

✧ *Testing of ovulatory function*

BBT
- clearcut stepwise shift of temperature
- 12+-day luteal interval

Endometrial biopsy and serum progesterone
- progesterone level greater than 15 ng/mL is more than 80% accurate
- biopsy results initially thought to be 80% accurate
  - interpretation variable dependent of histopathologic assessment

Hormonal profiles (Fig. 39-1)
- gold standard
- not practical for screening purposes

Salivary and vaginal electrical resistance
- easier to perform
- 80% correlation with more intensive schemes

Urinary LH kits
- based on monoclonal antibodies to LH
- results from kits are variable

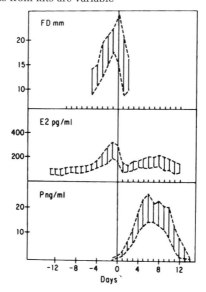

Figure 39-1. Normal cycle profiles of follicular diameter (FD), estradiol (E2), and progesterone (P) in 20 spontaneous ovulatory cycles. The 95% confidence intervals are shown. From the midluteal point onward, n = 12 days since conceptions occurred in 8 of the 20 cycles. (Hughes CL. Monitoring of ovulation in the assessment of reproductive hazards in the workplace. Reprod Toxicol 1988;2:163.)

✧ *Etiology and correction of dysfunction*

Systemic illness

Subtle hyperprolactinemia or hypothyroidism
- correction with bromocriptine can normalize ovarian function

Ovarian failure → donor eggs required

Hypothalamic amenorrhea
- GnRH pump
- hMG

Polycystic ovarian disease
- clomiphene
- ovulation induction with hMG
  - begin between cycle days 2 and 5
  - monitor with estradiol and ultrasound from day 6 onward
  - hCG given when follicles are greater than 18 mm for ovulatory release
  - premature luteinization can occur
    - prevented with GnRH agonist therapy

Progesterone supplementation
- treatment for luteal phase deficiency
  - controversial entity
    - diagnostic criteria difficult to assess
  - LH secretion is increased in cycles with subnormal progesterone production
    - follicular phase progesterone normalizes LH pattern
  - progesterone may serve to normalize LH pulse pattern for recruitment in the following cycle

FEMALE GENITAL TRACT LESIONS

◆ Lower Genital Tract

If coital frequency is at least two times per week and true intromission is occurring, vaginal infertility factors do not exist

Cervical factors
- suggested by poor sperm motility or survival on postcoital test
- most common cause is poor timing of test within cycle
- second most common cause is male factor (e.g., oligiospermia)

Immunologic factors
- antisperm antibodies (relevant vs. irrelevant)

Inflammatory processes (cervicitis)

Iatrogenic
- clomiphene use
  - antiestrogen effect on mucus
    - use between cycle days 3 to 7 instead of days 5 to 9
    - probably not a profound effect given the significant conception rate

✧ *Therapy*

No specific therapy available
Washed intrauterine insemination (IUI) or ART
The present trend leans away from postcoital testing
- treatment options independent of results of postcoital test

◆ Upper Genital Tract

Most efficiently accomplished by laparoscopy and hysteroscopy
- allows direct examination of peritoneal services
- assess mobility and patency of fallopian tubes
Hysterosalpingogram can be a useful adjunct

✧ *Tubal occlusion*

Proximal
- can consider resection with end-to-end reanastomosis
- reimplantation results are much poorer (10% conception rate after 2 years)
Distal
- fimbrioplasties variable in efficacy
- 25% pregnancy rate in first 2 years

✧ *Adhesions*

Laparoscopy or possible laparotomy required
Reformation occurs to some extent in all patients
Advancement to ART may be best option

✧ *Endometriosis*

Severe forms may have very low cycle fecundity
Milder forms have one fifth to one half normal fecundity
- probably different mechanism
Intraperitoneal inflammatory process
Medical therapy improves pain scores
- does not clearly improve fecundity
Surgical therapy
- treatment improvement in moderate endometriosis
- no long-term improvement in pregnancy outcome
Consider medical therapy prior to conservative surgery
Further options
- IUI and ovulation enhancement
- GIFT
- IVF

MULTIFACTORIAL INFERTILITY

Infertility factors often coexist in the infertile couple (Table 39-3)

UNEXPLAINED INFERTILITY

Incidence of 5% to 20%
- inversely correlated with the severity of the criteria used

TABLE 39-3. Infertility Diagnosis, Tests, and Therapies

Diagnosis	Incidence* (%)	Common Tests	Diagnostic Results	Initial Therapy	Advanced Therapies
Multifactorial	40	Complete survey†	See individual tests	Treat one or more specific factors	IUI, GIFT, IVF-ET
Endometriosis	17	Laparoscopy	Characteristic implants and adhesions	Prospective observation, suppression with medication or conservative resection at laparotomy	IUI, GIFT, IVF-ET
Male factor	12	Semen analysis	<20 million normal motile sperm per ejaculate	Prospective observation or donor insemination	IUI, GIFT, IVF-ET
Ovulatory dysfunction	11	Midluteal serum progesterone; late-luteal endometrial biopsy	Progesterone <15 ng/mL is suspect; <10/mL is abnormal. Biopsy lag ≥2 days	Directed therapies for endocrine diseases; otherwise, clomiphene	Human menopausal gonadotropin or gonadotropin-releasing hormone
Tubal factor/pelvic adhesions	8	Laparoscopy with hydrotubation; HSG	Tubal occlusion/presence of adhesions at laparoscopy. HSG does now show adhesions	Laser laparoscopy or lysis of adhesions and tuboplasties at laparotomy	IVF-ET

372

Cervical factor	1	Postcoital test	<5 motile sperm/hpf in late follicular phase mucus	Prospective observation	IUI, GIFT, IVF-ET
Uterine factor	1	Hysteroscopy; HSG	Septum, polyp, fibroid seen; HSG has a significant false-negative rate	Hysteroscopic resection	Metroplasty at laparotomy
Idiopathic	10	Complete survey	See individual tests	Prospective observation, empirical therapy Clomiphene or empirical antibiotics	IUI, GIFT, IVF-ET

*Approximate.
†Minimum of semen analysis, midluteal serum progesterone, and laparoscopy or hysteroscopy with hydrotubation.
GIFT, gamete intrafallopian transfer; HSG, hysterosalpingography; IUI, washed intrauterine insemination with husband's sperm, usually in superovulation cycles; IVF-ET, in vitro fertilization with embryo transfer.
Soper J, Clarke-Pearson D, Hughes C. Gynecologic surgery. In: Liechty RD, Soper RT, eds. Fundamentals of surgery. 6th ed. St Louis: CV Mosby, 1989:526.

Empirical therapy
- conservative
  - observation for 6 to 12 months
- minimally aggressive
  - precise timing of coital behavior
  - condom use for several cycles followed by discontinuation of barrier contraception
  - empiric antibiotic therapy
  - consider other options after 6 to 12 months
- aggressive therapy
  - IUI and ovulation enhancement
  - IVF
  - GIFT
  - see Chapter 40 for review in greater detail

40

◆ Assisted Reproductive Technology

INTRODUCTION

Assisted reproductive technology (ART) began earnestly in mid-1970s

New options now available
- in vitro fertilization-embryo transfer (IVF-ET) (Fig. 40-1)
- gamete intrafallopian transfer (GIFT) (Fig. 40-2)
- donor gametes
- micromanipulation

Future directions
- gene therapy
- preimplantation genetic diagnosis

ART CYCLE PARAMETERS

◆ Patient Selection

Originally reserved for tubal factor infertility only
- now expanded to essentially all categories of infertility and beyond
- peri- and premenopausal women with donor eggs
- gestational surrogates
- preimplantation genetic diagnosis

Future evaluation prior to ART may involve only
- uterine evaluation hysterosalpingogram (HSG)
- cycle day 3 follicular stimulating hormone (FSH) level
- semen analysis
- further expansion now includes synchronized cycles for gestational surrogacy and embryo biopsy for preimplantation genetic analysis

◆ Ovarian Stimulation

Most commonly involves pituitary downregulation with gonadotropin-releasing hormones (GnRH) analog followed by high-dose gonadotropins

Immeasurable variations
- use of pure FSH
- flare cycles
- use of growth hormone

After ovarian stimulation human chorionic gonadtropin (hCG) given as LH substitute
- administer 35 to 36 hours prior to planned retrieval

Luteal support
- hCG in divided doses
- progesterone
- no adjunctive support

◆ Monitoring

Evolved from urine lutenizing hormone (LH) to serum estradiol and transvaginal ultrasound

Use of GnRH analogs has greatly reduced risk of premature LH surge

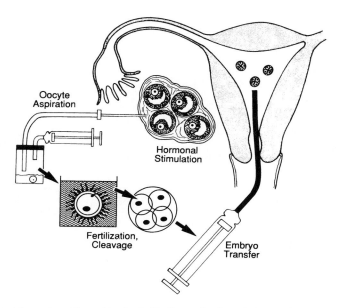

Figure 40-1. Steps of in vitro fertilization and embryo replacement are ovarian stimulation, monitoring, ultrasound or laparoscopy, oocyte retrieval, in vitro fertilization, and uterine preembryo replacement.

- also useful for coordinating patient's cycles
- increases necessary gonadotropin dose

Protocols have become simpler

- some satellite center programs have been very successful

◆ Oocyte Retrieval

Laparoscopic retrieval originally the standard method
Some programs combine oocyte retrieval and diagnostic laparoscopy (Fig. 40-3)
Current standard is transvaginal aspiration

◆ Gamete and Embryo Replacement

Standard approach is uterine replacement

- at four- to six-cell stage
- after 48 hours in culture

GIFT, zygote intrafallopian transfer (ZIFT) avoid need for rigorous in vitro culture

- use patient's tube as incubator
  - sacrifices information regarding fertilization
  - ZIFT and tubal embryo transfer (TET) attempt to resolve this aspect of GIFT
    - no improved pregnancy rate over that with GIFT or IVF

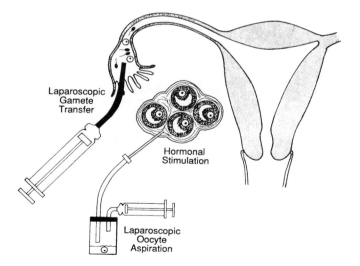

Figure 40-2. Steps of gamete intrafallopian transfer are ovarian stimulation, monitoring, laparoscopic oocyte retrieval, and transfer of the gametes to the fallopian tube.

OPTIMIZING REPRODUCTIVE EFFICIENCY

◆ Oocyte Quality

Reproductive age and ovarian reserve
- reproductive performance with ART correlates with age
  - better correlation with ovarian reserve
  - cycle day 3 FSH
    - clomiphene or GnRH analog stimulation test
      - not more information than baseline cycle day 3 FSH
- FSH levels and ART
  - >25 mIU/mL essentially no successful cycles
  - 20 to 25 mIU/mL markedly diminished success
  - age and FSH levels independent variables

Oocyte quality decreases but cycles can remain regular
- donor oocytes very successful
  - use estrogen/progesterone to synchronize recipient
  - preembryo transfer on third day of progesterone
    - artificially set at day 18 of cycle
  - GnRH agonist useful to suppress endogenous gonadotropins in recipient
  - oocyte cryopreservation would minimize need for synchronized cycles

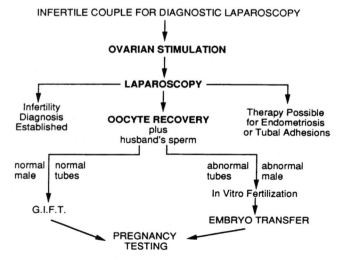

Figure 40-3. Flow diagram of the components of a program for oocyte retrieval and diagnostic laparoscopy that combines assisted reproductive technology with diagnostic infertility laparoscopy.

SPERM QUALITY

◆ Andrology Assessment

One of the greatest advances in ART was treatment of male-factor infertility
- IVF requires only 50,000 to 100,000 motile sperm/per oocyte
  - can be obtained from compromised specimens

◆ Microsurgical Fertilization

Wide range of techniques (Fig. 40-4)
Sperm selection still problematic
More advanced techniques
- intracytoplasmic sperm injection (ICSI)
  - may be successful with extremely low counts/motility
Can always consider donor insemination

PREEMBRYO QUALITY

◆ Morphologic Assessment

Criteria are qualitative and subjective
- cell number
  - four- to eight- cell stage at 48 hours usually a goal
- symmetry and roundness of blastomeres
- lack of fragmentation or vacuoles
Coculture systems may improve quality
Assisted hatching in cases of zona pellucida thickness

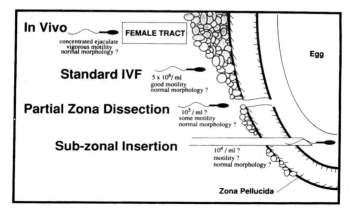

Figure 40-4. Therapy for male factor infertility using in vivo and in vitro fertilization and microsurgical fertilization techniques. (Courtesy of J. Cohen.)

◆ Biochemical Assessment

Analysis of preembryo conditioned media may allow insight into
preembryo health
- oncofetal fibronectin
- platelet-activating factors
- pregnancy-associated plasma protein A (PAPP-A)
- integrins

◆ Chromosomal Evaluation

Blastomere biopsy
PCR to amplify genome
Transfer only selected preembryos
Gene therapy
- cloning (artificial twinning)
  - use of artificial zona
  - could be combined with preimplantation genetic diagnosis

IMPLANTATION CAPACITY

◆ Hormone Environment

Implantation rates in most IVF programs 10% to 15% of
preembryos
- may be higher in artificial cycles with estrogen/progesterone
Natural (unstimulated cycle IVF)
- cost savings
- minimize risk of multiple gestation
- no difference in implantation rate
GIFT
- allows more physiologic incubation
- decreased fertilization probably offsets improved implantation rate
ZIFT/TET
- also demonstrate no significant advantage over IVF

◆ Uterine Receptivity

Anatomic defect should be corrected
Gestational surrogacy
- failed treatment of uterine defect
- hysterectomy patient
- mullerian agenesis
- severe maternal disease
- Rh incompatibility
- cardiac disease
- diabetes
- hypertension

41

◆ Endometriosis

DEFINITION

Clinically defined as the presence of both endometrial glands and stroma outside the uterine cavity

◆ Epidemiology

Almost exclusively seen in women of reproductive age
- age range of 10 to 80 years
- 2% to 4% post menopausal

Relatively common in women less than 20 years-of-age
- 50% incidence in patients with pelvic pain or dyspareunia

Family history is a risk factor
- threefold to tenfold increase in patient with first degree relatives with endometriosis
  - polygenetic inheritance pattern

PREVALENCE

Wide range of estimates based on operative procedure performed at time of diagnosis (10% overall)
- tubal reanastomosis (1%)
- laparoscopic tubal ligation (2%)
- abdominal hysterectomy (11%)
- operative laparoscopy (31%)

PATHOLOGY

Many different appearances
- bluish-gray powder burns
- nonpigmented clear vesicles
- white plaques
- reddish petechiae or flame-like areas

Scarring is a frequent feature

Adhesions are common
- cul-de-sac obliteration

- anterior uterovesicle fold
- ovary to posterior leaf of broad ligament
- sigmoid colon to left pelvic sidewall

Peritoneal pockets
- seen in 18% of women with endometriosis
- two thirds have endometriosis around rim or at base of lesion
- most likely a development defect in pelvic peritoneum

Endometriomas
- occur frequently in the ovary
- filled with chocolate brown fluid

Microscopic appearance
- glands and stroma
- glands frequently cystic
- majority of implants do not exhibit cyclicity

Ultrastructural evaluation
- may or may not exhibit cycle-dependent changes
  - giant mitochondria
  - appearance of nuclear channel system

PATHOGENESIS

◆ Histogenesis

Three major theories: coelomic metaplasia, ectopic transformation, induction hypothesis

◇ *Coelomic metaplasia*

Metaplastic transformation of pelvic peritoneum
Observations have shed doubt on this theory
- only a few cases in men
- no increase with age (typical of metaplastic processes)
- usually found in pelvis not abdominal peritoneum or pleura
- no scientific evidence to confirm that metaplasia can result in endometriosis

◇ *Ectopic transplantation of endometrium*

First proposed in 1921 by Sampson
Some supportive evidence of retrograde flow
- hypotonia of uterotubal junction
- increased incidence in müllerian anomalies

Direct evidence still lacking
Some women predisposed to retrograde flow as detailed above
Best empirical data seems to support this hypothesis

◇ *Induction hypothesis*

Substances released from shed endometrium induce formation of endometriosis
Support from rabbit model
Overall evidence still lacking

◆ Immune Response

Evidence suggests decreased T-cell response

Also possible defects in natural killer cell activity, β-cell function and dysfunctional complement pathway

◆ Growth Factors

Various growth factors may be integral to the development of endometriosis
- epidermal growth factor (EGF)
- insulin-like growth factor 1 (IGF-1)
- platelet-derived growth factor (PDGF)

Protooncogene activation (c-erb-2 and c-*myc*)

SYMPTOMS AND SIGNS

Most common symptom is pain
- secondary dysmenorrhea
- worsening primary dysmenorrhea
- dyspareunia
- noncyclic diffuse pelvic pain

Infertility frequently seen
- prevalence unclear secondary to selection bias

Unusual location may produce unusual symptoms
- gastrointestinal involvement
- urinary tract disease
- pulmonary disease
- nervous system disease

Physical findings
- no pathognomonic physical findings
- cul-de-sac tenderness
- uterosacral ligament nodularity and tenderness
- endometrioma as a palpable adnexal mass

DIAGNOSIS

Serum testing
- CA-125
  - insufficient sensitivity or specificity
- placental protein 14
  - may be increased in deeply infiltrating endometriosis
  - clinical value undemonstrated
- endometrial antibodies
  - insufficient sensitivity and specificity

Imaging techniques
- ultrasound
  - can be helpful in identifying potential endometriomas
  - sensitivity of 11% in diagnosis of focal endometriosis
- MRI

- highly sensitive for endometriomas
  - 90% sensitive, 98% specific
- identification of focal lesions is poor
- surgery (Fig. 41-1)
  - gold standard is direct visualization by laparoscopy (Fig. 41-1)
  - excision may be necessary to confirm diagnosis

PATHOPHYSIOLOGY

◆ Pain

Mechanism remains speculative
- local irritation of peritoneum
- retraction of adhesions
- displacement of pelvic organs
- stretching of peritoneum

Increased tissue penetration associated with increased pain

Medical therapy can diminish pain

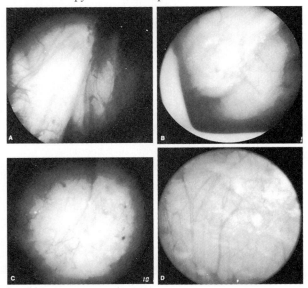

Figure 41-1. Laparoscopic appearance of endometriosis lesions. (**A**) A classic blue-black powder burn lesion on the left broad ligament. (**B**) A white-appearing endometriotic lesion in the cul-de-sac. (**C**) A variety of endometriotic lesions: white, clear vesicular, black, and red. (**D**) Clear, pale areas of endometriosis in the cul-de-sac. (David B. Redwine, M.D., Bend, OR.)

◆ Infertility

Clear association in presence of adhesions
Implants alone may not adversely affect fertility
Infertility may contribute to development of endometriosis, not vice-versa

CLASSIFICATION

American Fertility Society staging system deals with fertility prognosis (Fig. 41-2)
* no correlation with pelvic pain
* predictions of fertility may not be reliable
New classifications and staging systems under development

TREATMENT

Must be individualized to patient's symptoms
* pain vs. fertility

◆ Medical treatment

✧ *Danazol*
Isoxazol derivative of 17-α-ethinyl testosterone
* results in attenuated mid-cycle LH surge
* inhibits multiple enzymes in steroidogenic pathway
* increases free testosterone
Causes chronic anovulation and hyperandrogenism
Side effects
* weight gain
* acne
* deepening of voice
* increased muscle mass
Effective at decreasing both endometriosis and pain relief
No effect on fertility

✧ *Progestins*
Produce decidualization
Side effects
* abnormal bleeding
* fluid retention
* depression
* nausea
Usually medroxyprogesterone 20 to 30 mg daily
Effective at reduction of disease and at pain control
No improvement in fertility

✧ *Oral contraceptives*
Few data to support routine use
No controlled or comparative trials

Patient's Name _____ Date_____

Stage I (Minimal) · 1-5
Stage II (Mild) · 6-15
Stage III (Moderate) · 16-40
Stage IV (Severe) · >40
Total_____

Laparoscopy_____ Laparotomy_____ Photography_____
Recommended Treatment_____

Prognosis_____

PERITONEUM	ENDOMETRIOSIS		<1cm	1-3cm	>3cm
		Superficial	1	2	4
		Deep	2	4	6
OVARY	R	Superficial	1	2	4
		Deep	4	16	20
	L	Superficial	1	2	4
		Deep	4	16	20

	POSTERIOR CULDESAC OBLITERATION	Partial		Complete	
		4		40	

	ADHESIONS		<1/3 Enclosure	1/3-2/3 Enclosure	>2/3 Enclosure
OVARY	R	Filmy	1	2	4
		Dense	4	8	16
	L	Filmy	1	2	4
		Dense	4	8	16
TUBE	R	Filmy	1	2	4
		Dense	4*	8*	16
	L	Filmy	1	2	4
		Dense	4*	8*	16

*If the fimbriated end of the fallopian tube is completely enclosed, change the point assignment to 16.

Additional Endometriosis: _____   Associated Pathology: _____
_____   _____
_____   _____

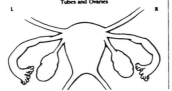
To Be Used with Normal
Tubes and Ovaries
L _____ R

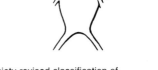
To Be Used with Abnormal
Tubes and/or Ovaries
L _____ R

Figure 41-2. The American Fertility Society revised classification of endometriosis, 1985. (American Fertility Society. Revised American Fertility Society classification of endometriosis. Fertil Steril 1985;43:351.)

♦ GnRH agonist

Modification of native GnRH
- causes down regulation of pituitary gonadotropins
  - medical oophorectomy

Side effects
- menopausal symptoms
- osteoporosis

As effective as others at disease regression and pain relief
No improvement in fertility rates

✧ *Surgical intervention*

Most common approach
- vaporize, coagulate, cauterize, excise lesions

Recurrence rate of 28% at 18 months, 40% at 9 years

Efficacy of pain relief unclear

Pregnancy rates in severe cases can be significantly improved with surgery

Definitive surgery is hysterectomy with bilateral salpingo-oophorectomy
- pain eliminated in up to 90%
- one third of patients with advanced disease and ovarian preservation will require further treatment

✧ *Symptomatic treatment*

Nonsteroidal antiinflammatory agents
- tolfenamic acid
- naproxen sodium

Surgical ablation
- laparoscopic uterosacral nerve oblation (LUNA)
- presacral neurectomy (PSN)
  - may have high recurrence rates

Fertility treatments
- controlled ovarian hyperstimulation and IUI
  - pregnancy rate increased threefold compared with expectant management
- in vitro fertilization also significantly increases fecundity (14%)

42

◆ Climacteric

INTRODUCTION

U.S. population is aging
- >50 million women have reached the climacteric

Approximate age of menopause is 51 years
- mean life expectancy is 85 years-of-age
- most women will live more than one third of their lives without estrogen production

CAUSE OF MENOPAUSE

Exhaustion of gonodotropin-responsive follicular units in ovary results in cessation of menses

Age of menopause not affected by
- race
- socioeconomic status
- number of pregnancies
- oral contraceptive use
- education
- physical characteristics
- alcohol consumption
- age of menarche
- date of last pregnancy
- only cigarette smoking has conclusively been shown to hasten follicular exhaustion

OVARY AND MENOPAUSE

Ovary develops on medioventral border of urogenital ridge

Indifferent until 42 days of gestation
- contains large primordial germ cells
  - migrate from yolk sac to genital ridge

300 to 1300 primordial germ cells
- undergo mitosis to form oogonia
  - 600,000 by eighth week of gestation
  - 6 to 7 million by twentieth week

- meiosis initiated between the eighth and thirteenth week
  - converts oogonia to primary oocytes
    - surrounded by precursors of granulosa cells thus creating primordial follicles
  - conversion not completed until sixth month after birth
  - primary oocytes that do not form primordial follicles degenerate
- primordial follicles present at birth are lost by ovulation or atresia
  - total number of oocytes at puberty and efficiency of atresia may determine age of menopause

Gross and microscopic changes occur with age
- weight declines from 14 to 5 g
- stroma more prominent
- remaining primordial follicles undergo atresia

SYSTEMIC CHANGES WITH AGING

Senescence is the process or condition of aging
Many organ systems affected by the aging process

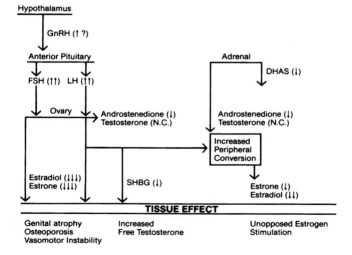

Figure 42-1. Schematic diagram of hormonal changes after menopause. Arrows refer to direction of change in menopausal women. (DHEAS, dehydroepiandrosterone sulfate; FSH, follicle-stimulating hormone; GnRH, gonadotropin-releasing hormone; LH, luteinizing hormone; N.C., no change.) (Hammond CB, Maxson WS. Physiology of the menopause. Monograph in Current Concepts. Kalamazoo, MI: Scope Publications, 1983.)

REPRODUCTIVE ENDOCRINE CHANGES IN CLIMACTERIC WOMEN

◆ Hypothalamus-Pituitary

Changes in hypothalamus-pituitary axis responsible for menstrual irregularity of perimenopause (Fig. 42-1)
Follicular phase lengthens
- diminished supply of gonodotropin-sensitive follicles

Anovulatory cycles result if estrogen levels are insufficient
FSH levels often are >40 mIU/mL in premenopause
- values >100 indicate follicular exhaustion
- maximal levels 2 to 3 years after menopause
  - increase more rapidly (20 days) in surgical menopause

Estrogen will lower LH and FSH levels but not to premenopausal levels
- possibly result of loss of inhibin from granulosa cells

Abnormal LH pulse patterns
- pulse frequency of 10 to 20 minutes

Loss of opioid inhibition
Probably an overall increase in GnRH

◆ Estrogen Production

Principle circulating estrogen is estradiol-17β
- produced by direct secretion or peripheral conversion of testosterone and estrone
- 80 to 500 µg daily during reproductive years
- two-cell theory
  - theca produces C-19 steroids
  - granulosa cell layer converts these to estrogens

In postmenopausal patients the principle estrogen is estrone
- biological potency is one third that of estradiol
- most formed by peripheral conversion of androstenedione
- daily production
  - 40 µg/day estrone
  - 6 µg/day estradiol
- only 0.1% of testosterone converted to estradiol

◆ Androgen Production

Diminished concentration of androgens probably due to estrogen deprivation
Estrogen is noncompetitive inhibitor of 3β-hydroxysteroid dehydrogenase
- relative block would augment DHEA, DHEAS production

Androstenedione production decreases
Postmenopausal ovary produces larger percentage of testosterone (50%)

THE MENOPAUSE SYNDROME

Hormone related
- genitourinary atrophy
- vasomotor instability
- osteoporosis

Probably hormone related
- atherosclerotic cardiovascular disease
- psychosocial symptoms
- insomnia, fatigue, and depression

◆ Vasomotor Symptoms

Experienced by 75% to 85% of perimenopausal and postmenopausal women

37% to 50% of premenopausal women also develop hot flashes
after bilateral oophorectomy

80% have symptoms >1 year

Less than 25% have symptoms >5 years

✧ *Etiology*

Not a peripheral cause

No difference in the ratio or absolute levels of LH to FSH or in
total estrogens in those with or without flashes

Do not occur in women with gonadal dysgenesis who have not
been exposed to estrogen

Temporal relationship with LH pulse

Hypothalamic factors probably responsible
- four neurotransmitters in preoptic and anterior hypothalamic
  nuclei
  - GnRH
  - norepinephrine
  - dopamine
  - β-endorphin

Estrogen deficiency primary abnormality
- dependent on biologically available estrogen

Drug of choice: estrogen
- other options
  - medroxyprogesterone acetate, 10 mg or more PO daily or
    100 mg IM monthly
  - bellergal (ergot alkaloid)
  - clonidine, 0.1 to 0.2 mg BID

◆ Genitourinary Atrophy

Atrophy at different rates

Most common vulvar symptom is pruritus

Vagina becomes pale and thin
- increased vaginitis

Cervical lesions more common
- erosion, ectropion, ulcer

Increased incidence of prolapse
Urethral syndrome common
- no increase in true stress urinary incontinence

Increased rate of bacteriuria 7% to 10%

◆ Osteoporosis

Primary osteoporosis (senile)
- women between 55 and 70 years-of-age
- most common fracture: vertebrae, long bones

Secondary osteoporosis
- bone loss and fracture caused by a specific disease

One third of women will develop some complication of osteoporosis

◆ Menopause and Bone Loss

Maximal skeleton mass at 35 years-of-age
By 50 years-of-age, generalized bone loss
Natural menopause
- 1% to 2% bone loss per year

Surgical menopause
- 3.9% per year for the first 6 years, then 1% to 2% per year

30% to 50% loss of skeletal mass by 80 years-of-age
Associated factors
- dietary calcium
- alcohol, caffeine, tobacco use

◆ Estrogen and Bone Mineral Metabolism

Bone remodeling cycle takes 100 days
Osteoblast and osteoclast
PTH increase in response to hypocalcemia
Vitamin D deficiency also causes substantial bone loss

◆ Diagnosis

30% to 35% will develop symptomatic osteoporosis
Many different techniques to measure bone mass (Table 42-1)
Limited as screening tools but may provide useful information
  to a patient
Extreme reduction in bone mass should be further assessed with
  laboratory tests

◆ Estrogen Therapy to Prevent Osteoporosis

Significant reduction in bone loss if initiated within 3 years of
  loss of ovarian function
Role of estrogen in established osteoporosis is less clear
- may prevent further complications

Dose of 0.625 mg of conjugated estrogen is adequate protection
  in most patients

TABLE 42-1. Techniques to Measure Bone Mass

Technique	Site of Measurement	Corticotrabecular Ratio	Accuracy (%)	Precision (%)	Radiation Dose
Single-photon absorptiometry	Midshaft radius	95 : 5	4	2-4	5 mrem
	Distal radius	75:24	5	2-4	
Dual-photon absorptiometry	L2, L3, L4	40:60	5-7	2-5	5-15 mrem
	Femoral neck	75 : 25	?	?	5-15 mrem
	Total skeleton	80 : 20	2-4	2-4	10-40 mrem
Dual-energy computed tomography	Vertebral body	5 : 95	?	?	200 mrem

Lindsay R. Prevention of osteoporosis: In: Muir Gray JA, ed. Prevention of disease in the elderly. New York: Longman (Churchill Livingstone), 1985:102.

TABLE 42-2. Commonly Used Estrogens for Replacement Therapy

Generic or Chemical Name	Commercial Preparation	Doses Available (mg)	Usual Starting Dose (mg)
Estradiol	Transdermal patch	0.5; 0.1	0.05
	Estrace	1; 2	1
Conjugated Estrogens	Premarin	0.3; 0.625; 0.9; 1.25; 2; 5	0.625
Estropipate	Ogen	0.625; 1.25; 2.5; 5	1.25
Esterfied Estrogens	Estratab	0.3; 0.625; 1.25; 2.5	0.625

London SN, Chihal HJ. Menopause: clinical concepts. Durant, OK: Essential Medical Information Systems, 1989.

ATHEROSCLEROTIC CARDIOVASCULAR DISEASE

500,000 women die annually from cardiovascular disease
Increasing data that estrogen replacement therapy reduces risk
Risk factors
- age
- family history
- hypertension
- cigarette smoking
- total cholesterol level

Lipids and coronary heart disease
- 3 major density classes of lipoproteins
  - very-low-density lipoproteins (VLDL)
  - low-density lipoproteins (LDL)
  - high-density lipoproteins (HDL)
- LDL is cholesterol rich
  - accumulation can lead to atherosclerosis
- HDL aids liver in removal of cholesterol
  - prevents atherosclerosis

PSYCHOSOCIAL PROBLEMS

Insomnia and fatigue in 30% to 40%
- may be result of nocturnal hot flashes

Estrogen may combat depression
No direct evidence to support hormonal deprivation as cause of diminished sexual response
- sexual decline probably one of circumstance, not potential

ESTROGEN THERAPY

◆ Definite Risks

✧ *Endometrial carcinoma*

Progression from adenomatous hyperplasia to cancer depends on intensity and duration of estrogen stimulation
Unopposed estrogen therapy will increase risk
- lack of progesterone

Progesterone therapy
- duration as important as the dose
- 5 to 7 days insufficient
- 10 days will reverse 98% of all endometrial hyperplasias
- 13 days reduces risk to near zero

✧ *Cholelithiasis*

Relative risk of 2.5
Mechanism unknown
Possibly alteration in bile salts

◆ Possible Risks

✧ *Breast cancer*
A multifactorial disorder
Addition of progestin to protect against development of breast
cancer is controversial
- three studies suggest decreased risk

Prognosis may be better for estrogen users later diagnosed with
breast cancer
Decreased mortality rate

✧ *Thromboembolism*
No evidence of increased risk
Use caution in case of recent thromboembolic disorder

✧ *Hypertension*
No adverse affect on existing hypertension
Unresolved relationship between estrogen therapy and devel-
opment of hypertension

ESTROGEN PHARMACOLOGY

90% of circulating estrogen protein associated with transport
protein
- 38% SHBG
- 60% albumin
- 2% to 3% free

Free estrogen is biologically active form
Many preparations available (Table 42-2)
Most commonly prescribed
- conjugated estrogens
  - 48% estrone sulfates
  - 15% 17α-dihydroequilin sulfate

Other choices: estradiol (orally or transdermally)

PROGESTIN PHARMACOLOGY

Secreted by corpus luteum for 14 days
- deceases receptor content and mitotic activity of endometrium
- induces estradiol dehydrogenase
- facilitates endometrial shedding

Oral activity
- modifying progesterone at C-17 (17-acetoxyprogestins)
- removing C-19 from testosterone and placing ethinyl group at
  C-17 (19-norprogestins)
  - large variations in oral absorption

Native progesterone can be administered by suppositories
All affect lipid metabolism adversely
- elevated LDL, lower HDL

Oral micronized progesterone devoid of lipid effects

MANAGEMENT OF ESTROGEN THERAPY IN MENOPAUSE

Absolute contraindications
- known or suspected estrogen-dependent neoplasia
- undiagnosed genital bleeding
- active thrombophlebitis
- active liver disease
- known or suspected pregnancy

Should be considered in all women with symptoms of estrogen deficiency
- traditionally given in cyclical manner but may be given continuously
  If cyclic
  - estrogen on days 1 to 25
  - progestin on days 16 to 25
  - 5 days free
- more recently given estrogen continuously with monthly progestin therapy on the first 10 to 14 days of the month
  - bleeding before day 10 suggest need for higher progestin dose
- continuous estrogen and progestin
  - no bleeding in 70%
  - irregular bleeding in 30%
  - doses usually estrogen, 0.625 mg, and medroxyprogesterone, 2.5 mg
- calcium supplementation, 1500 mg daily
- cancer screening (Table 42-3)

TABLE 42-3. Cancer Screening for the Climacteric Woman

Type of Cancer	Screening Test
Laryngeal cancer	Examination with persistent hoarseness. Stop tobacco products.
Lung cancer	No screening available. Stop smoking.
Breast cancer	Annual physician examination, monthly patient self-examination, mammography every 1 to 2 years.
Skin cancer	Check skin. Have any suspicious lesions removed.
Colorectal cancer	Stool samples (2 to 3 per year) for occult blood.
Vulvar cancer	Yearly pelvic examination. Evaluation of persistent vulvar itching.
Cervical cancer	Annual Pap smear.
Endometrial cancer	Aggressively investigate any abnormal vaginal bleeding.
Ovarian cancer	Yearly pelvic examination.

London SN, Chihal HJ. Menopause: clinical concepts. Durant, OK: Essential Medical Information Systems, 1989.

43

◆ Perioperative Care

PREOPERATIVE PREPARATION

◆ General Condition

Surgery is a situation of stress for anyone
Patient must have clear understanding of several aspects
- nature of the procedure
- other options for therapy
- risks and benefits of each procedure discussed

Physician should always volunteer to involve family members in these discussions
Nature of these discussions and their scope should be stated in the medical record

◆ Operative Permit

Informed consent
- signing of the paper is irrelevant
- the patient's understanding of the content of the procedure determines informed consent

Educating without anxiety
- possible complications
- realistic appraisal of positive results
- lethal complications
  - dependent on the nature of the procedure
    - hysterectomy mortality rates
      - benign disease: 6/10,000
      - pregnancy-related: 29/10,000
      - cancer: 38/10,000

Signing the consent
- should be witnessed
- summary documented by progress note in patient's chart

◆ History and Physical Examination

Useful diagnostic information
- 70% from history
- 20% from physical examination

- 10% from special laboratory tests

Physician should listen in a sympathetic and unhurried fashion

Operative risk
- best indicator of cardiopulmonary status is routine activity level

Full review of systems necessary
- drug, alcohol, tobacco use
- complete physical examination

◆ Laboratory Studies

Routine testing should be discouraged

Suggested tests
- healthy young patient for elective gynecologic surgery
  - pap smear
  - pregnancy test
  - hematocrit
  - >40 years-of-age (Roizen Guidelines)
    - hematocrit
    - electrocardiogram (EKG)
    - blood urea nitrogen (BUN), serum glucose
  - >60 years-of-age (Roizen Guidelines)
    - add chest x-ray

Known medical illnesses may lead to more intensive evaluation

Routine barium enema and intravenous pyelogram (IVP) with pelvic masses should not be performed

Use in specific cases only
- barium enema
  - >50 years old
  - gastrointestinal symptoms
    - blood in stool
  - left-sided mass suggestive of diverticulitis
- IVP
  - fixed solid mass suggestive of malignancy
  - pelvic kidney
  - unexplained renal insufficiency
    - can substitute renal ultrasound if necessary

DETERMINING SURGICAL RISKS

◆ Operative Mortality

American Society of Anesthesiologists has adopted Dripps physical status classification systems (Table 43-1, Table 43-2)
- emergency surgery doubles mortality risk for levels I, II, and III

Most common causes of operative mortality
- myocardial infarction
- pulmonary embolism
- infection
- heart failure

TABLE 43-1. American Society of Anesthesiologists
Physical Status Classification

Category	Description
I	Healthy patient
II	Mild systemic disease—no functional limitation
III	Severe systemic disease—definite functional limitations
IV	Severe systemic disease that is a constant threat to life
V	Moribund patient unlikely to survive 24 hours without operation

Schneider AJL. Assessment of risk factors and surgical outcome. Surg Clin North Am 1983;63:1113.

TABLE 43-2. American Society of Anesthesiologists
Physical Status Classification and Overall
Death Rates

Physical Status	Number	Deaths	Mortality Rate (%)
I	50,703	43	0.08
II	12,601	34	0.27
III	3,626	66	1.82
IV	850	66	7.76
V	608	57	9.38

Vacanti CJ, Van Houten RJ, Hill RC. A statistical analysis of the relationship of physical status to postoperative mortality in 58,388 cases. Anesth Analg 1970; 49:564.

PREOPERATIVE PREPARATION

Need for preoperative admission
Blood bank
- autologous and donor-directed
Bowel preparation
- clear liquid 1 day prior to surgery
- mild cathartic 1 to 2 days prior to surgery
- use of antibiotics is controversial
- alternative for rapid cleansing of the bowel: GoLYTELY
Shaving and cleansing
- unwise to shave skin in advance of surgery
- may increase skin infection through formation of micro-abscesses
- douching before vaginal surgery is intuitive, but has never been tested

Hydration
- nothing-by-mouth (NPO) 8 to12 hours prior to surgery

Prophylactic antibiotics
- recommended for vaginal hysterectomy
- possibly beneficial for abdominal hysterectomy
  - presence of bacterial vaginosis or trichomoniasis may increase rate of infections and complications in hysterectomy patients
    - treat 1 month prior to surgery if possible
- unnecessary for adnexal surgery unless evidence of previous infection or vaginal contamination
- use of antibiotics in infertility procedures is common by physician preference
- drug of choice
  - usually cefazolin, 1 g IV prior to surgery
  - consider anti-embolic prophylaxis
    - low-dose heparin
    - pneumatic compression devices
    - elastic stockings (TED hose)

Medications
- hypertensive patient
  - antihypertensive should be taken on morning of surgery with sip of water
- diabetics
  - oral agents
    - stop 1 to 3 days prior to surgery
  - insulin (three methods)
    1. withhold all glucose and insulin perioperatively for short procedures
    2. give one half usual dose of long-acting insulin and start IV with D5W with 100 cc/hour
    3. maintain continuous drips of insulin and D5W
  - previous steroid treatment (greater than 1 week of duration during the preceding year)
    - stress doses should be used
      - hydrocortisone, 100 mg evening before surgery, morning of surgery, and then every 8 hours
    - no tapering if duration of therapy is short

IMMEDIATE POSTOPERATIVE CARE

Most crucial period is the first 72 to 96 hours after surgery

◆ Pain Control

Intravenous or intramuscular narcotics
Patient-controlled analgesia
Epidural analgesia

◆ Prophylaxis

Deep venous thrombosis (DVT) prophylaxis
- low-dose heparin or external pneumatic compression devices

Atelectasis and pneumonia prophylaxis
- incentive spirometry

Infectious prophylaxis
- antibiotics as deemed appropriate

◆ Physical Examination

Should be routinely performed
- cardiovascular system
  - neck veins
- wound examination
- extremities

◆ Fluid Management

Careful management is necessary to avoid fluid overload
Oliguria demands evaluation
- determine volume status
  - may require central venous pressure (CVP) monitoring
- check bladder catheter (or place catheter)
- consider laboratory studies
  - urinary electrolytes (prior to diuretic therapy)
  - urine osmolarity and creatinine

◆ Bowel Function

Normal bowel sounds and no distention → clear liquid diet
Flatus or bowel movement → regular diet
Distention and vomiting without normal bowel sounds may represent ileus
- nasogastric (NG) tube may be necessary for patient comfort

◆ Fever

First 24 hours usually represents atelectasis
>48 hours after surgery should be further assessed
- often surgical site infection
  - pelvic abscess
  - cuff cellulitis (diagnosis of exclusion)
  - wound infection
    - often late complication

Treatment
- clindamycin and aminoglycoside
  - add ampicillin or penicillin if patient fails to improve after 24 hours to cover enterococcus
- further failure may be result of septic pelvic thrombophlebitis
  - treat with full heparinization
  - fever should resolve within 24 to 48 hours

◆ Pulmonary Complications

Preoperative pulmonary compromise is the major risk factor
- other risk factors
  - advanced age
  - smoking
  - obesity
  - prolonged anesthesia
  - preexisting pulmonary disease

Prevention is the key
- incentive spirometry
- bronchodilation therapy and chest physiotherapy as needed

Pulmonary embolism
- onset can be dramatic (Table 43-3)
- EKG, arterial blood gas measurements (ABG), and chest x-ray should be performed
  - pulmonary arteriography is most accurate and most morbid test
  - pulmonary ventilation perfusion scan can be reassuring

Differential diagnosis
- myocardial infarction
- pneumonia
- pneumothorax
- pulmonary edema
- pericardial tamponade

Treatment
- heparin for 7 days
- warfarin for last 2 to 3 days
  - total of 3 to 6 months of systemic anticoagulation

◆ Wound Complications

Dehiscence; disruption of any of the layers of the incision, usually used to describe breakdown of all layers except peritoneum

Evisceration; breakdown of all layers with protrusion of intra-abdominal contents

---

TABLE 43-3. Signs and Symptoms of Pulmonary Embolus

Signs	Symptoms
Tachypnea	Dyspnea
Rales	Pleuritic chest pain
Increase in second heart sound	Anxiety
Tachycardia	Cough
Cyanosis	Hemoptysis

Use of Smead-Jones type closure can reduce wound disruption (Fig. 43-1)
- especially useful in high-risk patients
  - previous history of wound infection
  - obesity
  - diabetes
  - chronic obstructive pulmonary disease (COPD)
  - steroid therapy
  - peritonitis
  - malignancy
  - previous radiation therapy

◆ Urinary Tract Complications

Urinary retention
- diagnosed by placement of catheter
- use of suprapubic catheter may be helpful to prevent this complication

Urinary fistula
- leakage of clear fluid from vagina should raise suspicion of fistula
- diagnose vesicovaginal fistula with indigo carnine dye placed in bladder
  - if no dye passes to vagina could be ureterovaginal fistula
    - inject dye intravenously
- treatment
  - vesicovaginal
    - immediate repair if tissue is healthy or 2 months later
  - ureterovaginal
    - reoperation
    - nephrostomy
    - anterior or retrograde stent placement

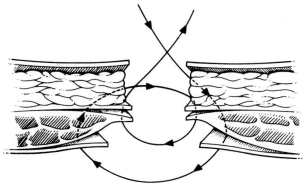

Figure 43-1. Modified Snead-Jones abdominal wall closure.

44

◆ Pelvic Organ Prolapse

PELVIC FLOOR AND THE NATURE OF GENITAL PROLAPSE

Pelvic floor forms a supportive layer that prevents abdominal and pelvic organs from falling through the opening in the pelvic bones (Fig. 44-1)

Prolapse develops as a result of increasing intraabdominal forces, not uterine weight

Factors important for support
- suspension of the genital tract by the ligaments in fascia
- closure of the pelvic floor by the levator ani

ANATOMY AND PATHOPHYSIOLOGY

◆ Basic Anatomy of the Pelvic Floor

◇ *Viscerofascial layer*
Uterus and vagina attach to pelvic walls by fibrous tissue (endopelvic fascia)
- parametria (cardinal and uterosacral ligaments)
- paracolpia (Fig. 44-2)

Suburethral endopelvic fascia attaches to the arcus tendineous from pelvis and to the medial border of the levator ani
- crucial for urinary continence

◇ *Levator ani muscles*
Lie below the uterus, vagina, bladder, and rectum
Medial portion is puborectalis (pubococcygeus)
Horizontal orientation
Closes urethra, vagina, and rectum by compressing them against the pubic bone

◇ *Interaction between the muscles and fascia*
If pelvic floor muscles are damaged, connective tissue can hold vagina in place only for limited time

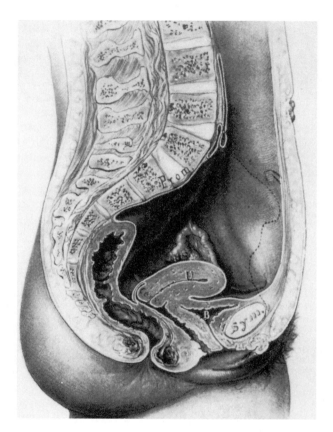

Figure 44-1. A sagittal section of the abdomen and pelvis shows the relation of the pelvic floor to the abdominal cavity. (Kelly HA. Gynecology. Baltimore: Appleton and Co., 1928.)

CAUSE OF PELVIC FLOOR DAMAGE

Several factors influence the development of prolapse (Table 44-1)

DIAGNOSIS AND CLASSIFICATION

◆ Technique of Examination

Two major principles
1. examination must be made with patient straining forcefully enough so that the prolapse is at its greatest.

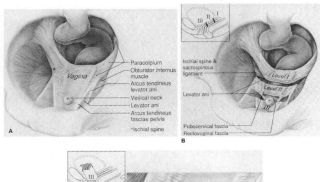

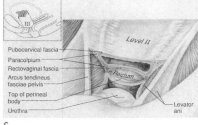

Figure 44-2. Support structures of the vagina after hysterectomy. The bladder has been removed to expose the vagina. (**A**) The paracolpium. (**B**) The different levels of support structures. (**C**) The details of the pubocervical and rectovaginal fasciae after a wedge of vagina and urethra has been removed (*inset*). (DeLancey JOL. Anatomic aspects of vaginal eversion after hysterectomy. Am J Obstet Gynecol 1992; 166:1717.)

  2. examination of individual elements of support must be made
     independently.
  Many different classification systems exist
  Anatomic descriptions are most reliable and more meaningful

EVALUATION OF INDIVIDUAL ELEMENTS OF SUPPORT

◆ Anterior Vaginal Wall

  Establish both urethral and bladder support
  • urethrocele
  • cystocele
  Urethrovesical crease is the line of demarcation
  Descent of the vagina past the hymenal ring is abnormal
  • may or may not be associated with stress urinary incontinence

---

TABLE 44-1. Factors Involved in Pelvic Organ Prolapse

Inborn strength of connective tissue and muscle
Loss of connective tissue strength
    Damage at childbirth
    Deterioration with age
    Poor collagen repair
Loss of levator function
    Neuromuscular drainage during childbirth
    Metabolic diseases that affect muscle function
Increased loads on the supportive system
    Prolonged lifting
    Chronic coughing from chronic pulmonary disease
Disturbance of the balance of the structural parts
    Alteration of vaginal axis by urethral suspension
    Failure to reattach the cardinal ligaments at hysterectomy

---

◆ Uterus and Vaginal Apex

Severity of prolapse gauged by cervical location
- descent to within 1 cm of hymenal ring indicates significant loss of support
- cervical elongation can occur

◆ Posterior Vaginal Wall

Site of both enterocele and rectocele
- rectocele
  - anterior rectal wall and overlying vagina protrude below hymenal ring
- enterocele
  - cul-de-sac becomes distended with intestine and bulges the posterior wall outward

✧ Enterocele

Cul-de-sac usually kept closed by suspension of upper vagina and intact levator plate
Pulsion enterocele
- may occur with vaginal apex or uterine walls suspended
Traction enterocele
- no bulging of cul-de-sac discovered until time of vaginal hysterectomy
- represents a potential enterocele
Must be detected by close inspection
- rectovaginal examination is very helpful

✧ Rectocele

Hallmark is the formation of a pocket which allows anterior rectal wall to bulge below introitus
Stool can become trapped in this pocket

◇ *Prolapse subsequent to hysterectomy*

Special care should be taken to identify apex of the prolapse

Significant deficit in support is present if apex decends to lower one third of vagina

◆ Symptoms

Dragging sensation

Sacral backache

Perineal wetness or ulceration

Cystourethrocele can be associated with retention and incontinence

Evacuation of stool may be made difficult

◆ Candidates for Surgery

Prolapse above the hymenal ring
- repair only for symptoms attributive to prolapse
- consider "pessary test"

Prolapse below the hymenal ring
- symptomatic
- asymptomatic may be associated with recurrent UTI and ureteral dilation

SURGICAL PROCEDURES

◆ Preoperative Consideration

Careful preoperative evaluation determines specific elements of the prolapse

Fleet enema night before surgery

Prophylactic antibiotics

Current Pap smear

Endometrial biopsy if associated symptoms of abnormal bleeding

◆ Technique of Vaginal Hysterectomy

Derived from operation originally described by Heaney (Fig. 44-3)

◆ Management of the Cul-de-Sac and Suspension of the Vaginal Apex

Reconstructive phase of operation actually addresses the problem of prolapse

Goal is closure of the peritoneum with suspension of vaginal apex

◆ Anterior Colporrhaphy

Performed in patients with cystocele

Vaginal mucosa identified (Fig. 44-4)

Plication of suburethral fascia should be done with care

◆ Posterior Colpoperineorrhaphy

Requires the most skill and judgment
- reconstruct rectovaginal septum
- normalize size of introitus

Endopelvic fascia reapproximated to midline (Fig. 44-5)
Assess adequacy of vagina for intercourse at the end of the procedure

◆ Posthysterectomy Prolapse

Correct by sacrospinous ligament suspension (Fig. 44-6) or abdominal sacral colpopexy
Need to address all components of prolapse
Colpocleisis can be considered in patient who is not sexually active

◆ Conservative Measures

Vaginal pessaries are the oldest effective treatment
May not function well if pelvic floor muscle is damaged
- cannot be held in place

Estrogen often is a useful adjunct to prevent mucosal erosion

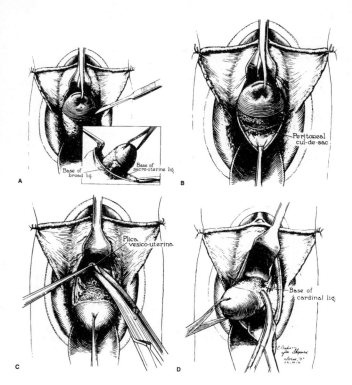

Figure 44-3. (**A**) Vaginal hysterectomy is initiated by circumscribing the cervix at the cervicovaginal junction. (**B**) The posterior cul-de-sac is opened. (**C**) The peritoneum of the anterior cul-de-sac is incised. (**D**) The base of the uterosacral and cardinal ligament is usually clamped in two bites. (**E**) The upper cardinal ligament is clamped prior to its transection. (**F**) The uterine fundus is delivered, and the connections between the adnexal structures and uterine corpus are clamped. (**G**) Ligaments and vaginal cuff as they appear after hysterectomy. The posterior cuff is whip-stitched (*inset*). (**H**) Technique for resuspension of the vaginal cuff and obliteration of the cul-de-sac. (1, placement of suture through exteriorized ligaments and vaginal wall; 2, reefing sutures placed in peritoneum; 3, modified internal McCall suture; 4, high purse-string suture to close the cul-de-sac.) (Mattingly RF, Thompson JD, eds. TeLinde's operative gynecology. 6th ed. Philadelphia: JB Lippincott, 1985.)

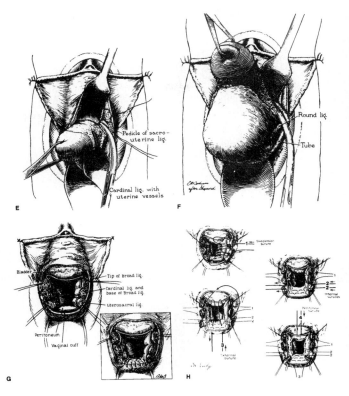

Figure 44-3. cont'd.

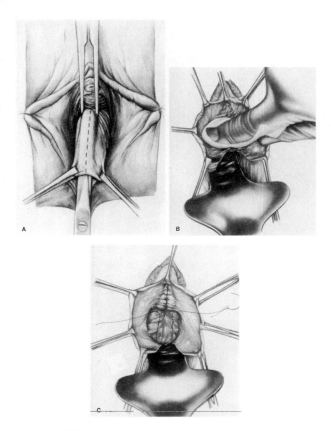

Figure 44-4. (A) The vaginal mucosa is undermined when commencing anterior colporrhaphy. **(B)** The fascia is separated from the mucosa. **(C)** The fascia is sutured together in the midline. Special care should be taken to ensure that the support at the urethrovesical junction is adequate. **(D)** Excess mucosa is trimmed. **(E)** The mucosa is closed. A bite of the underlying fascia is included to minimize dead space. (Mattingly RF, Thompson JD, eds. TeLinde's operative gynecology. 6th ed. Philadelphia: JB Lippincott, 1985.)

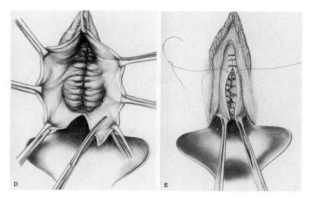

Figure 44-4. cont'd.

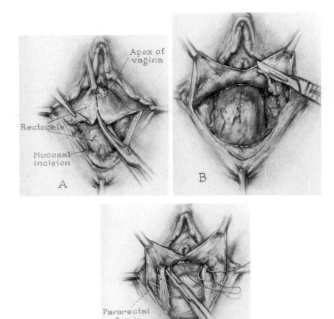

Figure 44-5. (A) To begin posterior colporrhaphy, a transverse incision is
made in the perineal body, and a vertical incision is extended toward the
vaginal apex. **(B)** The perirectal fascia are mobilized from the mucosa.
(C) The perirectal fascia is sutured, beginning above the site of the
rectocele. **(D)** The inner surface of the levator ani muscles are approxi-
mated in the perineal body, and redundant mucosa is excised. **(E)** The
mucosa and perineal skin are closed. (Mattingly RF, Thompson JD, eds.
TeLinde's operative gynecology. 6th ed. Philadelphia: JB Lippincott, 1985.)

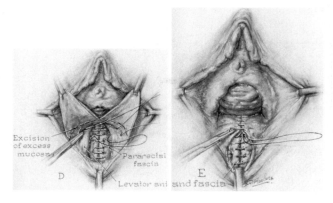

Figure 44-5. cont'd.

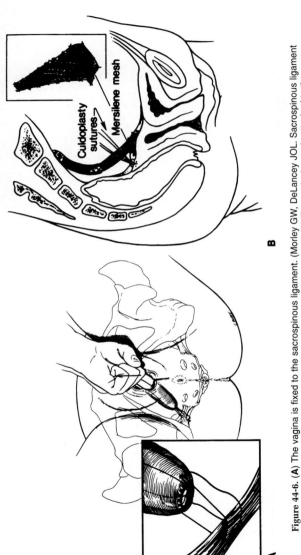

Figure 44-6. (A) The vagina is fixed to the sacrospinous ligament. (Morley GW, DeLancey JOL. Sacrospinous ligament fixation for eversion of the vagina. Am J Obstet Gynecol 1988;158:872.) **(B)** The vaginal apex is attached to the sacrum with an intervening graft. (Addison WA, Timmons MC, Wall LL, Livengood CH. Failed abdominal sacral colpopexy, observations and recommendations. Obstet Gynecol 1989;74:480.)

45

◆ Endoscopic Surgery

INTRODUCTION

New uses and more complicated procedures are constantly being developed
Potential advantages
- shortened hospital stay
- reduced expense, pain, morbidity, and recovery time
- improved cosmesis
- better patient acceptance

Cost savings may be offset by higher fees and equipment costs
Proof of efficacy is lacking in many procedures presently being performed

TRAINING

Training should include didactic and hands-on experience
- residency
- high-caliber postgraduate courses

Competency should be confirmed by proctor system
- further monitoring by peer review

OPERATING ROOM SETUP

Major complications can occur
- vascular, urologic, intestinal

Operating room must meet requirements for general surgery suite
Familiarity with instrumentation is crucial
- organize into major group or modules
  - laparoscopic cart
  - video cart
  - vaginal instrument table
  - hysteroscopy cart
  - hysteroscopy instrument table
- pneumoperitoneum with Verres needle
- four pelvic punctures

LAPAROSCOPIC SURGICAL PROCEDURES

◆ Adhesiolysis

Association between adhesions and chronic pelvic pain uncertain
  • empirical treatment
Relationship of adhesions to infertility evident in some cases
Adhesions usually re-form despite careful technique and adjuvant treatment

◆ Ovarian Tumors

Must avoid unnecessary surgery on functional cysts and overaggressive surgery in cases of potential malignancy
Only 5% of ovarian cysts in reproductive-age women are malignant
Risk rises dramatically between 40 and 60 years-of-age
Presence of benign characteristic does not always preclude malignancy

◇ *Ancillary diagnostic techniques*

Preoperative diagnosis of etiology of pelvic masses incorrect 50% of time from pelvic examination alone
Ultrasound best initial imaging modality
Benign
  • anechoic
  • smooth walled
  • thin or no septations
Malignant
  • solid
  • papillary excrescences
  • thick septations
  • ascites
Both cystic and solid components in dermoids, hemorrhagic corpus luteum, or endometrioma
MRI is costly but may be more accurate than ultrasound or CT
CA-125
  • may be elevated in benign conditions as well as malignancies
  • if used in combination with ultrasound and pelvic examination, more ovarian carcinomas can be recognized
  • elevation of CA-125 in postmenopausal women carries high positive predictive value

◇ *Surgical procedures*

Patient selection
Younger than 40 years-of-age with lack of regression after one menstrual period or 1 month of suppressive treatment
Older patients with no suggestion of malignancy by other tests
Unilocular cysts
  • aspiration alone associated with 30% recurrence risk
    • excision of entire cyst lining is necessary

Dermoids and complex cysts
- remove mass intact
  - colpotomy
  - endoscopic lap-sac

Postmenopausal patients
- cyst benign on ultrasound, CA-125 negative, and less than 3 cm
  - repeat examination in 3 months
- cyst larger and CA-125 positive
  - exploration

Laparascopic oophorectomy on large benign cyst possible

◆ Presacral Neurectomy

Intractable dysmenorrhea
- unresponsive to medical treatment

Needs steep Trendelenburg
Identify uterus and iliac vessels
Incise peritoneum over sacral promontory
- attention to hemostasis crucial
- isolate superior hypogastric nerve plexus
- excise 3 to 4 mm segment of nerve

Relief in 70% of patients

◆ Laparoscopic Uterosacral Nerve Ablation (LUNA)

Indications and results more controversial
Neither may be useful in dyspareunia, central pain from endometriosis, other mixed pelvic pain disorders

◆ Hysterectomy

650,000 hysterectomy procedures performed annually
- only 30% vaginal

Laparoscopy may convert some from abdominal to vaginal
No utility in performing laparoscopy if vaginal hysterectomy can be performed easily
Laparoscopic hysterectomy (LH)
- entire broad ligament divided laparoscopically

Laparoscopic-assisted vaginal hysterectomy (LAVH)
- lower uterine pedicles clamped from below

Several surgical techniques
- bipolar cautery and scissors
- laser
- multifire stapling instruments
  - expensive
  - may predispose to ureteral injury if used incorrectly

Unorthodox variations
- laparoscopic supracervical hysterectomy
- radical hysterectomy
- bladder suspension

◆ **Myomectomy**

Can be used in selected cases of symptomatic pedunculated or subserous myomas

Satisfactory uterine closure difficult

May result in poorly healed uterine scar

◆ **Appendectomy**

Indications
- acute appendicitis
- endometriosis involving appendix
- adhesions of appendix to the pelvic viscera

Several techniques
- electrocautery
- endoloop sutures
- automatic stapling devices

HYSTEROSCOPIC SURGERY

Oldest gynecologic endoscopic procedure

No longer only diagnostic

Therapeutic approaches are replacing former abdominal techniques

◆ **Endometrial Ablation**

20% of hysterectomies performed for menorrhagia

In 1981, successful endometrial ablation with Nd:YAG laser was described

◇ *Patient selection*

Intractable menorrhagia unresponsive to conservative therapy

Uterine malignancy or premalignant changes must be ruled out first

Large irregular uterus or desire for future fertility are reasons for exclusion

◇ *Technique*

Preoperative treatment
- danazol, 400 mg/BID 4 to 8 weeks prior to surgery
- GnRH analogs
  - depot leuprolide acetate, 7.5 mg 1 month prior

Distention medium
- 32% dextran 70 (Hyskon)
- ringers lactate
- 5% dextrose in water
- 1.5% glycine
- 3% Sorbital

Contact lasers
- touch and blanching methods

Electrocautery
- roller ball (Fig. 45-1)
- resectoscope

General anesthetic

Preoperative antibiotics

Usually well tolerated with out-patient treatment

✧ *Safety*

Most serious complication is fluid overload

Need to pay careful attention to amount of absorbed fluid

Other complications
- perforation
- hemorrhage
- infection

Long-term safety issues still need to be addressed

✧ *Effectiveness*

Amenorrhea, 40% to 50%

Hypomenorrhea or normal menses, 40% to 50%

Failure, 5% to 10%

Electrocautery may be more successful than laser

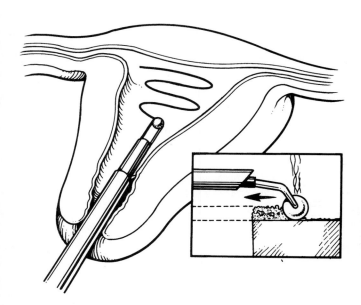

Figure 45-1. The intrauterine roller-ball technique for endometrial ablation.

◆ Submucous Myomas

Treatment via hysteroscopy is now possible
Goal is to shave myoma down to level of surface
- less successful if less than 60% of myoma extends into cavity

Menorrhagia is cured in over 90% of patients for at least 1 year

◆ Intrauterine Synechiae

Intrauterine adhesions (Asherman syndrome)
- typically occurs postpartum or postabortal with retained products of conception and often infection

Treat with scissors under direct visualization
May place pediatric foley in uterus for postoperative bleeding
Most surgeons use postoperative conjugated estrogens (5 mg per day for 3 months or until bleeding occurs) followed by progesterone for 10 days
Normal menstrual function in 90%
- 75% achieve pregnancy
  - 80% term pregnancies
  - 18% spontaneous abortions
  - 3% ectopic pregnancies
- long-term problems with placental separation may occur

◆ Uterine Septum

Operative hysteroscopy has replaced metroplasty
Perform with simultaneous laparoscopy
Pregnancy in 70% to 90%

46

◆ Urogynecology

NORMAL LOWER URINARY TRACT

◆ Anatomy

Urethra adheres closely to vaginal wall
Urethrovesicle junction (UVJ) usually in high retropubic location
Maintained by
- pubourethral ligaments

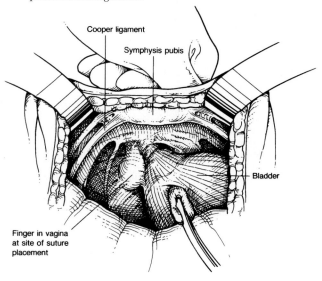

Figure 46-1. This surgeon's view of the retropubic space demonstrates the Cooper ligaments, the pelvic floor, and movement of the bladder away from the site where sutures will be placed. (Burch JC. Cooper's ligament urethrovesical suspension for stress incontinence. Am J Obstet Gynecol 1968;100:764.)

- endopelvic fascia
- urogenital diaphragm

Primary surgical procedures designed to resuspend the UVJ
- retropubic space developed during surgical treatment (Fig. 46-1)
- necessary to avoid large veins present in the fat pad

◆ Neurology

Bladder is the only smooth muscle under voluntary control
Parasympathetic innervation (S2 to S4)
- stimulates vesicular contraction
- inhibits urethral musculature

Sympathetic enervation (T10 to T12 down to L2)
- bladder is β-adrenergic
- urethra is α-adrenergic

Volitional control by means of four loops of control
- stress urinary incontinence may be a disease of the nervous system rather than an anatomic disorder

EVALUATION OF THE LOWER URINARY TRACT

◆ Triage of Patients with Lower Urinary Tract Symptoms

After obtaining a detailed history, diagnostic evaluation limited to a series of steps (Table 46-1)

◆ History and Physical Examination

Detailed evaluation of symptoms (Table 46-2)
24-hour urolog helpful

✧ *Physical examination*

Neurologic evaluation
- bulbocavernosus reflex
- anal reflex
- clitoral reflex

Vaginal examination for estrogen effect, prolapse (anterior and posterior)
- Urethral palpitation for tenderness
- Rectal examination to evaluate tone

✧ *Testing*

Q-tip test (Fig. 46-2)
Uroflow testing
- postvoid residual
- urine culture
- screening cystometry by backfilling bladder

TABLE 46-1. Evaluation of Lower Urinary Tract

Step 1: Urinalysis and culture
Step 2: Office evaluation, including history and physical examination, neurologic screen, urolog summary, uroflowmetry, residual urine, Q-tip test, urethral calibration
Step 3: Dynamic cystourethroscopy, stress test, screening cystometrography
Step 4: Multichannel urodynamic assessment, including urethral closure pressure profiles, rest and stress; voiding mechanism; electromyography

---

TABLE 46-2. Questions To Ask Patients With Urinary Incontinence

Do you lose urine in spurts during coughing, lifting, or aerobic activity?
Is the urge to void ever strong enough that you would leak if you do not reach the bathroom in time?
Have you leaked urine because you could not reach the bathroom in time?
How frequently do you urinate during the day?
How many times do you get up from sleep to urinate?
Have you wet the bed in the past year?
When you are passing urine, can you stop the flow?
Do you wear protection (pads) to protect your clothing from the loss of urine?
How severe a problem do you consider your urinary leakage to be?
Do you leak urine during intercourse?

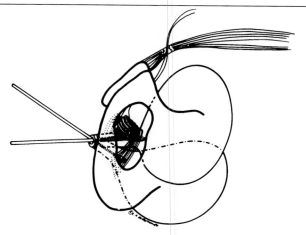

Figure 46-2. Q-tip test. At rest, the Q-tip is in a horizontal position, but with straining and coughing, it shows a positive deflection because of inadequate support at the urethrovesical junction.

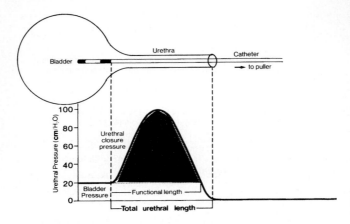

Figure 46-3. Urethral closure pressure profile. A dual-sensor catheter is slowly withdrawn from the bladder. The distal sensor measures the bladder pressure constantly, while the proximal sensor measures the urethral pressure. The urethral closure pressure and functional urethral length are shown in the shaded portion of the graph. (American College of Obstetricians and Gynecologists and Bent AE, ed. Urogynecologic evaluation, endoscopy, and urodynamic testing in the symptomatic female. Washington, DC: ACOG Audiovisual Library, 1990.)

◆ Urethral Pressure Profiles

Functional urethral length is a measure of the length of the urethra over which the urethra pressure exceeds the bladder pressure (Fig. 46-3)

◇ *Normal values*
Urethral closure pressure, 40 to 60 cm H_2O
Functional urethral length, 2.5 to 3.5 cm

◇ *Indications*
Previously failed surgery
Clinically severe incontinence
Continuous incontinence
Stress urinary incontinence after 65 years-of-age
Genital prolapse
Symptomatic patients with no demonstrable urine loss
Urethral diverticula

◇ *Results*
During coughing, when the bladder pressure is greater than urethral pressure, the urethral closure pressure is 0 (pressure equalization)

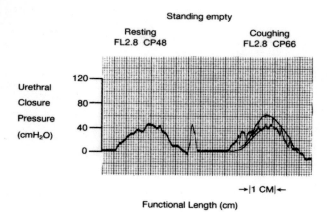

Standing empty

Resting
FL2.8 CP48

Coughing
FL2.8 CP66

Urethral
Closure
Pressure
(cmH₂O)

→|1 CM|←

Functional Length (cm)

Figure 46-4. Genuine incontinence. Although the resting profile in this patient appears normal, there is pressure equalization during coughing, while the detrusor pressure remains low.

Establishes diagnosis of genuine stress urinary incontinence (Fig. 46-4)

May be helpful in patients prior to correction of prolapse

◆ Radiographic Examination

Plain x-ray film in cases of suspected neurologic deficit
IVP in patients with possibly difficult surgery
Voiding cystogram (bead-chain)
May give information about UVJ

TREATMENT OF LOWER URINARY TRACT DISORDERS

◆ Urethral Syndrome

Chronic symptoms in absence of positive urine culture

◇ *Causes*
Periurethral gland inflammation
Hypoestrogenism
Spasticity
Chemical irritation

◇ *Diagnosis*
No specific findings
Differential diagnosis
• acute urethritis

- urinary tract infection
- interstitial cystitis
- hypotonic bladder with high residual
- diabetes insipidus
- urethral diverticulum
- vaginal infection
- acute and chronic vulvitis
- atrophic vaginitis
- urethral caruncle

✧ *Treatment*
Estrogen for perimenopausal and postmenopausal patient
- one quarter to one third of an applicator of vaginal cream nightly for 2 weeks, then 2 to 3 times per week
Behavioral modification
Chronic antibiotic therapy
- 50 mg nitrofurantoin daily or 1 tablet of TMP-SMX daily for 3 to 6 months
Urethral dilation
- less often used as first line therapy
Periurethral steroid injection

✧ *Outcome*
Relapse can occur

◆ **Fistula**

Constant urinary drainage
Often after surgical or obstetric delivery
Vesicovaginal fistula is diagnosed by placement of methylene blue into bladder
- suspicion of ureterovaginal fistula
- indigo carmine dye injected intravenously
Treatment
- ureterovaginal fistula
  - abdominal approach with reimplantation
  - Boari flap or Psoas hitch
- vesicovaginal fistula
  - insert suprapubic catheter and wait 6 weeks
  - spontaneous healing in 20%
- failure of spontaneous healing requires transvaginal repair
Urethrovaginal fistula
- primary closure of defect

◆ **Diverticula**

Clinical findings are suburethral tender swelling
Many are asymptomatic
Treatment usually consists of Spence procedure
- division of urethral vaginal septum up to diverticula with repair

◆ Lower Urinary Tract Infection

Generally defined as bacterial inflammation of urothelium in the bladder with associated symptoms
- 100,000 colonies/mL midstream urine
- 1000 colonies/mL catheterized specimen

Very common
Asymptomatic bacteria can often be seen
- 1% preschool-aged children
- 5% reproductive-aged women
- 10% postmenopausal women

Atrophic vaginitis predisposes to this condition

◇ *Organisms*
E Coli present in 80%

◇ *Treatment*
Best to obtain culture first
Single dose
- three double-strength TMP-SMX
- 3 grams ampicillin

Multiple day dosing
- one double-strength TMP-SMX BID for 5 days
- 100 mg nitrofurantoin QID for 4 days, 50 mg QID for 4 days
- sulfamethoxazole for 7 days
- gentamycin 80 mg, IM single dose

Other options
- cephalosporins
- fluoroquinolones

Recurrent infection (3 or more times per year)
- postcoital or continuous prophylaxis
- nitrofurantoin, 50 mg qhs
- single-strength, TMP-SMX

Adjunctive therapy
- pyridium
- hydration

◆ Detrusor Instability

Frequency, urgency, nocturia, sudden loss of urine with or without urgency
Many causes
- idiopathic
- cerebrovascular insufficiency
- outflow obstruction
- local irritation or infection
- psychosomatic or psychogenic condition

◇ *Differential diagnosis*
Severe genuine stress urinary incontinence
Fistula

Interstitial cystitis
Severe UTI or urethral syndrome

✧ *Evaluation*
History
Voiding diary
Urine culture
Cystometrogram (Fig. 46-5)

✧ *Treatment*
Behavioral modification
Biofeedback
Functional electrical stimulation
Medication
- oxybutynin, 5 mg BID to QID
- dicyclomine hydrochloride, 20 mg BID to QID
- flavoxate hydrochloride, 200 mg BID to QID
- imipramine hydrochloride, 25 to 75 mg daily to BID

◆ Stress Incontinence

Involuntary loss of urine associated with increased intraabdominal pressure in absence of detrusor activity
Incidence <10% of reproductive-aged women, 10% to 20% of
postmenopausal women

✧ *Pathophysiology*
Disruption of internal urethral sphincter
Abnormal structural muscle component of external urethral
sphincter
Disruption of fascial and muscular support to proximal urethra

✧ *Evaluation*
As previously described
Urethral closure pressure
- suggested prior to surgery
- recommended for patients >65 years-of-age

✧ *Treatment*
Topical estrogens
α-androgeneric stimulation
- phenylpropanolamine, 75 to 150 mg daily
- imipramine hydrochloride 50 to 150 mg daily
Kegel exercises (Table 46-3)

◆ Interstitial Cystitis

Chronic inflammation of all layers of bladder wall
Diagnosis based on clinical symptoms with cystoscopic finding
- Hunner ulcers
Treatment
- overdistention with fluid

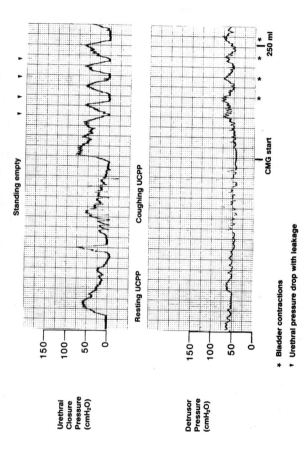

Figure 46-5. This patient with detrusor instability has pressure equalization with coughing. During bladder filling, regular bladder contractions occur with coincident urethral relaxation, followed by urinary leakage. The patient cannot inhibit the activity of an usntable bladder.

Standing empty

Urethral
Closure
Pressure
(cmH₂O)

Resting UCPP   Coughing UCPP

Detrusor
Pressure
(cmH₂O)

CMG start   250 ml

* Bladder contractions
▼ Urethral pressure drop with leakage

- steroids, heparin, Benadryl, and bicarbonate, combined with DMSO
- surgical therapy rarely indicated

SURGICAL TREATMENT OF STRESS INCONTINENCE

Selection of surgical procedure based on objective parameters (Fig. 46-6)

TABLE 46-3. Basics of Pelvic Floor Muscle Training

Repetition: graded activity to a desired maximum
Regular program: every other day or three times each week for 3 to 6 months.
Maximum intensity: squeeze pelvic floor muscles for 12 seconds and relax for 15 seconds (i.e., use resistance training)
Maintenance program: 15 repetitions performed one to three times each day
Follow-up: written record and weekly or biweekly visits to a therapist, who evaluates success

---

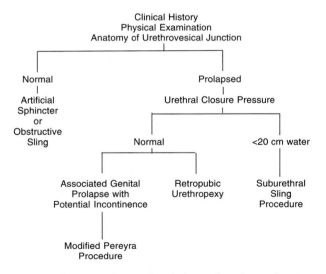

Figure 46-6. Objective selection of surgical procedures for genuine stress incontinence. The schema can assist in selecting the appropriate surgical procedure for stress incontinence based on urethral pressure and the presence or absence of hypermobility of the urethrovesical junction.

◆ Vaginal Approach (Fig. 46-7)

Anterior vaginal repair first described by Kelly in 1914
Success rates 50% to 60% 2 years after surgery

◆ Retropubic Urethropexy

Requires dissection of retropubic space (Fig. 46-1)
- paravaginal fascia identified

◇ *Burch procedure (Fig. 46-8)*

Permanent suture used
Figure-of-eight suture is placed at level of UVJ, 2 cm lateral to
  the midline
Second suture is more inferior, 2 cm lateral to urethra
- purpose is eventual fusion of paravaginal fascia and pelvis
  sidewall
- occurs during 3 months following surgery

◇ *Marshall-Marchetti-Krantz*

Similar to Burch procedure
Use absorbable suture

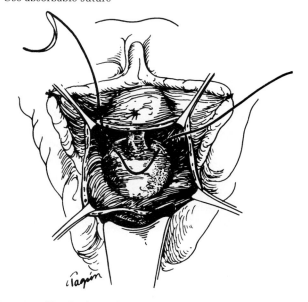

Figure 46-7. The classic anterior vaginal repair. After disection of the
anterior vaginal wall from the paravesical fascia, plication sutures are
placed under the urethrovesical junction in an attempt to elevate it. (Green
TH Jr. Am J Obstet Gynecol 1975;122:368.)

Place in periosteum of symphysis pubis as opposed to Cooper's ligament

Evaluate ureters at end of procedure

◆ *Postoperative care*

Continuous drainage for 2 to 3 days

Suprapubic catheter until postoperative residual is <100 cc

• may take several weeks

Success rates 80% to 90% after 1 year

◆ Combined Retropubic and Vaginal Approaches

First popularized by Pereyra in 1956

Better suited to treatment of potential incontinence in cases of genital prolapse

Less successful as a primary therapy of incontinence

◆ *Technique (Fig. 46-9)*

Identification of endopelvic fascia (Fig. 46-10)

Sutures then anchored to intraabdominal wall (Fig. 46-11)

◆ *Stamey procedure (Fig. 46-12)*

Retropubic space not entered from below

Bladder perforation can occur

Cystoscopy should be performed

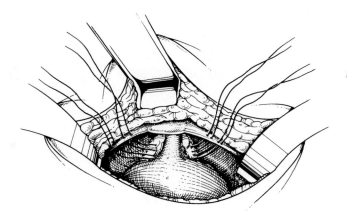

Figure 46-8. In the Burch retropubic urethropexy, sutures are placed lateral to the urethrovesical junction and lateral to the midurethra and brought to the Cooper ligament bilaterally. (Tanagho EA. Colpocystourethropexy: the way we do it. J Urol 1976;116:751.)

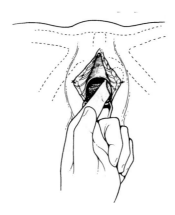

Figure 46-9. A modified Pereyra procedure is used to obtain entry into the retropubic space. Using blunt or a combination of blunt and sharp dissection, the index finger is insinuated through the urogenital diaphragm into the retropubic space. (Ostergard DR, ed. Gynecologic urology and urodynamics, theory and practice. 2nd ed. Baltimore: Williams & Wilkins, 1985.)

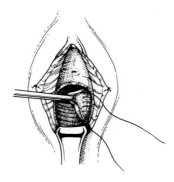

Figure 46-10. The helical permanent suture is placed on the paravaginal fascia in the modified Pereyra procedure. (Ostergard DR, ed. Gynecologic urology and urodynamics, theory and practice. 2nd ed. Baltimore: Williams & Wilkins, 1985.)

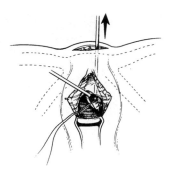

Figure 46-11. The ligature carrier is used to withdraw the ends of the sutures to the anterior abdominal wall in the modified Pereyra procedure. (Ostergard DR, ed. Gynecologic urology and urodynamics, theory and practice. 2nd ed. Baltimore: Williams & Wilkins, 1985.)

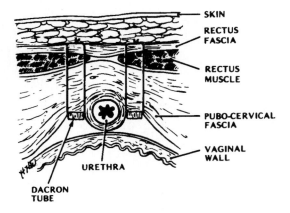

Figure 46-12. In the Stamey procedure, buttresses are used under the urogenital diaphragm to protect the fascia after elevation with the sutures attached to the anterior rectus fascia. (Stamey TA. Endoscopic suspension of the vesical neck for urinary incontinence in females: report on 203 consecutive patients. Ann Surg 1980;192:465.)

47

◆ Vulvar and Vaginal Diseases

BENIGN LESIONS OF THE VULVA

Vulvar skin is of ectodermal origin
- subject to genital-specific and general diseases

Biopsy should be used freely for suspicious lesions
Inspection with large magnifying lens after application of 5% acetic acid can be helpful

◆ Inflammatory Lesions of the Vulva

✧ *Contact dermatitis*
Most common benign affliction
- avoid irritants
- apply local fluorinated hydrocortisones (0.025% to 0.1%)

✧ *Intertrigio and seborrheic dermatitis commonly seen in diabetics*
Acute problem may be treated with corn starch and topical fluorinated hydrocortisones

✧ *Psoriasis*
Usually multifocal
Erythematous patch on the vulva without scales usually seen

✧ *Fungal infections*
Very common
- candidiasis often associated with vaginal infection
- tinea cruris
  - topical antifungals are effective

✧ *Vestibular adenitis*
Severe pain on vestibular contact
Patients may have suffered for years
Coitus may be impossible
Treatment
- interferon injection
- surgical excision (cure rate 60% to 80%)

◆ Ulcerative Lesions

Crohn disease especially important
- fistula formation
- treatment with prednisone and possibly the addition of metronidazole

Behçet disease
- vulvar ulcerations
- buccal ulcers
- iritis
- treatment
  - prednisone

◆ White Lesions

Vitiligo is common
- often appears in puberty
- seldom symptomatic
- purely a cosmetic defect not a systemic disease

Hyperkeratosis
- protective phenomenon
- clinical process of various etiology

Leukoplakia
- name applied to any white lesion
- a nonspecific term which should be eliminated

✧ *Lichen sclerosis*

Nonspecific, patchy, white alteration of the labial skin

✳ *Microscopic picture*

Moderate hyperkeratosis
Thinning of epithelium with loss of the rete pegs
Underlying collagenization
Inflammatory infiltrate

✳ *Treatment for symptomatic relief*

Prepubertal
- local hydrocortisone
  - long-term use can produce fibrosis

Postmenopausal
- topical testosterone

✧ *Hyperplastic dystrophy*

Gross lesions consist of white or gray firm patches
Increase in cellular elements of epithelium
- some underlying chronic infiltrates

Biopsy should be used freely
Treatment
- fluorinated hydrocortisone
- topical or subcutaneous injection

✧ *Atypical hyperplastic dystrophy*

Usually white but can be red or pigmented

Atypical maturation with intraepithelial pearl formation

⬦ ***Mixed dystrophy***
Combination of lichen sclerosis and hyperplasia
Biopsy to determine malignant potential

◆ Solid Tumors

Occur very rarely

◆ Other Tumors

⬦ ***Vascular tumors***
Congenital variety can appear at 2 to 3 months of age
Often disappear spontaneously

⬦ ***Hidradenoma***
Rare lesion
Intricate adenomatous pattern which has been confused with
    malignancy
Treat by local excision

⬦ ***Pigmented lesions***

✳ *Nevi*
Intradermal: no malignant potential
Junctional: greatest malignant potential
Compound: some malignant potential
Risk factors for development of melanoma (Table 47-1)

✳ *Papillary lesions*
Condylomata from HPV infection
May present a recurring therapeutic problem
Treatment
• podophyllin, TCA, 5-FU
• surgical ablation or excision

✳ *Cystic lesions*
Sebaceous cyst most common
• infected lesions usually respond to incision and drainage
Bartholin duct cyst

TABLE 47-1. Risks for Developing Melanoma

Family history of melanoma in blood relatives
Poor or no tanning ability, often with a history of sunburn in
    adolescence
Unusual moles with any of the following characteristics:
    Dark (i.e., blue-black) color
    Speckled or splotchy color pattern
    Jagged or fuzzy border
Recent change in size, shape, or color of a mole
Any mole larger than a dime

- if symptomatic, can marsupialize cyst under local anesthetic with placement of Word catheter

Labia majora cyst

BENIGN LESIONS OF THE VAGINA

◆ Inclusion Cyst

Usually occur at site of previous laceration or episiotomy
Treatment rarely needed

◆ Gartner (Mesonephric) Duct Cyst

Common but rarely symptomatic
Rarely undergoes malignant transformation

◆ Endometriosis

Biopsy to rule out malignancy
Often result of penetrating cul-de-sac endometriosis

◆ Adenosis

Usually result of aberrant ectopic cervical glands
Increased incidence in DES-exposed women
May represent risk of development of clear cell vaginal adeno-
carcinoma
Close follow-up indicated for at-risk patients

MALIGNANT TUMORS OF THE VULVA

3% to 4% of all primary malignancies of the genital canal
Delay in diagnosis can be extreme

◆ Carcinoma in Situ

Most commonly diagnosed during third and fourth decades of
life
Appearance varies greatly
- bowenoid lesion is scaly, red, blackened with white lesions
- other lesions are almost entirely white or red

Biopsy crucial to accurate diagnosis

Therapy
Surgical excision
- localized lesion→ wide local excision
- multifoci lesions→ skinning vulvectomy

◆ Paget Disease

Fiery red background mottled with white hyperkeratotic areas
Solely intraepithelial in 90%

Can recur locally
Treatment
- simple vulvectomy vs. local excision
- invasive disease should dictate inguinal and femoral lymph node dissection

◆ Invasive Carcinoma

Most common: squamous cell carcinoma
- 65% to 70% are mature, pearl-forming tumors
Average age of patients is 60 to 65 years-of-age
Symptoms
- pruritus
- lump
- local irritation

◆ Melanoma

Site of 2% to 3% of malignant melanomas
Survival rate related to depth of invasion
Treatment of choice is surgical
Lymphatic spread is common in more advanced disease

◆ Treatment of Squamous Cell Cancer

Sample superficial inguinal nodes if central lesion is <1 cm diameter and 5 mm depth
- if nodes are negative, wide local excision is acceptable
Verrucous carcinoma is unique
- no nodal metastases
Basal cell carcinoma
- wide local excision

MALIGNANT TUMORS OF THE VAGINA

2% to 4% of de nova genital canal anaplastic disease

◆ In Situ Epidermoid Carcinoma

Occurs in three situations
  1. regional response to a carcinogen
  2. after treatment for carcinoma in situ of the cervix
  3. after radiation therapy for invasive carcinoma of the cervix
Treatment
- local excision or laser vaporization
- 5-FU cream

◆ Invasive Epidermoid Carcinoma

Most common invasive neoplasm of the vagina
Two thirds of patients are over 50 years-of-age
Symptoms

- bloody vaginal discharge
- can be associated with total vaginal prolapse

Staging (see Appendix)

◇ *Treatment*

Radiation therapy
- external irradiation and brachytherapy

Improved survival rates now noted

    Stage I: 90%
    Stage IIA: 58%
    Stage IIB: 32%
    Stage III: 40%
    Stage IV: 0%

Lymphatic spread from lower one third of vagina similar to vulva (Fig. 47-1)

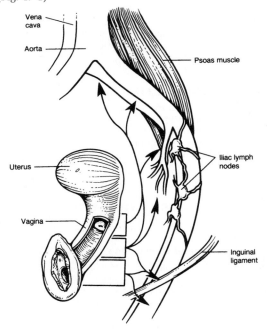

Figure 47-1. Lymphatic spread of carcinoma of the vagina. Lymphatic channels from the lower one third of the vagina drain into femoral and external iliac nodes (1). Channels from the middle one third of the vagina drain into the hypogastric nodes (2). Channels from the upper one third of the vagina drain into the common iliac, presacral, and hypogastric nodes (3). (Plentl AA, Friedman EA. Lymphatic system of the female genitalia. Philadelphia: WB Saunders, 1971.)

48

◆ Disorders of the Uterine Cervix

BENIGN LESIONS

ANATOMY AND PHYSIOLOGY OF THE CERVIX

◆ Normal Findings

2 to 4 cm long

Contiguous with inferior aspect of uterine corpus
- point of juncture is the isthmus

Internal os is the point of histologic transition from endocervical to endometrial tissue

Cervical mucus
- produced by secretory cells of endocervical glands
- under hormonal control

◆ Abnormal Findings

✧ *Stenosis*

Congenital stenosis is rare

Usually result of surgical or radiation therapy

May result in uterine distention
- hematometra (blood)
- hydrometra (fluid)
- pyometra (inflammatory exudate)

✧ *Polyps*

Vary from a few millimeters to 3 cm

Pedunculated, soft, smooth, red or purple

Hyperplastic condition of endocervical epithelium

Treat by excision after ligation of base

✧ *Hyperplasia and metaplasia*

Frequently found in surgical specimens

No definitive neoplastic potential

Microglandular hyperplasia
- related to oral contraceptive use
- benign lesion

Squamous metaplasia
- part of the picture of erosion healing

◆ Inflammatory Lesions

✧ *Acute cervicitis*
Most commonly caused by gonococcus
- squamous epithelium of the portio may become involved
- usually spreads as superficial inflammation

Diagnosis made by smears and cultures

Purulent discharge present

Treat with systemic antibiotics
- no role for local therapy

✧ *Chronic cervicitis*
90% to 95% of parous women have some evidence of chronic cervicitis

Most commonly seen as cervical erosion
- loss of superficial stratified squamous epithelium

Reparative attempts result in sealing of the gland necks
- may result in formation of nabothian cysts

Symptoms include:
- yellowish-white, thick discharge
- intermenstrual bleeding
- backache
- trigone irritation (honeymoon bladder)

Treatment
- exclude malignant process
- electrocautery, laser, or cryotherapy

✧ *Herpetic lesions*
Similar in appearance to vulvar lesion

May be associated with leukorrhea

Vaginal pain

Dyspareunia

Warm water douches may help symptoms

✧ *Condylomata acuminata*
Warty growth caused by human papillomavirus (HPV) (usually types 6, 11)

Lesions grow during pregnancies

Small biopsy done prior to therapy

Therapy
- podophyllin (not in pregnancy)
- tricholoracetic acid (TCA)
- laser, electrocautery, or cryotherapy

Recurrence is common
- consider treatment with 5-fluorouracil (5-FU)

◆ Noninflammatory Benign Lesions

◇ *Leiomyomas*
May present aborting through cervical canal
Treat by excision or hysterectomy
- may result in difficult surgical procedure
- myoma may fill the entire pelvis on occasion

◇ *Hemangioma*
Usually asymptomatic
Biopsy may result in heavy bleeding
Removal indicated based on symptoms

◇ *Endometriosis*
Presents as reddish or bluish lesion
- usually associated with pelvic endometriosis

◇ *Vestigial mesonephric structures and adenosis*
Ductal remains of the mesonephric (Wollfian) ducts
May be noted in surgical specimens
Adenosis refers to adenomatis proliferation
- tissues of müllerian origin
- diethylstilbestrol (DES) exposure may result in malignant transformation

◇ *Diethylstilbestrol-related cervical changes*
50% to 60% of DES-exposed female offspring have anomalous cervical changes
- recessed ring around external os
- portio covered with columnar epithelium
- endocervical gland hypertrophy
- anterior lip cervical protuberance (cock's comb)
May result in cervical incompetence, reduced fertility

◇ *Leukoplakia*
Hyperkeratosis
Wide range of histologic diagnosis found in these patients
Biopsy or further evaluation appropriate

◇ *Cervical pregnancy*
1/10,000 pregnancies
May result in life-threatening hemorrhage
Mortality rates may approach 5%
Hysterectomy may be required in face of excessive bleeding

MALIGNANT LESIONS OF THE UTERINE CERVIX

◆ Squamous Cell Carcinoma

◇ *Epidemiology*
Seventh most common cancer of women in the United States
- worldwide it is still the leading site of cancer in women

- 500,000 cases annually

Practically never encountered in virgins
- promoting factor or carcinogen likely sexually transmitted

✧ *Precursors of squamous cell carcinoma*

600,000 U.S. women annually diagnosed with cervical intraepithelial neoplasia (CIN)
- aggressive treatment of dysplasia has contributed to decrease
in cervical cancer deaths

Dysplasia divided into three grades
- CIN I (mild)
- CIN II (moderate)
- CIN III (severe, carcinoma in situ)

✧ *Screening*

Pap test has proven to decrease incidence and mortality

Annual Pap smear for all women once they become sexually active or at age 18

After three years of normal exams Pap smears may be performed
less frequently at physician's discretion

Risk factors
- early onset of sexual activity
- multiple sexual partners
- smoking

Screening important for all age groups
- death rates higher for women over 55

Pattern of spread
- endocervical canal
- through basement membrane (carcinoma)

Other changes
- loss of normal maturation process
- dyskeratosis

✧ *Cytologic characteristics*

Pap smear only a screening test
- false-negative rate 10% to 35%
- may approach 50% in invasive disease

Bethesda system describes a range of abnormalities (Table 48-1)

◆ Early Invasive Phase

Microinvasion
- depth <3 mm from basement membrane
- no vascular or lymphatic space involvement
- incidence of lymph node involvement <1%
- may treat with simple hysterectomy or possibly cone biopsy

Microcarcinoma (1987 FIGO)
- depth <5 mm
- horizontal spread <7 mm
- vascular space involvement ignored

TABLE 48-1. Bethesda System to Describe Range of Cervical Cytologic Abnormalities

Bethesda System	Classic System		Modified Papanicolaou System
Within normal limits	Normal		I
Infection (organism should be specified)	Inflammatory atypia		II
Reactive and reparative changes			
Squamous cell abnormalities			
• Atypical squamous cells of undetermined significance	Squamous atypia of uncertain significance		
• Low grade squamous intraepithelial lesion (SIL)	HPV atypia	CIN 1	IIR
	Mild dysplasia	CIN 2	III
• High grade squamous intraepithelial lesion (SIL)	Moderate dysplasia		
	Severe dysplasia	CIN 3	
	Carcinoma in situ		IV
• Squamous cell carcinoma	Squamous cell carcinoma		V

✧ *Histologic characteristics*

Squamous cell carcinoma represents 85% to 95% of cervical cancers

Can be divided into three histologic grades

Grade I
- 5% of squamous cell cancers
- well-differentiated
- keratin, pearl formation
- few mitoses

Grade II
- 85% of squamous cell cancers
- no intracellular bridges and little keratin, pearl formation
- increasing number of mitotic figures

Grade III
- 10% of squamous cell cancers
- rapid growth rate
- numerous mitoses
- difficult to identify as squamous cell in origin

✧ *Gross appearance*

Exophytic growth (64%)
- friable, granular, red and yellow fungating mass
- usually ulcerative and bleeds freely

Endophytic tumors
- may be deceptive on examination
- may only present as cervical enlargement (barrel lesion)

✧ *Spread of tumor beyond the cervix*

Vaginal extension

Lateral extension
- occurs frequently

Endometrial extension
- rare

Lymphatic spread (Fig. 48-1)
- involved even in early disease
  Stage I, 15%
  Stage II, 30%
  Stage III, 50%
  Stage IV, >60%

Blood vessel invasion
- allows spread to distant parts
- liver, lungs and spleen

✧ *Diagnosis*

Regular bimanual examination

Biopsy of lesion

Staging must be performed to allow correct therapy

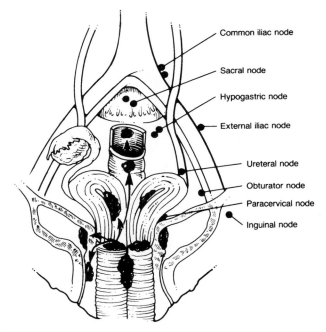

Figure 48-1. Possible sites of direct extension of cervical cancer to adjoining organs or regional nodes. The uterus, cervix, and vagina are depicted as bisected and opened to reveal the possible sites of tumor implantation.

◆ Clinical Staging

✧ *International conventions*
Based on physical examination, biopsy, radiographic evaluation
FIGO classification revised in 1987 (See Appendix)

◆ Treatment

✧ *Preinvasisve phase*
Based on reproductive desires (Fig. 48-2)
Techniques vary
Cryotherapy
• no tissue for pathologic diagnosis
• may be of limited efficacy in CIN III
Laser therapy
• also precludes tissue sampling

Electrosurgical excision (LEEP, LLTZ)
- edge artifact may be present
- repeat treatments may result in removal of significant degree of cervical stroma

◇ *Carcinoma in situ during pregnancy*
Follow during pregnancy with colposcopy
Postpartum reassessment for definitive therapy

◇ *Invasive phase*
Two treatment options for Stage I or IIA lesions
Radiotherapy
Radical hysterectomy
- young patient
- appropriate body habitus

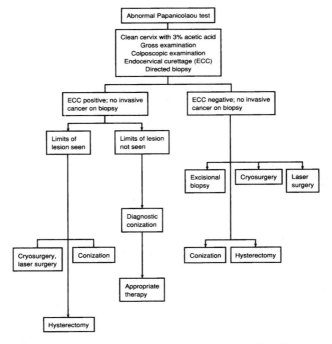

Figure 48-2. Evaluation and management of abnormal cytology. Patients with an abnormal Pap smear are given a colposcopic examination, and areas consistent with dysplasia or more advanced disease must be biopsied and an endocervical curettage (ECC) performed. Further therapy is determined on the basis of these results.

- good general health
- skilled surgical team in a hospital facility

More advanced disease
- radiotherapy
- chemotherapy
  - 50% response rate to cisplatin

Central recurrent disease
- pelvic exenteration

✧ *Prognosis*

Highly favorable for early stages
    Stage 0, 100%
    Stage IB, 85%
    Stage IIA, 70% to 75%
    Stage IIB, 60% to 65%
    Stage IIIB, 25% to 40%
    Stage IV, 5% to 10%

90% of recurrences occur within 24 months
- pelvis
- periaortic lymph nodes
- liver
- lungs

Death usually from uremia, infection, hemorrhage
- uremia most common (50%)
- infection (40%)
- hemorrhage (2% to 7%)

◆ Adenocarcinoma

10% to 15% of cervical cancers
Approximately the same prognosis and clinical behavior as squamous cell carcinoma
Staging and treatment are the same

COLPOSCOPY

◆ Correlation of Colposcopic and Histologic Findings (Table 48-2)

Vascular pattern is one of the most important diagnostic features

◆ Clinical Applications

Cytology and colposcopy both have advantages and disadvantages (Table 48-3)
Use of both will increase detection and rates

TABLE 48-2. Correlation of Colposcopic and Histologic Findings

Colposcopic Term	Colposcopic Appearance	Histologic Correlate
Original squamous epithelium	Smooth, pink Indefinitely outlined vessels No change after application of acetic acid	Squamous epithelium
Columnar epithelium	Grape-like structures after application of acetic acid	Columnar epithelium
Transformation zone	Tongues of squamous metaplasia Grand openings Nabothian cysts	Metaplastic squamous epithelium
White epithelium	White, sharp-bordered lesion visible only after application of acetic acid No vessels visible	Minimal dysplasia to carcinoma in situ
Punctation	Sharp-bordered lesion Red stippling Epithelium whiter after application of acetic acid	Minimal dysplasia to carcinoma in situ
Hyperkaratosis	White patch Rough surface Visible before application of acetic acid	Usually hyperkeratosis or parakeratosis; seldom carcinoma in situ or invasive carcinoma
Atypical vessels	Horizontal vessels running parallel to surface Constriction or dilatation of vessels Atypical branching, winding course	Carcinoma in situ to invasive carcinoma

TABLE 48-3. Advantages and Disadvantages of Colposcopy and Cell Study

Advantages	Disadvantages
Cell Study	
Ideal for mass screening	Cannot localize lesion
Economical	Inflammation, atrophic changes, folic acid deficiency may produce suspicious changes
Specimen can be obtained by any medical personnel	
Detects lesions in endocervical canal	Many steps between patient and cytopathologist allow misdiagnosis
Detects adenocarcinoma	Value of single smear is limited
Colposcopy	
Localizes lesion	Inadequate for detection of endocervical lesions
Evaluates extent of lesion	Difficult training
Differentiates inflammatory atypia from neoplasia	
Differentiates invasive from noninvasive cervical lesions	
Enables follow-up	

49

◆ Disorders of the Uterine Corpus

BENIGN LESIONS OF THE UTERINE CORPUS

BENIGN LESIONS OF THE ENDOMETRIUM

◆ Endometrial Hyperplasia

A confusing entity with differing opinions as to malignant potential

◇ *Pathology*

Hyperplasia may not represent a continuum ending with neoplasia

- cytologic atypia distinguishes one from the other

Kurman categorization of hyperplasia (no malignant potential)

- simple hyperplasia: increased number of glands
- cystic hyperplasia: glands are dilated
- adenomatous hyperplasia: irregular glands with crowding
- complex hyperplasia: complex growth, back-to-back crowding but no atypia

Atypical hyperplasia

- proliferation of glands with varying degrees of nuclear atypia and loss of polarity (cytologic atypia)
  - mild to moderate grading
  - malignant risk is present

◇ *Patient profile*

Hyperplasia related to unopposed estrogen (endogenous or exogenous)

- two thirds occur before 50 years-of-age

Abnormal bleeding is most common symptom

◇ *Treatment*

After diagnosis with endometrial biopsy, proceed with formal D&C to rule out malignancy

- no additional therapy needed in many cases

Patients with continually unopposed estrogen should be treated with progesterone

- 10 to 12 days at end of each month
  - resample in 3 to 6 months
  Atypical hyperplasia in the perimenopausal or postmenopausal patient should result in consideration of hysterectomy

◆ Endometrial Polyps

Sessile or pedunculated projections of endometrium
- most are asymptomatic
- can present with nonspecific abnormal bleeding
Incidence unknown
Most prevalent in women 30 to 59 years-of-age
Pathology
- less than one third show functional endometrium
- may show cystic hyperplasia
- can protrude through cervix
Diagnosis and treatment
- usually diagnosed at curettage, hysteroscopy, or hysterectomy
- may co-exist with carcinoma in 10% of postmenopausal women

BENIGN LESIONS OF THE MYOMETRIUM

◆ Leiomyomas

Well-circumscribed, nonencapsulated benign uterine tumor
Smooth muscle with some fibrous connective tissue elements

◇ *Incidence*

Most common pelvic tumor
One quarter to one fifth of women over 35 years-of-age have myomata
Most produce no symptoms
60% of laparotomies in women are for myomas
More common in African-Americans than Caucasians

◇ *Location*

Classified by uterine location
- submucous, intramural, subserousal
May become parasitic

◇ *Pathology*

Corpus is most common site of origin
- may distort the cavity (Fig. 49-1)
Gross appearance is smooth and glistening white with a whorled and fasciculated pattern
Microscopic appearance is interlacing pattern or smooth muscle

◇ *Histogenesis*

Origin and development not well understood
Clearly estrogen responsive

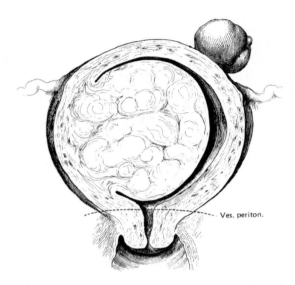

Figure 49-1. Large submucous myoma. Great distortion of uterine cavity shows futility of attempted curettage in such a circumstance. (Kelly HA. Operative gynecology, vol. 2. New York: Appleton, 1903.)

✦ *Degeneration and complications*
Variety of degenerative phenomena
Necrosis can occur and may present with acute pain
- gross appearance may be confused with sarcoma

✦ *Physical signs*
Uterine enlargement with abdominal displacement
Pelvic examination often very revealing

✦ *Symptoms*
Most produce no symptoms
Bleeding
- often excessive or prolonged menses
- exact mechanism unknown

Pressure
- voiding difficulties
- constipation
- urethral compression

Pain
- may result from degeneration
- sensation of pelvic heaviness or bearing down may occur

Abdominal distention

Infertility

- always evaluate for other potential causes

◇ *Treatment*

* *Observation and reassurance*

May be appropriate for asymptomatic patients, patients with small lesions, or postmenopausal patients

Active intervention may be chosen for usually large tumors, symptomatic tumors or when the diagnosis is unclear

* *Surgery*

Myomectomy may be performed on submucous myoma by vaginal or by abdominal approach

Multiple myomectomy has a high risk of postoperative complications

- adhesions
- small bowel obstruction
- recurrence

Surgical techniques should emphasize hemostasis and multilayer uterine closure

- preoperative hormone manipulation has been advocated by some
- GnRH agonist

* *Medical management*

Increased interest in GnRH agonist

- works through pituitary down regulation
- estradiol reduced to <20 pg/mL
- long-term use restricted by cost and risk of osteoporosis

◇ *Myomas in pregnancy*

Incidence varies from 0.3% to 7.2%

- usually increase in size during pregnancy

Increased frequency of spontaneous abortion

Degeneration in second or third trimester may produce symptoms similar to acute adomen

- best treated by bedrest, symptomatic relief, and careful observation

May result in dystocia during labor

◆ Adenomyosis

Presence of endometrial glands within myometrium

◇ *Clinical picture*

Usually diagnosed by pathologist as an incidental finding

- found in 20% of hysterectomy specimens

Correctly diagnosed only 10% of the time prior to surgery

Symptoms

- progressively heavy menstrual flow
- increasing dysmenorrhea
- enlarging tender uterus

✧ *Pathology*
    Endometrial gland foci separated from the basal layer of lining endometrium by greater than one low power microscopic field
    Adenomyoma has no cleavage plane or pseudocapsule

✧ *Treatment*
    Hysterectomy is treatment of choice

◆ Stromal Adenomyosis
    Also referred to as endolyphatic stromal myosis, stromatosis, stromal endometriosis, stromal adenomyosis
    Morphologically similar to adenomyosis but only endometrial stromal present, no glands
    Hysterectomy is adequate treatment in truly benign variety (no vascular involvement)
    Other unusual tumors
- hemangioma, lymphangioma, lipomas and mesonephric cysts

MALIGNANT LESIONS OF THE UTERINE CORPUS

◆ Carcinoma of the Endometrium
    Most common female pelvic malignancy in the United States
    33,000 cases annually
    Increasing incidence observed worldwide

✧ *Epidemiology*
    Primarily a disease of postmenopausal women
- median age 61 years

    Risk factors
- obesity
- nulliparity
- late menopause

    Associated medical problems
- diabetes and hypertension

✧ *Estrogens in endometrial cancer*
    Oral contraceptives are protective
- probably prevent 2000 cases of endometrial carcinoma per year in the United States

    Unopposed exogenous estrogens increase risk of carcinoma
- survival rates are excellent
- addition of progesterone offers protective effect

    Tamoxifen may increase risk of endometrial carcinoma

✻ *Spread*
    Invades adjacent endometrium then myometrium
    Lymphatic spread and vascular invasion increase with increasing grade (Table 49-1)
    Staging now changed to surgical staging since 1988

TABLE 49-1. Risk of Lymph Node Metastasis, Deep Muscle Invasion, and Recurrence in Stage I Endometrial Cancer by Tumor Grade

Grade	Lymph Node Metastasis (%)	Deep Muscle Invasion (%)	Recurrence (%)
1	2	4	4
2	11	15	15
3	27	39	42

TABLE 49-2. Five-Year Survival Rates in Patients With Stage I Endometrial Cancer by Histologic Subtype

Subtype	Number of Patients	Survival Rate (%)
Adenocanthoma	192	87.5
Adenocarcinoma	501	79.8
Papillary	34	67.6
Adenosquamous	49	53.1
Clear cell	43	44.2

◇ *Diagnosis*

Abnormal bleeding is most important symptom

Diagnosis made by sampling endometrium

- curette biopsy 90% accurate
- vacuum curettage approximately 100% accurate
- pap smear is not a helpful screening test

Screening for endometrial carcinoma with transvaginal ultrasound has been suggested

- endometrial thickness <5 to 6 mm usually atrophic
- exceptions have been reported

◇ *Prognostic factors*

Staging

Grade

Age

- younger patients have early well differentiated lesions in most cases

Pathologic subtypes (Table 49-2)

Myometrial invasion

Adnexal metastasis present in 10% of patients with clinical stage I disease

Peritoneal cytology

◇ *Surgery*
Stage I lesions managed based on grade and operative finding (Fig. 49-2)

Stage II lesions over-diagnosed preoperatively in 50%
- preoperation radiation therapy has been used but would be unnecessary in 50% of these patients

◇ *Adjunctive therapy*

✳ *Radiation*
Occult stage II lesions usually receive postoperative radiotherapy as for stage I, G2, G3 lesion

Same is for occult stage II without pelvic lymphadenectomy

✳ *Progestins*
One third of recurrent patients respond
- high response rate in those with well-differentiated lesion

Also better response rate in those in presence of both estrogen and progestin receptors

✳ *Chemotherapy*
Results have been disappointing in general
- 30% response rate with single agent cisplatin
- 50% response rate with multiagent chemotherapy
  - cisplatin, cytoxan, doxorubicin

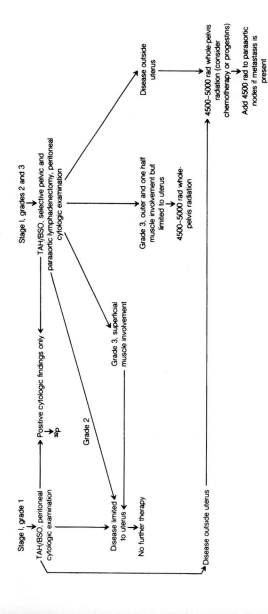

Figure 49-2. Primary surgical management of stage I adenocarcinoma of the endometrium. (^{32}P, radioactive phosphorus; DiSaia PJ, Creasman WT. Clinical gynecologic oncology. St. Louis: CV Mosby, 1984.)

50

◆ Tumors of the Fallopian Tubes and Broad Ligament

BENIGN LESIONS

Cysts of the broad ligament are of mesonephric or paramesonephric origin

Classified by character of epithelial lining

◆ Hydatids of Morgagni

Pedunculated cysts (Fig. 50-1)

Rarely >1 cm diameter

◆ Interligamentous Cysts

Can reach 15 cm

Separate ovary from cyst

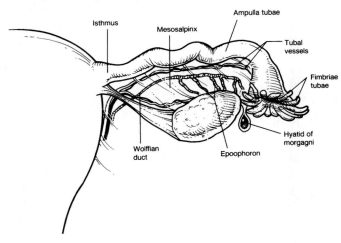

Figure 50-1. Anatomy of the fallopian tube.

◆ Walthard Cysts Rests

Most common tumor-like lesion of the oviduct
Probably arise from coelomic epithelial

◆ Salpingitis Isthmica Nodosa (SIN)

Discrete acini within thickened smooth muscle
Inflammatory or congenital etiology
May be associated with infertility

◆ Rare Tumors

Teratoma
Hemangioma
Adenomatoid tumors
Myomata (Fig. 50-2)
Adrenal rests
• usually diagnosed microscopically
• rarely functionally active

MALIGNANT LESIONS

◆ Primary Carcinoma of the Fallopian Tube

✧ *Epidemiology and cause*

One of the rarest malignancies of the female genital tract (0.3%
of gynecologic cancers)

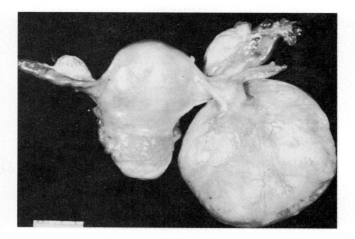

Figure 50-2. Myoma of round ligament. The uterus, oviducts, and ovaries
are normal.

1200 cases reported
Primarily affects older women; average age is 55 years
Etiology unknown

✧ *Clinical presentation*
Most are asymptomatic
Hydrops tubae profluens
• abnormal discharge (bloody or watery) with colicky pain
Abdominal or pelvic mass is the most common finding

✧ *Pathology*
Usually 80% unilateral
Ascites is rare
Microscopic pattern is papillary adenocarcinoma
May metastasize via lymphatics
• aortic nodes involved in one third of cases

✧ *Staging*
Established in 1991 (see Appendix)
Often difficult to distinguish from ovary

✧ *Management*
Surgical staging (total abdominal hysterectomy, bilateral salpingo-
oophorectomy, omentectomy) with follow-up (Fig. 50-3)
Use of chemotherapy seems appropriate but little data is available

✧ *Sites of failure and prognosis*
Distant recurrence common site of failure
5-year survival rates are approximately 40%
  Stage I: 50% to 88%
  Stage II: 25% to 35%
  Stage III: 15% to 20%

◆ Other Malignancies

✧ *Metastatic disease*
Much more common (80% to 90% of malignancies in the ovi-
duct)
Epithelium usually intact

✧ *Sarcoma*
Less than 50 cases reported

✧ *Choriocarcinoma*
Extremely rare
Treated with combination therapy

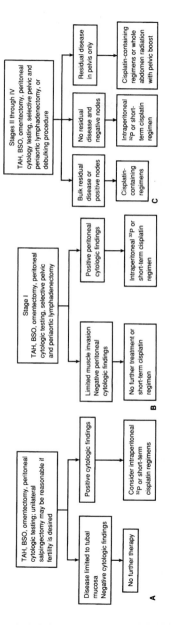

Figure 50-3. Algorithm for the suggested management of carcinoma in situ with mucosal involvement only of the fallopian tube. (BSO, bilateral salpingo-oophorectomy; TAH, total abdominal hysterectomy; adapted from DiSaia PJ, Creasman WT. Clinical gynecologic oncology. St Louis: CV Mosby, 1993.)

51

◆ Ovarian Neoplasms

BENIGN LESIONS

◆ Embryology

Primitive germ cells originate in dorsal part of epithelium lining the hindgut
- migrate to posterior portion of gonad

Organ development
- formation of primary cell cords from local mesenchyme after migration of germ cells
- later, cell aggregates form from surface epithelium and fuse with primary sex cords
- germinal sex cords partition into islands
  - each contains two or more germinal cells
  - segmentation completed when each oocyte is surrounded by single layer of prospective granulosa cells

Cellular proliferation followed by liquefaction forms graafian follicle
- 12% to 15% graafian follicles are present in fetal ovary during 36th week of gestation
- network of connective tissue develops in medullary and subepithelial layers
- forms tunica albuginea

◆ Anatomy

✧ *Follicular development*

Well-developed graafian and atretic follicles can be seen in newborn and infant

Number of ovum in newborn, 50,000 to 400,000
- only 300 to 400 proceed to ovulation

Primordial follicles decrease in number from birth

Follicular growth
- increase number of granulosa cells
  - follicular fluid (liquor folliculi) accumulates
    - etiology uncertain
      - cell secretion
      - cellular degeneration
      - vascular transudate

- ovum begins to project into cavity of follicle
  - cumulus oophorus
- cells around the ovum increase in number (corona radiata)

Outer layers around follicle
- theca interna and externa become delineated

✧ *Ovulation and corpus luteum formation*
Exact trigger of human ovulation unknown
- ovum is extruded into two or the peritoneal cavity

Corpus luteum development in four stages
1. proliferative
2. vascularization
3. complete development
4. regression
   - begins on day 26 of cycle

Corpus albicans requires 70 days to develop

✧ *Follicular atresia*
All primordial follicles do not reach maturity
- most degenerate (atresia)

Ovum degenerates first followed by follicular epithelial necro-biotic changes

◆ Functional Cysts

✧ *Follicular cyst*
Result of failure of ovulation
Usually multiple, occurring in both ovaries
Average size 2 cm, occasionally >3 cm
Rarely produce symptoms
Usually spontaneous regression in 8 weeks (Fig. 51-1)

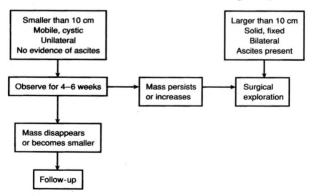

Figure 51-1. Management of a premenopausal woman with an adnexal mass. (DiSala PJ, Creasman WT. Clinical gynecologic oncology. 4th ed. St Louis: CV Mosby, 1993.)

TABLE 51-1. Symptoms of a Ruptured Corpus Luteum

Symptom or Feature	Number of Patients (%)
Location	
Right ovary	114 (66)
Left ovary	56 (32)
Unknown	3 (2)
Abdominal pain	173 (100)
Onset with intercourse	29 (17)
Right ovary	21 (72)
Left ovary	8 (28)
Duration	
<24 h	94 (54)
1-7 d	40 (23)
>7 d	14 (8)
Unknown	25 (15)
Nausea, vomiting, or diarrhea	60 (35)

Hallatt JG, Steele CH, Snyder M. Ruptured corpus luteum with hemoperitoneum: a study of 173 surgical cases. Am J Obstet Gynecol 1984;149:6.

✧ *Corpus luteum cyst*
Rarely >4 cm and usually asymptomatic
Protrudes from ovarian surface
• can be filled with blood
Symptoms related to size or complications of torsion, rupture, or hemorrhage
Spontaneous regression usually within 8 weeks
Hemoperitonium can occur with rupture (Table 51-1)

✧ *Theca lutein cyst*
Least common
Can occur in 50% to 60% of women with hydatidiform mole
• 5% to 10% of women with choriocarcinoma
Increased cyst formation probably from increased production of chorionic gonadotropins
Almost always bilateral
• may exceed 15 cm
May produce symptoms but usually an incidental finding in patient with molar pregnancy
Complete regression occurs after termination of pregnancy or evacuation of mole

◆ Hyperplastic Conditions
✧ *Polycystic ovaries*
Part of a complex of symptoms and endocrine abnormalities related to anovulation
• enlarged tense and oval ovary (Fig. 51-2)
  • thick fibrous capsule

- prominent hyperplasia of theca interna
- atretic follicles are numerous
- morphologic appearance similar, regardless of etiology of anovulation
  - prepubertal
  - Stein Leventhal syndrome (polycystic ovary syndrome)
- menstrual abnormalities
- hirsutism (hyperandrogenism)
- other endocrinopathies

✧ *Luteoma*
Hyperplastic nodules of lutein cells
Can be associated with androgen manifestations
- lipid-cell tumors
Luteoma of pregnancy
- bilateral in 50% of cases
- may be as large as 20 cm
- one quarter of all patients have androgen manifestations
- regresses after delivery

✧ *Serous inclusion cysts*
Nonfunctional cyst
Probably results from trapping of surface epithelium after ovulation
May be the origin of epithelial neoplasms

◆ Endometrial Cysts
Vary in size from powder burn to 10 to 12 cm diameter lesions
Dense adhesions common
Can be associated with infertility, dysmenorrhea, dyspareunia
Not all chocolate cysts are endometrial in origin
- bleeding into any cystic cavity yields decomposed blood later
Treatment is surgical excision

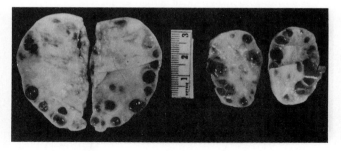

Figure 51-2. Gross appearance of the cut surfaces of bilateral polycystic ovaries.

◆ Ovarian and Tuboovarian Abscess

Salpingitis or pelvic peritonitis can result in inflammatory masses
- can be large as 15 cm

Severe pelvic pain and tenderness are typical
- antibiotics, analgesics, and occasional local heat are useful in alleviating symptoms

BENIGN OVARIAN NEOPLASMS

◆ Epithelial Neoplasms

✧ *Serous cystadenoma*

Constitutes 15% to 25% of all benign ovarian tumors

Occurs commonly in patients between 20 to 50 years-of-age

Usually 5 to 15 cm diameter

Solid portions suggestive of malignancy

Bilateral in 12% to 50%
- more common with papillary projections

Malignant change greater in papillary tumors

Derived from surface epithelium of the ovary
- unilocular, parvilocular, or multilocular
- lined with epithelium that resembles mucosa of the oviduct
- external papillary projections occur in 10% to 30% of tumors
- psamomma bodies can be found in stroma adjacent to epithelium
  - calcific concretions
  - may be visible in x-rays

Often asymptomatic

Treatment
- beyond childbearing years: hysterectomy and bilateral salpingo-oophorectomy
- in reproductive years: conservative treatment is recommended

✧ *Mucinous cystadenoma*

Constitutes 16% to 30 % of all benign neoplasms

Bilateral in only 5% to 7%

Rarely become malignant

Most common in patients between 20 to 40 years-of-age

Histogenesis
- differentiation of ovarian surface epithelium to endocervical type of müllerian duct epithelium
- monophyletic teratoma of intestinal origin

Often very large
- most 15 to 30 cm

Completely cystic and multilocular
- no extracystic papillary growths
  - intracystic papillary processes in 10% to 25%
    - more common in malignant types

Epithelial lining: tall, columnar cells resembling secretory cells of endocervix

Treatment
- young patient: unilateral oophorectomy
- older women: hysterectomy and bilateral salpingo-oophorectomy are preferrable

◈ *Pseudomyxoma peritonei*
Results from spillage of mucinous contents into peritoneal cavity
- biologically malignant, histologically benign
  - can result in progressive malnutrition
    - repeated laparotomies may be necessary in cases of bowel obstruction

◈ *Cystadenofibroma*
Variant of serous cystadenoma
- less common
Partially cystic and partially solid
Usually benign and unilateral
Surface with broad papillae or deep sulci
Treatment varies with age and associated findings

◈ *Brenner tumor*
Fibroepithelial tumor with gross characteristics similar to fibroma
Constitutes 1% to 2% of all ovarian tumors
Rarely malignant
5% to 13% are bilateral
Usually in patients >50 years-of-age
Histogenesis
- arise from Walthard cell rests
  - can coexist with mucinous cystadenomas
Usual size 10 to 15 cm
Usually solid
Can be associated with Meigs syndrome (ascites and hydrothorax)
Treatment
- excision or oophorectomy

◆ **Gonadal Stromal Tumors**

Tumors of each morphologic type may demonstrate clinical features of androgen and estrogen production or both
Histogenesis
- arises from mesenchymal ovarian stroma

◈ *Thecoma*
12% of feminizing mesenchymomas
2% of all ovarian tumors
Uncommon in women <35 years-of-age
- most common in postmenopausal women
Arises from ovarian cortical stroma
Unilateral and almost never malignant
Size may be 15 to 20 cm
Some tumors show marked luteinization

- no hormone activity in 25%

Most frequent symptom is postmenopausal bleeding

Can be associated with Meigs syndrome

Treatment: oophorectomy in young patients and hysterectomy and bilateral salpingo-oophorectomy in older patients

✧ *Hilus cell tumor*

Extremely rare

- only 50 cases described in literature

Symptoms are usually masculinization

- produces high levels of testosterone

Treatment: unilateral oophorectomy is recommended

◆ Nonintrinsic Connective Tissue Tumors

✧ *Ovarian fibroma*

Most frequent in middle-aged patients (average age of 48 years)

Histogenesis

- connective tissue of ovarian cortical stroma or possibly inactive endstage thecoma

Bilateral 2% to 10%

Average size is 6 cm

Can be associated with Meigs syndrome

Treatment: removal of tumor

◆ Germ Cell Tumors

✧ *Benign cystic teratoma (dermoid)*

Constitutes 18% to 25% of all ovarian neoplasms

Peak incidence in patients 20 to 40 years-of-age

- almost always benign

Malignant elements usually squamous epithelium

Bilateral in 12%

Average size 5 to 10 cm

Histogenesis

- arises from primordial germs cells
- contains sebaceous material, teeth, sweat glands, nervous tissue, skin
- often solid portion at one end containing cellular elements
  - 30% to 50% of cysts contain formed teeth
    - can be seen on x-ray

Treatment

- excision of cyst with ovarian conservation

✧ *Struma ovarii*

Unique benign cystic teratoma with thyroid tissue

- not distinguishable externally from dermoid cyst

5% produce signs of thyrotoxicosis

✧ *Gonadoblastoma*

Most common neoplasm of abnormal gonads

- abnormal sexual development

- 80% of patients are phenotypic females
  - 90% have Y chromosome
  - some patients are virilized

Large range of tumor size

Histogenesis
- mixture of germ cells and gonadal stroma cells
  - 50% are overgrown by germinoma

Treatment
- any patient with gonadal dysgenesis and Y chromosome runs risk of developing germ cell tumor
  - prophylactic removal of gonadal tissue in these patients seems prudent after puberty
  - 25% incidence of malignancy

Total abdominal hysterctomy and bilateral salpingo-oophorectomy indicated for treatment of gonadoblastoma

◆ Treatment of Benign Lesions

Management is surgical
- exclude malignancy
  - ovarian enlargement >7 cm are probably neoplastic
  - 93% of ovarian cysts <5 cm are nonneoplastic
  - solid tumors have greater probability of malignancy (even <7 cm)

Observation with close follow-up may be indicated in some cases
- oral contraceptives have been used by some to increase rate of involution
- infants and young girls demand surgical evaluation
- probably true for postmenopausal women with cysts >5 cm
  - unilocular cysts <5 cm may be followed by ultrasound

Surgical technique
- options dictated by operative findings and patient's desire for fertility
- tapping large cysts will result in peritoneal spillage
- bivalving of contralateral normal appearing ovary not advisable

◆ Torsion

More common in right ovary

May occur in up to 12% of patients with ovarian tumors
- Incomplete or complete torsion may occur

More common in pregnancy and in children

Untwisting the pedicle is safe
- may allow for conservative surgery with ovary sparing cystectomy

◆ Rupture

Cyst may rupture as result of hemorrhage, torsion, or trauma
- symptoms may intensify
  - chemical peritonitis with dermoid spillage

- rupture should initiate immediate surgical evaluation

Intraoperative rupture of malignant neoplasm should be avoided

◆ Concomitant Pregnancy

Most ovarian enlargements in pregnancy are follicular or corpus luteum cysts
- 99% disappear by 18 weeks

Surgical intervention
- cystic masses remain unchanged in second trimester
  - torsion can occur in postpartum period in cystic lesions that persist to third trimester
- any solid ovarian masses
- cystic mass >10 cm

MALIGNANT LESIONS

Most frequent cause of death among all genital tract cancers
Overall 5 year survival only 30%

◆ Classification

Over 30 types of neoplasms identified in the ovary
Most of malignant neoplasms fall into three broad categories
1. epithelial tumors
2. gonadal stroma tumors
3. germ cell tumors

◆ Epidemiology and Etiology

18,500 to 22,000 new cases per year
11,500 to 15,000 deaths per year
Fifth most frequent type of cancer in women
Fourth leading cause of cancer deaths (after lung, breast, and colon cancer)
Worldwide variation
- highest in Scandinavia (11/100,000 age-adjusted death rate)
- lowest in third world and Japan 2/100,000
- United States 7/100,000

Average age 50 to 59 years
- increased incidence with age

Epithelial neoplasms most common (greater than 90%)
Most ovarian cancers in children are germ cell
Etiology
- environmental factors or diet
- genetic factors
  - one first-degree relative raises risk ratio
- endocrine milleau
  - reduced risk with oral contraceptive pill users
  - protective effect of pregnancy

◆ Diagnosis

Physical examination
- empty bladder and rectum
- check for presence of acities
- uterine displacement

Laboratory studies, imaging techniques, and laparoscopy cannot substitute for careful history and physical examination

◆ Symptoms

Early diagnosis is difficult
- vague or absent symptoms
  - pelvic or abdominal discomfort
  - urinary frequency
  - gastrointestinal alteration
  - abdominal fullness, early satiety with larger lesions
  - abnormal vaginal bleeding occurs in 15% of patients
- endocrine abnormalities
  - menstrual irregularities
  - estrogen production with granulosa cell tumors
    - postmenopausal bleeding
    - precocious puberty
  - testosterone secretion
    - virilization in 50% of patients with Sertoli-Leydig tumors

◆ Physical Findings

Vary with the nature of the tumor
- bilaterality, mobility, consistency
- abdominal distention
  - huge masses
  - ascites
- uterine displacement

◆ Preoperative Evaluation

Plain film of abdomen, chest x-ray, complete blood count, serum chemistries, (including liver functions tests)
Intravenous pyelogram
Barium enema
Upper gastrointestinal tract (GI) series in some high-risk patients (Japanese)
Pap smear
Endometrial biopsy

◆ Ultrasound

Rarely necessary
Management not influenced by findings
- CT and ultrasound may be useful in advanced or recurrent disease

Fine-needle aspiration should not be used for primary diagnosis
Appropriate to document recurrence

◆ Staging

Staging is the most important determinant in prognosis (Fig. 51-3)
FIGO system revised in 1987 (See Appendix)
- proper staging requires vertical mid-line incision
- sample subdiaphragmatic areas
Diffuse spread is common

◆ Patterns of Spread

Several pathways of spread
- transabdominal dissemination most common
- lymphatic spread most common (50% in advanced disease) (Fig. 51-4)

◆ Epithelial Tumors

Constitute more than 60% of all ovarian neoplasms and more than 90% of malignant tumors
Probably derived from ovarian surface epithelium within epithelial inclusion cysts in cortex
Classified by predominant pattern and differentiation
Degree of cellular proliferation, atypia, and stromal invasion determines benign low malignant potential or carcinoma

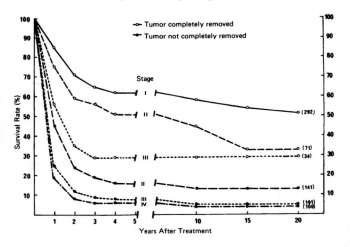

Figure 51-3. Survival rates for patients with ovarian carcinoma in relation to the stage and operability of the tumor. The numbers of patients are given in parentheses.

- lesions of low malignant potential (LMP)
    - 70% have localized disease
    - 95% five-year survival rate in stage I
    - even with advanced disease mean survival rate is much better than with invasive carcinoma

◆ Serous Tumors

38% of malignant epithelial tumors
- twice as frequent as serous LMP
Frequently bilateral
- 35% in LMP

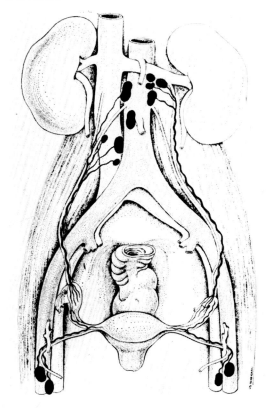

Figure 51-4. Diagram of the lymphatics of the ovary shows the drainage to paraaortic lymph nodes. There is inconstant drainage toward the external iliac and inguinal nodes.

- 40% to 60% in carcinoma

Extraovarian spread

- 30% in low malignant potential (LMP)
- 85% in carcinoma

✧ *Gross pathology*

Large unilocular, multilocular

50% greater than 15 cm

- most 5 to 15 cm

Cystic lining with papillary excrescences

- solid areas suggest carcinoma

✧ *Microscopic pathology*

Tumors of LMP have features intermediate between cystadenoma and carcinoma

- mild to moderate nuclear atypia
- psamomma bodies found in in 50%
- tufts of micropapillae
- no invasion

Carcinoma

- papillae with increased mitotic activity
- stromal invasion
- poorly differentiated in most cases
- trabecular or solid pattern of growth

◆ Mucinous Tumors

Account for 10% to 20% of all malignant epithelial tumors

- 5% to 10% for both LMP and carcinoma

Average age of patients is 50 to 55 years

- bimodal age distribution

Extraovarian spread less common

- 15% of LMP
- 40% of mucinous carcinomas

✧ *Gross pathology*

Large neoplasms (16 to 17 cm)

Multilocular

Thick viscous mucin

Solid areas, hemorrhagic, necrosis present in both LMP and carcinoma

✧ *Microscopic pathology*

LMP epithelium 2 to 3 cell layers, mild to moderate atypia, moderate mitotic activity, no invasion

Carcinoma

- glands and cysts back-to-back
- numerous mitotic figures
- stromal invasion
- desmoplastic response

Appearance may vary within the same tumor

⬦ *Pseudomyxoma peritonei*
  Progressive accumulation of mucin within abdominal cavity
  Does not develop as consequence of intraoperative rupture
  • can develop secondary to mucocele of the appendix
  50% of patients will die of this condition, usually after a long
    illness

◆ **Endometrioid Tumors**

  Histogenesis appearance identical to adenocarcinoma of
    endometrium
  Constitutes 15% to 20% of malignant epithelial tumors of the
    ovary
  • second most common type
  5% to 10% originate in endometriosis
  20% to 30% are bilateral
  • 15% at stage I
  Extraovarian spread in 40% to 50% of patients
  15% to 20% of patients have synchronous endometrium adeno-
    carcinoma
  • separate primary neoplasms

⬦ *Gross pathology*
  No specific appearance

⬦ *Microscopic pathology*
  LMP are rare (no deaths reported)
  Carcinoma characterized by
  • stratified columnar epithelium
  • mitotic figures
  • solid growth
  • squamous differentiation occurring in 25% to 50% of cases

◆ **Clear Cell Tumors**

  Accounts for 5% to 10% of malignant epithelial tumors of the
    ovary
  Closely related to endometrioid carcinoma
  • 25% of patients have pelvic endometriosis
  60% to 70% present with stage I tumors
  • fewer than 5% have bilateral disease

⬦ *Gross pathology*
  10 to 20 cm diameter
  Most are cystic
  Hemorrhage and necrosis are common

⬦ *Microscopic pathology*
  Rarely classified as low malignant potential (LMP)
  Carcinoma
  • varied appearance
    • two cell types

1. clear cell (glycogen-containing)
2. hobnail cells
   • line papillae, tubules, or cysts

◆ Other Types

Brenner tumors resemble transitional epithelium
• malignant transformation is rare
• LMP referred to as proliferation
   • follow benign course
Malignant mixed mesodermal tumors
• biphasic neoplasm
• histologically identical to mixed müllerian tumors of the uterus
• low grade variant is adenosarcoma
Undifferentiated
• 5% to 10% of epithelial tumors
• bilateral in 50% of patients

◆ Treatment of Epithelial Tumors

✧ *Surgery*

Carcinoma of the ovary
• total abdominal hysterectomy and bilateral salpingo-oophorectomy
• complete or partial omentectomy
• debulking
Exceptions to the above
• hysterectomy may be excluded if there is heavy involvement of the pelvic peritoneal surfaces, especially the cul-de-sac
   • could lead to significant serous vaginal discharge
• conservative therapy (unilateral salpingo-oophorectomy) (Table 51-2)
Cytoreductive surgery
• may improve survival
• can reduce symptoms from tumor burden
• can slow reaccumulation of ascitic fluid

TABLE 51-2. Requirements for Conservative Management of Epithelial Ovarian Cancer

---

Stage (IA preferred)
Well-differentiated lesions preferred
Young woman of low parity
Otherwise normal pelvis
Encapsulated and free of adhesions
No invasion of capsule, lymphatics, or mesovarium
Peritoneal washings negative
Bivalve of opposite ovary if abnormal
Omental biopsy negative
Close follow-up probable

Second-look surgery
- evaluation of response after chemotherapy
- laparoscopy may be useful if residual cancer is detected
- cytoreductive surgery at second look may also improve prognosis

✧ *Chemotherapy*
Stage I disease
- except stage I well-differentiated carcinoma
- cisplatin (Platinol) as a single agent

Combination chemotherapy in patients with bulky residual disease
- no survival advantage demonstrated
- complete clinical remission in 40% to 60%

Intraperitoneal chemotherapy
- may be useful in microscopic or minimal (less than 2 cm) residual disease
- cisplatin may be drug of choice

✧ *Radiation therapy*

✳ *Radioisotope therapy*
^{32}P chromic phosphate
- usual dose 15 mCi

Instilled into peritoneal cavity in fluid

No significant advantage demonstrated over systemic chemotherapy

✳ *External-beam radiotherapy*
Pelvic dose 4500 to 5000 cGy
Abdominal dose 2250 to 2800 cGy
Successful in cases of minimal residual disease
Overall results disappointing
- more morbid than chemotherapy

◆ Tumor Markers

Malignant germ cell tumors produce α-fetoprotein (AFP), human chronic gonadotropin (hCG)
- greatest use in detecting recurrence

Epithelial ovarian cancer
- CA-125
  - false-positives can occur (Table 51-3)
  - meaningful if it is positive
  - rising titers suggest recurrence

◆ Prognosis

Overall 5-year survival rate poor (30%)
  - Stage I: 70%
  - Stage II: 25%
  - Stage III: 12%
  - Stage IV: 5%

**TABLE 51-3. Conditions Associated With Elevated Serum
Levels of CA 125**

Benign Conditions	Malignant Conditions
Menstruation	Ovarian cancer
Pregnancy	Pancreatic cancer
Endometriosis	Lung cancer
Leiomyomata	Breast cancer
Adenomyosis	Large bowel cancer
Pancreatitis	Fallopian tube cancer
Peritonitis	Endometrial cancer
Chronic hepatitis	Cervical cancer
Renal failure	

◆ Germ Cell Tumors

Constitute 15% to 20% of all neoplasms
4% are malignant
- primarily in children and young women
  - 84% are malignant in children <10 years-of-age

◆ Dysgerminoma

Most common malignant germ cell tumor
- 50% of malignant germ cell tumors
- 2% of all malignant ovarian neoplasms
  - 75% of patients 10 to 30 years-of-age
2% of nonpregnant women have positive pregnancy test

✧ *Gross pathology*
Solid fleshy tumor
Median diameter 15 cm

✧ *Microscopic pathology*
Aggregates of large polygonal cells
- often infiltrated by lymphocytes
Syncytiotrophoblast may be present
- produce hCG

✧ *Prognosis and treatment*
5-year survival rate (63% for advanced cases to 96% for stage IA
   for tumors)
75% have stage I disease
- occasionally bilateral
  - 5% occult dygerminoma in contralateral ovary
Highly sensitive to radiation and chemotherapy
Chemotherapy preferred in patient desiring future fertility
- VP-16, blemoycin, cisplatin (VBP regimen)

◆ Endodermal Sinus Tumor

Second most common malignant germ cell tumor
- Constitutes 1% of all ovarian malignancies

Patients usually younger than 40 years-of-age
- frequently sudden presentation

70% of patients have stage I disease

✧ *Gross pathology*

Soft with smooth exterior
Median diameter 15 cm
Large areas of hemorrhage and necrosis

✧ *Prognosis and treatment*

Before chemotherapy 84% of patients with stage IA tumors died
- now 80% of women with stage I disease survive 5 years
- 50% with advanced disease survive 5 years

Unilateral salpingo-oophorectomy and chemotherapy recommended in young patients

◆ Embryonal Carcinoma

Relatively rare (accounting for 5% of malignant germ cell tumors)
Median age of patients is 15 years-of-age
Short duration of symptoms
- precocious puberty in 50% of prepubertal girls
- hCG levels often elevated

✧ *Gross pathology*

Large (17 cm tumor) and soft
Extensive hemorrhage and necrosis

✧ *Prognosis and treatment*

Unilateral salpingo-oophorectomy (USO) and chemotherapy

◆ Immature Teratoma

Third most common malignant germ cell tumor
- represents 25% of all malignant germ cell tumors in patients under 15 years-of-age

20% of patients are prepubertal
Symptoms of short duration

✧ *Gross pathology*

Large unilateral tumor
Median diameter 18 cm
Hair present in 20%

✧ *Prognosis and treatment*

70% are stage IA
Prognosis related to grade
- improved with new chemotherapy

Stage IA grade 1; USO

Higher stage or grade
- hysterectomy, BSO, and chemotherapy (VAC regimen)

◆ Choriocarcinoma

Rarely occurs in pure form
Admixed with teratoma, endodermal sinus tumor, embryonal carcinoma, or dysgerminoma

✧ *Gross pathology*
Soft and hemorrhagic

✧ *Treatment*
Surgical excision and combination chemotherapy

◆ Mixed Germ Cell Tumors

Represent 8% of malignant germ cell tumors

✧ *Gross pathology*
Large neoplasms (15 cm)
Appearance of cut surface depends on elements contained within neoplasm

✧ *Microscopic pathology*
Most common element is dysgerminoma, (80%)
- endodermal sinus tumor, (70%)
- embryonal carcinoma, (15%)

Most frequent combination is dysgerminoma and endodermal sinus tumor

✧ *Prognosis and treatment*
Two thirds of patients will have stage IA disease
Prognosis is dependent on elements and grade
USO acceptable
- occult contralateral involvement in <5%

◆ Gonadal Stromal Tumors

Constitute 6% of all ovarian neoplasms
90% are granulosa cell or thecoma
Histogenesis is uncertain
All have potential for steroid hormone production

◆ Granulosa Tumors

Account for 1% to 3% of all ovarian neoplasms
Wide age range
- 40% after menopause
- 5% before puberty

Most patients present with symptoms of functional tumor or mass
- <5% asymptomatic
- 75% demonstrate endocrine manifestations
- 10% with endometrial adenocarcinoma

✧ *Gross pathology*
  Circumscribed
  Consistency varies between tumors
  Areas of hemorrhage and necrosis common

✧ *Microscopic pathology*
  Small round cells
  • prominent longitudinal groove (coffee bean appearance)
  Most contain theca cells
  Variety of patterns
  • microfollicular → Call-Exner bodies
  • usually see admixture of patterns
  Juvenile granulosa cell tumor
  • numerous mitotic figures
  • cytologic atypia
  • only 15% metastasize
  Cystic granulosa tumor
  • usually associated with hirsutism or viralization
  • rarely has metastases

✧ *Prognosis and treatment*
  Low potential for malignant behavior
  90% are stage IA
  10-year survival rate 86% to 96% for stage I
  TAH/BSO is standard treatment
  • USO in young women
  Recurrences treated with surgery or radiation therapy

52

◆ Radiation Therapy

PHYSICAL AND CHEMICAL NATURE

Radiation produced by decay of atomic nuclei: gamma rays
Radiation originating outside the nucleus: x-rays
Collectively, gamma rays and x-rays are called photons
• energy of the photon is the important aspect, not the source
Ionizing radiation may initiate free-radical formation from water
(Fig. 52-1)

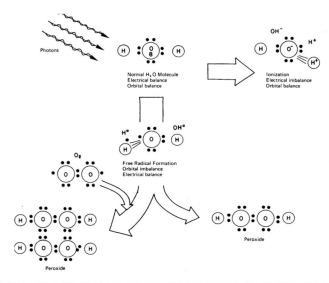

Figure 52-1. Effects of radiation on water. Ionizing radiation produces water ions and may initiate free radical formation, yielding peroxide. The latter process is enhanced by addition of pure oxygen. (Nolan JF. Clin Obstet Gynecol 1961;4:504.)

BIOLOGIC EFFECTS

Selective destruction of tissue forms the basis of therapeutic radiology
- neoplastic cells are killed more easily
- radiosensitivity and radiocurability are not identical
- cervical carcinoma is relatively radioinsensitive but curable

Unit of exposure (rad)
Unit of absorption (centigray cGy)
- 1 Gray = 100 rads = 100 cGy

CELL CYCLE EFFECTS

Cell cycle
- G1: presynthetic phase
- S: DNA synthesis
- G2: postsynthetic phase
- M: mitosis

Resistance to radiation varies over cell cycle: S >G2, M >G1

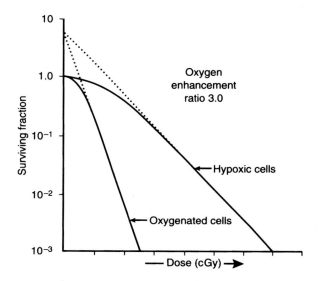

Figure 52-2. Survival curves for mammalian cells exposed to x-rays in oxygenated and hypoxic environments. The difference in radiation sensitivity is threefold.

TABLE 52-1. Average Radiation Dose to the Fetus and
             Maternal Gonads From Diagnostic
             Examinations

Examination	Dose to Fetus and Maternal Gonads $(1 \times 10^{-5}$ Gy)
Lower extremity roentgenography	1
Cervical spine roentgenography	2
Skull roentgenography	4
Chest roentgenography	8
Pelvimetry	750
Chest fluoroscopy	70
Cholecystography	300
Lumbar spinal roentgenography	275
Abdominal roentgenography	185/film
Hip roetengenography	100
Intravenous or retrograde pyelography	585
Upper gastrointestinal roentgenography	330
Lower gastrointestinal roentgenography	465

OXYGEN EFFECT

One of the most important in radiation biology
Functions as a radiosensitizer
Hypoxic cells may be radioresistant (Fig. 52-2)

GENETIC EFFECTS

Cannot assign a mutation rate to a specific radiation dose
No person from conception to 30 years-of-age should be exposed
    to greater than 10 cGy (Table 52-1)

EFFECTS ON THE FETUS

<25 cGy : no classic effects of radiation described
<10 cGy : inability to produce effects
Diagnostic x-ray procedures should be avoided unless clearly
    indicated in pregnant patient

PRINCIPLES OF RADIATION THERAPY

◆ External Irradiation

Energy and penetrating power are dependent on proton wave-
    length
Supervoltage radiation has a reduced skin effect compared with
    orthovoltage
Isodose curves represent tissue part receiving equivalent doses

Use of multiple fields in gynecologic radiation therapy reduces exposure of normal tissue with increased target doses
  * usually use two- or four-field technique

◆ Local Irradiation

Intensity of radiation decreases with distance (inverse square law)
Local application uses this law to its advantage
Minimization of dosage to local tissues depends on careful placement
Usually multiple discrete sources
Interstitial needles can be used (Fig. 52-3)

IONIZING RADIATION IN GYNECOLOGIC THERAPY

◆ Treatment of Cervical Cancer

Intracavitary radiation cannot deliver concentrated dose beyond 3 cm from external cervical os (Fig. 52-4)

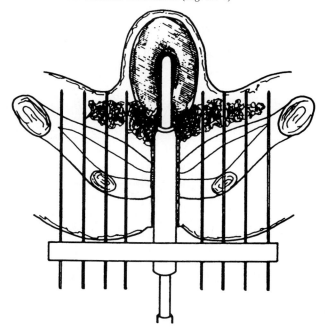

Figure 52-3. Diagram of an interstitial implant used to treat a stage IIIB cervical cancer with a Syed-Noblett applicator.

Goal is to sterilize the central lesion and destroy neoplastic cells
in parametrium and nodes
Often start with external beam
Several methods of intracavitary radiation application (Fig. 52-5)
• tumor dose of 7000 to 8000 cGy attempted

◇ *Techniques*

✳ *Stockholm*
Two intracavitary applications of radium (3 weeks apart)
Each application, 25 to 28 hours in duration
• 50 to 75 mg radium
Lower 2 cm of uterine tandem has no radium
Vaginal applicator consists of a series of boxes or cylinders
• 60 to 80 mg radium

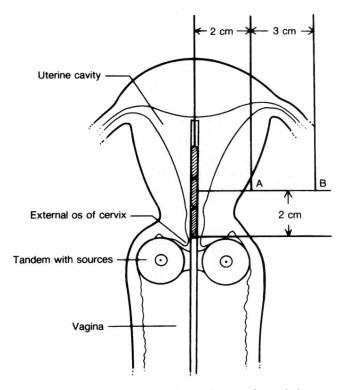

Figure 52-4. Diagram of a tandem and ovoid placement for cervical cancer
with points A and B identified.

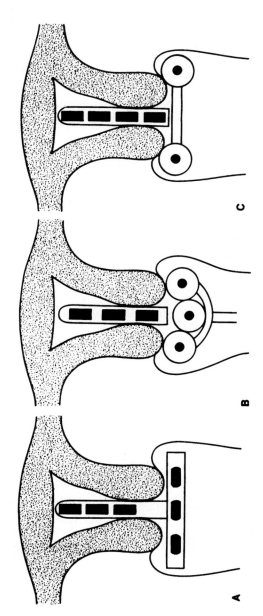

Figure 52-5. Application of radium in the treatment of cervical cancer. (**A**) Stockholm technique. (**B**) Paris technique. (**C**) Manchester technique.

Hot loading over a brief period
Point A: 6000 cGy, point B: 1900 cGy

✳ *Paris*
Uterine tandem
- 6.6 mg radium in canal, 2 cephalad sources
Pair of vaginal ovoids
Equivalent to Manchester technique (5700 cGy over 6 days)
One treatment for 96 to 200 hours

✳ *Manchester*
Modification of Paris system (tandem and pair of ovoids)
Designed to yield constant isodose patterns
Fletcher-Suit modification allows afterloading

✳ *External pelvic irradiation*
Whole pelvic radiation usually administered through an anterior and posterior field 15 to 18 cm^2
Small lesions may be treated best by parametrial irradiation to provide for optimal future intracavitary radiation
Survival rate has been very good
- 90% 5-year survival rate for stage I

◆ Carcinoma of the Vagina and Vulva

Initial external beam, then local therapy for vaginal carcinoma
Vulvar carcinoma not a good candidate for treatment
Severe pruritus and radiation necrosis can result

◆ Carcinoma of the Endometrium

◇ *Preoperative or postoperative external radiation*
Customary dose 4000 to 5000 cGy administered over 5 to 6 weeks
No evidence regarding improved survival
Clearly controls pelvic recurrences

◇ *Postoperative vaginal intracavitary application*
Intuitive and not based on documented improved outcome
See Chapter 49

◇ *Radiation treatment of recurrent cancer*
Unresectable localized recurrence can be treated with ^{125}I seed placement
External radiation also may be useful
- delineate lesion with surgical clips
Recurrences in the pelvis are often in fibrotic areas
- poor response often seen

◆ Carcinoma of the Ovary

External radiation is not useful in most cases
Dysgerminomas are radiosensitive, but most epithelial carcinomas are not very responsive

^{32}P intraperitoneal treatment may be appropriate in some stage I and II patients

IMPROVED THERAPEUTIC STRATEGIES

Hyperthermia may improve response rates in association with radiation

Newer techniques are being developed and may have clinical utility in the future

53

◆ Gestational Trophoblastic Neoplasms

INTRODUCTION

Unique group of benign and malignant tumors derived from human placenta

Malignant gestational torophoblastic neoplasms (GTN) are among the most sensitive human solid malignancies in regard to chemotherapy

PATHOLOGY

◆ Hydatidiform Mole

Two distinct types of molar gestation described (Table 53-1)
1. complete mole
2. partial mole
   • may represent extreme form of hydropic placental degeneration

TABLE 53-1. Complete and Partial Hydatidiform Moles

Feature	Partial Hydatidiform Mole	Complete Hydatidiform Mole
Karotype	Triploid paternal and maternal origin	Most 46.XX paternal origin
Pathology		
Fetus or amnion, fetal vessels	Present	Absent
Hydropic villi	Variable, often focal	Pronounced, generalized
Trophoblast proliferation	Focal	Variable, often marked
Clinical		
Mole clinical diagnosis	Rare	Common
Uterus large for dates	Rare	30% to 50%
Malignant sequelae	<10%	6% to 36%

✧ *Partial hydatidiform mole*
  Often associated with identifiable fetus
  Mixture of normal and hydropic villi
  Fetal vessels and red blood cells identified
  Almost always are haploid maternal and two haploid paternal
    sets of chromosomes
  • presumably a result of dispermic fertilization
  Less than 5% require chemotherapy for malignant GTN

✧ *Complete hydatidiform mole*
  Hydropic villi
  Lack of fetus and membranes
  All secrete hCG, which is a useful marker to monitor regression
  Almost all are uniformly diploid with paternal chromosome
    markers
  One third to one half of patients present with enlargement greater
    than expected for gestational dates
  20% have theca lutein cysts

✧ *Invasive mole*
  Also called chorioadenoma destruens
  Complete hydatidiform mole invading myometrium
  • usually diagnosed within 6 months of molar evacuation
  Probably underdiagnosed because most women with GTN now
    are treated without hysterectomy

◆ **Choriocarcinoma**

  Highly anaplastic malignancy derived from trophoblastic ele-
    ments
  • no villi are identified
  Rapidly invades and metastasizes
  • lung and vagina are most common metastatic loci
  Can follow any kind of pregnancy
  • one half preceded by hydatidiform mole
  • one half preceded by term gestation and abortion or by ec-
    topic pregnancy

◆ **Placental Site Tumor**

  Locally invasive neoplasm derived from intermediate cells of
    placenta
  Rare neoplasm
  Rarely shows systemic metastasis
  Much more resistant to chemotherapy than other forms of GTN
  • hysterectomy is initial treatment of choice

INCIDENCE AND EPIDEMIOLOGY

  Identified in 1/1500 to 1/2000 of pregnancies in the United States
  • 3000 molar pregnancies per year

- 500 to 750 malignant GTNs per year

Much more common (5 to 15 times higher) in Far East and South East Asia
- may represent reporting biases of referral centers
- racial differences exist

Previous molar gestation increases risk of developing a subsequent molar gestation by 4 to 5 times

Increased risk at both extremes of reproductive age

Nutritional factors may play a role

Incidence of partial mole unknown (probably 10% of all molar pregnancies)

Invasive mole follows 10% to 15% of complete moles

Choriocarcinoma complicates
- 1/40 moles
- 1/5000 ectopic pregnancies
- 1/15,000 abortions
- 1/150,000 normal pregnancies

MANAGEMENT OF HYDATIDIFORM MOLE

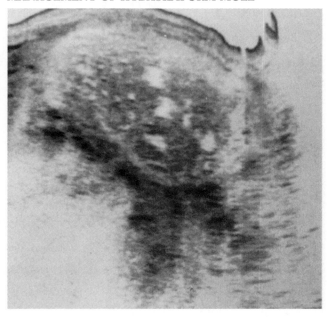

Figure 53-1. A longitudinal ultrasound reveals a hydatidiform mole. The mixed echoic pattern is caused by hydropic villi and focal intrauterine hemorrhage.

◆ Diagnosis

Ultrasound is diagnostic method of choice (Fig. 53-1)
Patient often presents with vaginal bleeding, uterine enlargement
in absence of fetal heart tones

◆ Evaluation

Complete physical examination
CBC
Blood chemistries (renal, liver, and thyroid function tests)
Baseline hCG level
Chest x-ray
Pelvic ultrasound

◆ Treatment

Suction curettage has low complication rate with uterine size
<16 weeks
Excessive uterine enlargement may predisposed to pulmonary
complications
- trophoblastic deportation
- preeclampsia
- fluid overload
Uterine size >16 weeks mandates further preoperative assessment
- EKG
- radionucleotide-gated heart pool scan for ejection fraction
- cardiac ultrasound to assess valvular function
Perform suction prepared to convert to laparotomy and obtain
central hemodynamic monitoring if needed
Primary hysterectomy
- patients who have completed childbearing and desire sterilization are good candidates
- reduces malignant sequelae from 20% to 5%

◆ Theca Lutein Cysts

Usually regress spontaneously over several weeks
Avoid manipulation
Can undergo torsion, infarction, rupture
Oophorectomy may be required

◆ Prophylactic Chemotherapy

May reduce malignant sequelae in high-risk patients
Not routinely recommended in cases of uncomplicated mole and
reliable patients

◆ Surveillance After Molar Evacuation

Sensitive hCG assays have greatly improved surveillance

✧ *Recommendations*

Baseline

- β-hCG
- physical examination with pelvic examination
- chest x-ray

Surveillance of hCG levels

- hCG every week until negative
- then every 2 to 4 weeks after negative to confirm spontaneous hCG regression
- then every 1 to 2 months for 6 to 12 months
- start contraception during surveillance
- oral contraceptives are best choice

MALIGNANT GTN

◆ Malignant Sequelae After Molar Evacuation

Wide spectrum

- molar proliferation without invasion (retained mole)
- invasive mole
- choriocarcinoma
- clinically identified metastatic GTN without histologic diagnosis

Initiation of treatment during surveillance (20%)

- rising hCG
- hCG plateau for 3 or more consecutive weeks
- appearance of metastases
- histologic evidence of invasive mole or choriocarcinoma

◆ Diagnosis

See above criteria for hCG surveillance

May be discovered in patients after nonmolar gestation with unusual symptoms

✧ *Evaluation*

Physical and pelvic examination

Baseline hCG

CBC and blood chemistries

Chest x-ray

Pelvic ultrasound

CT or radionucleotide brain scan

Abdominal and pelvic CT or liver scan with IVP

50% of patients with malignant GTN have lung metastases detected by chest x-ray

Role of MRI not yet defined

Occult CNS lesions may be determined by lumbar puncture for hCG assay

Thorough evaluation for metastic disease is crucial

Selection of therapy is dependent on staging

**TABLE 53-2. Clinical Classification of Malignant
Gestational Trophoblastic Neoplasia**

I. Nonmetastatic GTN
   A. Not defined in terms of good versus poor prognosis
II. Metastatic GTN
   A. Good prognosis (i.e., absence of high-risk factors)
      1. Pretreatment hCG level <40,000 IU/mL serum β-hCG
      2. <4-Month duration of disease
      3. No evidence of brain or liver metastasis
      4. No significant prior chemotherapy
      5. No antecedent term pregnancy
   B. Poor prognosis (i.e., any single high-risk factor)
      1. Pretreatment hCG level >40,000 IU/mL serum β-hCG
      2. >4-Month duration of disease
      3. Brain and/or liver metastasis
      4. Failed prior chemotherapy
      5. Antecedent term pregnancy

GTN, gestational trophoblastic neoplasms; hCG, human chorionic gonadotropin.

◆ Staging and Classification

Several systems developed to assess therapy and prognosis (Table 53-2, Table 53-3)
FIGO staging is simple
   Stage I: disease confined to uterine corpus
   Stage II: vaginal or pelvic metastases
   Stage III: lung metastases
   Stage IV: other metastases
WHO scoring system correlates well with survival

◆ Therapy

Methotrexate developed in 1950s
GTN is presently the most curable of human solid tumors

◇ *Chemotherapy*

Based on clinical classification (Table 53-4)
Many different choices all with excellent results (Table 53-5)
Poor-prognosis patients who fail standard chemotherapy are very challenging

◇ *Surgical and radiation therapy*

✳ *Hysterectomy*
Rarely indicated as initial treatment for malignant GTN
May decrease time to remission in some cases
Surgery performed during treatment cycle

✳ *Thoracotomy*
Has been used to remove drug-resistant disease, rarely
Always consider occult pelvic growth

TABLE 53-3. World Health Organization Prognostic Scoring System for Gestational Trophoblastic Neoplasia

Prognostic Factor	Score*			
	0	1	2	4
Age	≤39	>39		
Antecedent pregnancy	Hydatidiform	Abortion; ectopic	Term pregnancy	
Interval (months)†	<4	4-6	7-12	>12
hCG level (IU/L)	$<10^3$	10^3-10^4	10^4-10^5	$>10^5$
ABO blood groups (female/male)		O/A A/O	B AB	
Largest tumor (cm)	<3	3-5	>5	
Site of metastasis		Spleen, kidney	Gastrointestinal tract, liver	Brain
Number of metastasis		1-3	4-8	>8
Prior chemotherapy			Single drug	Multiple drugs

*Low risk, ≤4; intermediate risk, 5-7; high risk, ≥8. †Interval: time between antecedent pregnancy and start of chemotherapy.

TABLE 53-4. Chemotherapy for Malignant Gestational Trophoblastic Neoplasms

Type of Disease	Initial Treatment	Salvage Treatment
Nonmetastatic GTN	Single agent, methotrexate or MTX/FA	Single agent, dactinomycin Combination chemotherapy
Good-prognosis metastatic GTN	Single agent, methotrexate	Single agent, dactinomycin Combination chemotherapy
Poor-prognosis metastatic GTN	Triple therapy (MAC)	Other combination chemotherapy

GTN, gestational trophoblastic neoplasms; MTX/FA, methotrexate-folinic acid; MAC, methotrexate-dactinomycin chlorambucil.

✳ *Brain and liver metastases*
Whole brain and whole liver radiotherapy may be used in conjunction with chemotherapy
Other options include intrathecal methotrexate

✳ *Placental site tumors*
Serum hCG not as reliable
Often aggressive invading myometrium

◇ **Monitoring therapy**

✳ *Laboratory evaluations*
Careful monitoring of renal, hepatic, and hematologic indices
Withhold cycles for total leukocyte count <3000, platelets <100,000
Serial hCG levels crucial
  • consider changing chemotherapy if a 25% drop in hCG is not demonstrated after treatment cycle

---

TABLE 53-5. Results of Chemotherapy for Nonmetastatic Gestational Trophoblastic Neoplasms

Treatment	Number of Patients	Primary Remission Rate (%)	Final Remission Rate (%)
Methotrexate			
5-Day methotrexate			
Hammond et al, 1967	47	93	98
Smith et al, 1982	39	92	100
Methotrexate-folinic acid			
Berkowitz et al, 1986	163	90.2	100
Smith et al, 1982	29	72	100
Wong et al, 1985*	68	76	100
Mutch et al, 1986	39	74.6	100
Weekly methotrexate			
Holmesley et al, 1988	63	81	98
Dactinomycin			
5-Day dactinomycin			
Goldstein et al, 1975	12	84	100
Petrilli and Morrow, 1980	13	77	
Bolus dactinomycin			
Petrilli and Morrow, 1980	5	80	
Twiggs, 1983	12	100	
Petrilli et al, 1986	31	94	
5-Fluorouracil			
Sung et al, 1984	69	92.9	
Etoposide (VP-16)			
Wong et al, 1986*	60	98	100

*Includes low-risk metastatic gestational trophoblastic neoplasms.

✳ *hCG remission and surveillance*
Complete remission
• three consecutive weekly hCG levels within normal limits
Surveillance
• every 1 to 2 weeks for 3 months
• every 2 to 4 weeks for 4 months
• every 1 to 2 months for 6 months
• every 6 months for thereafter

◇ *Prevention of recurrent disease*
Recurrence rate is 3% to 26%
Treatment beyond first normal hCG level
• nonmetastatic disease: one cycle
• good-prognosis metastatic GTN: two cycles
• poor-prognosis metastatic GTN: three to four cycles

◇ *Reproduction after therapy*
Little or no added risk of congenital malformation in future pregnancies
Increased incidence of repeat mole, modest
After treatment for malignant GTN
• possibly increased risk for placenta accreta
• defer pregnancy for at least 1 year
• consider postpartum hCG after subsequent delivery to rule out choriocarcinoma

54

◆ Medicolegal Issues

OVERVIEW OF MEDICAL MALPRACTICE LAW

Area of law known as torts cover medical malpractice
Three types of torts
1. internal torts
2. negligence
3. straight liability (not imposed on physicians)

◆ Elements of Negligence

Difficult to prove as there are several requisite elements
- duty of due care
- breach of that duty
- compensable injury or damages
- causal link between breach of duty, injury and damages

◇ *The physician's duty*

Judge determines the existence of physician/patient relationship
Physician must enter into relationship with appropriately matched patients
The measure of the duty taken is based on prevailing standard of care in community
Informed consent
- professional practice rule
- materiality rule
  - determined by the jury

◇ *Breach of duty*

Not a simple task
Expert witnesses for both sides usually disagree
Juries reach their own conclusions, largely ignoring professional opinion

◇ *Proximate cause*

Need to establish that the act or omission of the physician was a substantial factor leading to the injury

✧ *Damages*
Economic
Noneconomic
- pain and suffering
- loss or consortium

◆ **Statute of Limitations**

Vary from state to state, patient to patient

◆ **Settlement of Claims**

90% settled before or during trial
50% dropped with no monetary payment
Physicians win most jury verdicts
Certain cases lead to nearly certain settlement
- neurologic deficit cases
- comatose, vegetative, blind patient
- injuries to eye, face, or heart
- scarring, especially over exposed area by seasonal dress
- defendant physician practicing outside his or her field
- startling surprises
- inappropriate changes made in the records
- arrogant, cold, hostile, or aloof physician

PROFESSIONAL LIABILITY CLIMATE

◆ **Epidemiology of Liability**

77% of obstetricians and gynecologists have been sued
35% have greater than three claims
17 million civil law suits filed in 1987

✧ *Why are obstetricians and gynecologists sued?*
General public assumes obstetrics to be relatively routine and
normal and that child birth is a simple natural act
Poor physician/patient relationship
Interdependence with other members of the health care team
Reluctance to consult or refer

FOCUS OF LIABILITY RISK IN MEDICAL PRACTICE

◆ **Motivation for Claims**

Concept of perception is often at the base of claim
- only 37% of patients express total satisfaction with their obstetric care
Reasons that patients file perinatal injury claims
- 33% advised to do so by "knowledgeable acquaintance"
- 24% recognized a cover-up
- 24% needed the money

TABLE 54-1. Office Risk Management Checklist

Appointment scheduling: does your current scheduling method often result in your getting behind in seeing patients?

Office location: is your office conveniently located for patients and easily accessible from the street, parking lot, or sidewalk?

Reception area: is it a comfortable, well-lighted environment with informative reading materials or simply a waiting room?

Examination rooms: do they ensure privacy from view and from sound

Office records: are they safe from casual reading by visitors?

Office appointments: do you have a system for tracking and following-up missed appointments?

History: is the patient questioned closely enough to ensure a complete record?

Prescription drugs: are you familiar with other drugs being taken by the patient. Do you know the contraindications of the drugs you prescribe? Do you renew prescriptions without reexamining the patient?

Informed consent: do you obtain consent in the office, where time is available for questions, answers, and exchange of information?

Office staff: are your office personnel involved in risk management to ensure that problems are anticipated and solved in a timely manner?

TABLE 54-2. Hospital Risk Management Checklist

Prehospitalization instruction: is your patient prepared for what to expect when she arrives at the hospital?

Initial progress notes and orders: are notes made promptly and standing orders adjusted to respond to the individual patient?

Consultations: are consultations sought appropriately and documented?

Cosigning, initialing: do you read everything before you sign it?

Checking standing or telephoned orders: do you periodically reconfirm and review orders?

Progress notes: are progress notes recorded immediately after the patient visit? Do you read progress notes before entering the room?

Correcting prior record entries: do you correct prior entries in the appropriate manner (i.e., chronologically, legibly, with explanations)?

Operating room responsibility: is there a clear protocol of operating room responsibility for the health-care team?

Health-care team: is interaction courteous, communicative, cooperative, and coordinated?

Incident management: are operative errors corrected quickly and documented appropriately, and are patients and their families appropriately counseled?

Operative report: is the operative report dictated within 24 hours?

Postoperative visits and discharge: do you plan adequate time for postoperative visits with the patient and prepare them for the first days at home after a hospital visit?

- 20% to get more information
- 19% to get revenge

Risk management check list (Tables 54-1, 54-2)

◆ Zones of Risk in Obstetrics and Gynecology

Diagnostic error
- failure to diagnose
- delay in diagnosis
- misdiagnosis

Documentation may reduce diagnostic error rates
- drug allergies
- signing off diagnostic reports
- alcohol, smoking, and drug use history
- appropriate management of labor

Particular areas of risk
- childbirth
- ectopic pregnancy
- breast cancer

IMPACT OF PROFESSIONAL LIABILITY ON OBSTETRIC PRACTICE

◆ Impact on Medical Education

Teaching of defensive medical practice

◆ Impact on Practice

Increasing malpractice premiums
Many obstetricians limiting their practice

◆ Impact on Patients

Poor availability of obstetricians
High-risk groups often have inadequate care

◆ Emotional Impact on Physicians

Cases often stretch out for years
Emotional toll can be devastating
- anger
- tension
- depression

Serious erosion of physician/patient relationship can occur

55

◆ Medical Ethics

FUNDAMENTALS OF MEDICAL ETHICS

◆ Legacy of Unethical Research

Nazi legacy of human experimentation
Nuremberg medical war crimes trials resulted in increased attention
Some notorious cases have occurred in the United States
- Jewish Memorial Hospital
  - cancer cells transferred to patients without their knowledge
- Tuskegee syphilis study
  - long-term follow up of untreated black patients with syphilis
- Willowbrook incident
  - induction of hepatitis in retarded patients

Complete disclosure and voluntary consent is crucial

◆ Government Commissions and Search for Ethical Principles

National Commission released the Belmont Report
- respect: respect of an autonomous person's wishes and interests and protection for those with diminished autonomy
- beneficence: do good and avoid harm
- justice: treat people fairly in selection for research and in making the benefits of research available

◆ Role of the Courts in Moral Dilemmas

Removal of life support in extreme cases
- Karen Ann Quinlen in 1975
Treatment of handicapped infants
- Baby Doe
  - can no longer withhold indicated treatment for fetus with correctable problem even if handicapped (Down syndrome)
- Baby Jane Doe
  - spina bifida placed in similar category to Down syndrome

◆ Advances in Technology Determine a Moral Agenda

These remain timely questions
- organ transplantation
- surrogate parenting
- gene therapy

◆ Social Assaults on Established Values and Institutions

Social unrest in the 1960s and 1970s resulted in the American Hospital Association patient Bill of Rights in 1973
- full disclosure
- truth telling
- patient's right to self-determination

ESSENTIAL NATURE OF MEDICAL ETHICS

Attribute moral agency only to humans capable of abstract thought
There is little that physicians do where they are not concerned with ethics
- attention to standards necessary in all aspects

◆ Objectivity, Competence, and the Science of Medicine

Must stay current with standard of care
Lack of intention is not an ameliorating condition if the doctor could have and should have known to avoid such behavior

◆ Physician-Patient Interaction

Previously a paternalistic relationship; now altered by empowerment of the patient
Compassion does not include lying
Obligation of confidentiality
- can be breached only to avoid a serious specific harm to others

◆ Ethics of the Social Limits and Uses of Medicine

Beneficence and nonmaleficence
- part of the Hippocratic tradition
  - physicians should do no harm

✧ *Beneficence*

Embraced by the National Commission
- the duty to do no harm and to help a patient
Risk-benefit analysis

◆ Autonomy and Informed Consent

Information, comprehension, voluntariness
A legal and ethical duty of the physician

◆ Abortion as a Paradigm for Moral Conflict

One of the most divisive ethical issues in the United States
- American public opinion split
  - 20% believe abortion should not be available on any grounds
  - 20% believe no restrictions should be present
  - 60% believe abortion should be restricted to specific instances

Pregnancy is a morally unique state

◆ Physician-Patient Conflict in the Delivery Room

Rarely arises that physician advises cesarean delivery and patient refuses
- courts have ruled both ways

Best choice is to obtain consultation and attempt to reason with the patient

◆ Ethical Concerns in Assisted Reproduction

Most members of society see no ethical problems in these procedures
- the Vatican is the exception

Surrogacy is the most troubling of the social arrangements

APPROACH TO ETHICAL ISSUES

Seldom present as a choice between right and wrong
Often involve conflicts between two obligations

Appendix

◆ Clinical Staging of Gynecologic Malignancies

STAGING OF BREAST CANCER

TX Primary tumor cannot be assessed
T0 No evidence of primary tumor
Tis Carcinoma in situ: intraductal carcinoma, lobular carcinoma in situ, or Paget disease of the nipple with no tumor
T1 Tumor 2 cm or less in greatest dimension
    T1a Tumor 0.5 cm or less in greatest dimension
    T1b Tumor more than 0.5 cm but not more than 1 cm in greatest dimension
    T1c Tumor more than 1 cm but not more than 2 cm in greatest dimension
T2 Tumor more than 2 cm but not more than 5 cm in greatest dimension
T3 Tumor more than 5 cm in greatest dimension
T4 Tumor of any size with direct extension to chest wall or skin
    T4a Extension to chest wall
    T4b Edema (including peau d'orange) or ulceration of the skin of the breast or satellite skin nodules confined to the same breast
    T4c Both T4a and T4b
    T4d Inflammatory carcinoma
NX Regional lymph nodes cannot be assessed (e.g., previously removed)
N0 No regional lymph node metastasis
N1 Metastasis to movable ipsilateral axillary lymph node(s)
N2 Metastasis to ipsilateral axillary lymph node(s), fixed to one another or other structures
N3 Metastasis to ipsilateral internal mammary lymph node(s)
M   Presence of distant metastasis cannot be assessed
M0 No distant metastasis
M1 Distant metastasis (including metastasis to ipsilateral supraclavicular lymph node(s))

Stage	Tumor size	Lymph node metastases	Distant metastases
0	Tis	N0	M0
I	T1	N0	M0
IIa	T0	N1	M0
	T1	N1*	M0
	T2	N0	M0
IIb	T2	N1	M0
	T3	N0	M0
IIIa	T0	N2	M0
	T1	N2	M0
	T2	N2	M0
	T3	N1,N2	M0
IIIb	T4	Any N	M0
	Any T	N3	M0
IV	Any T	Any N	M1

*Note: the progress of patients with N1a is similar to that of patients with pN0.

Am Joint Committee on Cancer. Manual for Staging of Cancer, 4th ed, Beahrs et al, eds, JB Lippincott Co, 1992.

FIGO STAGING OF INVASIVE CARCINOMA OF THE VULVA

Stage 0	Carcinoma in situ, intraepithelial carcinoma
Stage I	Tumor confined to the vulva or perineum, ≤2 cm in greatest dimension, no nodal metastasis
Stage II	Tumor confined to the vulva or perineum, >2 cm in greatest dimension, no nodal metastasis
Stage III	Tumor of any size with (1) Adjacent spread to the lower urethra, the vagina, or the anus, or (2) Unilateral regional lymph node metastasis
Stave IVA	Tumor invades any of the following: Upper urethra, bladder mucosa, rectal mucosa, pelvic bone, or bilateral regional node metastasis
Stage IVB	Any distant metastasis, including pelvic lymph nodes

STAGING OF CERVICAL CANCER
(cysto, procto, IVP, CXR permitted)

Stage 0	Carcinoma in situ, intraepithelial carcinoma (CIN)
Stage I	The carcinoma is strictly confined to the cervix
Stage IA	Invasive cancer identified only microscopically. All gross lesions even with superficial invasion are Stage IB cancers. Invasion is limited to measured stromal invasion with maximum depth of 5 mm and and a maximum width of 7 mm*
Stage IA1	Measured invasion of stroma no greater than 3 mm in depth and no wider than 7 mm

Stage IA2   Measured invasion of stroma greater than 3 mm and no greater than 5 mm in depth, and no wider than 7 mm

Stage IB   Clinical lesions confined to the cervix or preclinical lesions greater than Stage IA

Stage IB1   Clinical lesions no greater than 4 cm in size

Stage IB2   Clinical lesions greater than 4 cm in size

Stage II   The carcinoma extends beyond the cervix but not to sidewall, vaginal involvement upper two thirds only

Stage IIA   No obvious parametrial involvement

Stage IIB   Obvious parametrial involvement

Stage III   The carcinoma extends to the pelvic sidewall, on rectal examination there is no cancer-free space between the tumor and the wall. The tumor involves the lower one third of the vagina. All cases with hydronephrosis or a nonfunctioning kidney secondary to cancer = Stage III.

Stage IIIA   No pelvic sidewall extension

Stage IIIB   Extension to sidewall, and/or hydronephrosis or nonfunctioning kidney

Stage IV   The carcinoma has extended beyond the true pelvis or has clinically involved the mucosa of the bladder or rectum. Bullous edema does NOT = Stage IV.

IVA   Spread of growth to adjacent organs

Stage IVB   Spread to distant organs

*The depth of invasion should not be more than 5 mm taken from the base of the epithelium, either surface or glandular, from which it originates. Vascular space involvement, either venous or lymphatic, should not alter the staging.

Staging Announcement; Cancer Committee FIGO, 1995 Society of Gynecologic Oncologists

FIGO STAGING OF CARCINOMA OF THE UTERINE CORPUS

Stage IA   Endometrial adenocarcinoma without myometrial invasion

Stage IB   Less than 50% myometrial invasion

Stage IC   Greater than 50% myometrial invasion; grade should also be included: G1, G2, G3

Stage IIA   Endocervical mucosal involvement

Stage IIB   Cervical stromal invasion

Stage IIIA   Adnexal metastasis or positive peritoneal cytology

Stage IIIB   Pelvic nodal metastasis

Stage IIIC   Periaortic nodal metastasis or intraperitoneal disease

Stage IV   Invasion of bladder, rectum, or distant metastasis

G, grade of differentiation.
*The International Federation of Obstetrics and Gynecology has announced a major change in the staging of endometrial carcinoma. The committee has adopted a surgical staging system that will more accurately reflect patient prognosis. The stage of the disease will now be similar to ovarian carcinoma in that it will be based on the surgical-pathologic findings at the time of surgical exploration and hysterectomy.

FIGO STAGING OF FALLOPIAN TUBE CANCER

Stage 0	Carcinoma in situ limited to tubal mucosa
Stage I	Growth limited to the fallopian tubes*
Stage IA	Growth limited to one tube with extension into the submucosa or muscularis but not penetrating the serosal surface: no ascites
Stage IB	Growth limited to both tubes with extension into the submucosa or muscularis but not penetrating the serosal surface: no ascites
Stage IC	Tumor stage IA or IB, but with tumor extension through or onto the tubal serosa; or with ascites present containing malignant cells or with positive peritoneal washings
Stage II	Growth involving one or both fallopian tubes with pelvic extension
Stage IIA	Extension or metastasis to the uterus or ovaries
Stage IIB	Extension to other pelvic tissues
Stage IIC	Tumor stage IIA or IIB and with ascites present containing malignant cells or with positive peritoneal washings
Stage III	Tumor involves one or both fallopian tubes with peritoneal implants outside of the pelvis or positive retroperitoneal or inguinal nodes; superficial liver metastases equals stage III, and tumor appears limited to the true pelvis, but with histologically proven malignant extension to the small bowel or omentum
Stage IIIA	Tumor grossly limited to the true pelvis with negative nodes, but with histologically confirmed microscopic seeding of the abdominal peritoneal surfaces
Stage IIIB	Tumor involving one or both fallopian tubes with histologically confirmed implants of abdominal peritoneal surfaces, ≤2 cm in diameter; lymph nodes are negative
Stage IIIC	Abdominal implants >2 cm in diameter or positive retroperitoneal or inguinal nodes
Stave IV	Growth involving one or both fallopian tubes with distant metastases; for pleural effusion, there must be positive cytology to be stage IV; parenchymal liver metastases equals stage IV

*Staging for fallopian tube cancer is done by the surgical pathologic system. The operative findings designating stage are determined before tumor debulking.

FIGO STAGING OF OVARIAN CARCINOMA

Stage I   Growth limited to the ovaries

Stage IA   Growth limited to one ovary, no malignant ascites, no tumor on external surface, capsule intact

Stage IB   Growth limited to both ovaries, no malignant ascites, no tumor on external surface, capsule intact

Stage IC   Tumor IA, or IB, but positive for surface growth, or malignant ascites, or positive washings, or capsule ruptured at or prior to surgery

Stage II   Growth involving one or both ovaries with pelvic extension

Stage IIA   Extension and/or metastases to the uterus and/or tubes

Stage IIB   Extension to other pelvic organs

Stage IIC   Tumor IIA or IIB, but positive for surface growth, or malignant ascites, or positive washings, or capsule(s) ruptured at or prior to surgery

Stage III   Tumor involving one or both ovaries with peritoneal implants outside the pelvis and/or positive nodes (retroperitoneal or inguinal). Tumor limited to true pelvis but with histologically proven extension to small bowel and omentum. Superficial liver metastases = Stage III

Stage IIIA Tumor grossly limited to the true pelvis with negative nodes but microscopic seeding of abdominal peritoneal surfaces

Stage IIIB Tumor with abdominal peritoneal implants but none >2 cm, nodes negative

Stage IIIC Abdominal implants >2 cm, and/or positive retroperitoneal or inguinal nodes

Stage IV   Growth involving one or both ovaries with distant metastases. Pleural effusions must be tapped for cytology. Parenchymal liver metastases = Stage IV.

INDEX

Page numbers followed by a "t" indicate tabular material.
Page numbers in italics indicate figures.